Your steps to success. W9-BTE-999

EXPLORE PEARSON mynursingkit™

MyNursingKit is your one stop for online chapter review materials and resources. Prepare for success with additional NCLEX®-style practice questions, interactive assignments and activities, web links, animations and videos, and more!

Register your access code with the instructions below

STEP 1: Register

All you need to get started is a valid email address and the access code below. To register, simply:

1. Go to **www.mynursingkit.com**.
2. Click "**Students**" under "**First-time users**."
3. Find the appropriate book cover. Cover must match the textbook edition being used for your class.
4. Click "**Register**" beside your book cover.
5. Read the **License Agreement** and **Private Policy**. If you accept, click "**I Accept**."
6. Leave "**No**" selected under "**Do you have a Pearson account?**"
7. Using a coin scratch off the silver coating below to reveal your access code. Do not use a knife or other sharp object, which can damage the code.
8. Enter your access code in lowercase or uppercase, without the dashes.
9. Follow the on-screen instructions to complete registration.

During registration, you will establish a personal login name and password to use for logging into the Website. You will also be sent a registration confirmation email that contains your login name and password. Be sure to save this email.

Your Access Code is:

Note: If there is no silver foil covering the access code, it may already have been redeemed, and therefore may no longer be valid. In that case, you can purchase access online using a major credit card. To do so, go to www.mynursingkit.com. click "Students" under "First Time Users," find the cover of your textbook, then click "Buy Access," and follow the on-screen instructions.

STEP 2: Log in

1. Go to **www.mynursingkit.com** and click "**Students**" under "**Returning Users**."
2. Find the appropriate book cover. Click on "**Login**" next to your book cover.
3. Enter the login name and password that you created during registration. If unsure of this information, refer to your registration confirmation email.
4. Click "**Login**."

Got technical questions?

Customer Technical Support: To obtain support, please visit us online anytime at http://247pearsoned.custhelp.com where you can search our knowledgebase for common solutions, view product alerts, and review all options for additional assistance.

SITE REQUIREMENTS

For the latest updates on Site Requirements, go to www.mynursingkit.com. Click "**Students**" under "**Returning Users**". Pick your book and click "**Login**". Click on "**Need help**" at bottom of page for site requirements and other frequently asked questions.

Important: Please read the Subscription and End-User License agreement, accessible from the book website's login page, before using the *mynursingkit* website. By using the website, you indicate that you have read, understood, and accepted the terms of this agreement.

0135136113

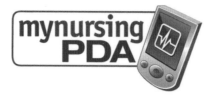

MyNursingPDA is the complete mobile solution for nursing professionals and students offering easy access to clinical information they need in the palms of their hands. Based on reliable nursing content from Pearson, this series of mobile products allows users to search across multiple titles seamlessly to find the right information about conditions, nursing management, drugs, labs, skills, and more.

- Exceptional cross-linking Technology provides faster access & greater ease of use
- Point & click navigation
- Smart-type searching by topic, disease, drugs, labs, and more
- Book-marking content
- Note-taking & highlighting
- Navigational history
- Updates (Drug Guide only)
- Links to web (wireless capability required)
- SD memory card support
- Landscape orientation for some content as needed
- Comprehensive table views of some content as needed
- Full-color images as needed

For more information visit
www.mynursingpda.com

Success in the Classroom, in Clinicals, and on the NCLEX-RN®

Classroom

- Detailed lecture notes organized by learning outcome
- Suggestions for classroom activities
- Guide to relevant additional resources
- Comprehensive PowerPoint™ presentations integrating lecture, images, animations, and videos
- Online course management systems complete with instructor tools and student activities

Clinical

- Suggestions for Clinical Activities and other clinical resources organized by learning outcome

Real Nursing Simulations Facilitator's Guide: Institutional Edition

- 25 simulation scenarios that span the nursing curriculum
- Consistent format includes learning objectives, case flow, instructions for set up, student debriefing questions and more!
- Companion online course cartridge with student exercises, activities, videos, skill checklists, and reflective questions also available for adoption

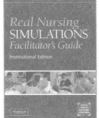

NCLEX-RN®

- Test Item Files with NCLEX®-style questions and complete rationales for correct and incorrect answers mapped to learning outcomes. *available in TestGen, Par Test, and MS Word*

Instructor Resources

Nursing Care at the End of Life

Ginny Wacker Guido

More *information and instructor resources*
visit www.mynursingkit.com

Brief Contents

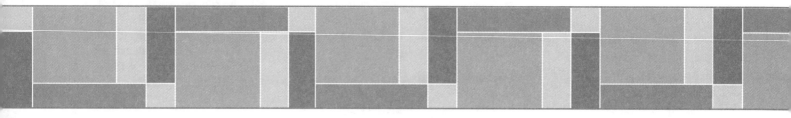

NURSING CARE AT THE END OF LIFE

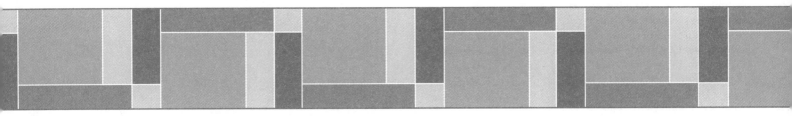

Ginny Wacker Guido

Ginny Wacker Guido, JD, MSN, RN, FAAN
Regional Director-Nursing and Assistant Dean
College of Nursing
Washington State University Vancouver
Vancouver, Washington

Pearson

Boston Columbus Indianapolis New York San Francisco Upper Saddle River
Amsterdam Cape Town Dubai London Madrid Milan Munich Paris Montreal Toronto
Delhi Mexico City Sao Paulo Sydney Hong Kong Seoul Singapore Taipei Tokyo

Library of Congress Cataloging-in-Publication Data
Guido, Ginny Wacker.
    Nursing care at the end of life / Ginny Wacker Guido.
        p. cm.
    Includes bibliographical references and index.
    ISBN-13: 978-0-13-513611-9
    ISBN-10: 0-13-513611-3
    1. Terminal care. 2. Hospice nurses. I. Title.
    [DNLM: 1. Nursing Care. 2. Terminal Care. 3. Palliative Care. WY 152 G948n 2009]
    RT87.T45.G85 2009
    616′.029—dc22

                                                    2009014126

Publisher: Julie Levin Alexander
Publisher's Assistant: Regina Bruno
Editor-in-Chief: Maura Connor
Executive Acquisitions Editor: Pamela Fuller
Development Editor: Pat Gillivan
Editorial Assistant: Jennifer Aranda
Managing Production Editor: Patrick Walsh
Production Liaison: Cathy O'Connell
Production Editor: Erin Melloy, S4Carlisle Publishing Services
Manufacturing Manager: Ilene Sanford
Art Director: Maria Guglielmo
Cover Design: Kevin Kall
Interior Design: Wee Design
Director of Marketing: Karen Allman
Senior Marketing Manager: Francisco Del Castillo
Marketing Specialist: Michael Sirinides
Marketing Assistant: Crystal Gonzalez
Media Project Manager: Rachel Collett
Composition: S4Carlisle Publishing Services
Printer/Binder: Edwards Brothers
Cover Printer: LeHigh-Phoenix Color/Hagerstown

Notice: Care has been taken to confirm the accuracy of information presented in this book. The authors, editors, and the publisher, however, cannot accept any responsibility for errors or omissions or for consequences from application of the information in this book and make no warranty, express or implied, with respect to its contents.

The authors and publisher have exerted every effort to ensure that drug selections and dosages set forth in this text are in accord with current recommendations and practice at time of publication. However, in view of ongoing research, changes in government regulations, and the constant flow of information relating to drug therapy and drug reactions, the reader is urged to check the package inserts of all drugs for any change in indications of dosage and for added warnings and precautions. This is particularly important when the recommended agent is a new and/or infrequently employed drug.

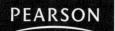

www.pearsonhighered.com

10 9 8 7 6 5 4 3 2 1
ISBN-10:   0-13-513611-3
ISBN-13: 978-0-13-513611-9

About the Author

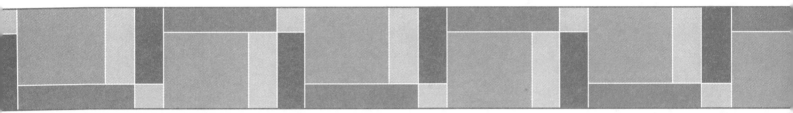

Ginny Wacker Guido has been active in legal and ethical issues in nursing for the past 30 years. She developed an interest in this area of nursing when she was teaching undergraduate nursing students in Texas, and this excitement for further knowledge and understanding of this content area encouraged her to pursue a doctorate of jurisprudence degree.

She is active in nursing education and is currently employed as the Regional Director for Nursing and Assistant Dean, College of Nursing, Washington State University Vancouver. Over the years, she has had numerous publications and presentations on legal and ethical issues with special emphasis in a variety of clinical practice settings.

DEDICATION

This text is dedicated to all nurses who care for persons at the end of life.

Thank You

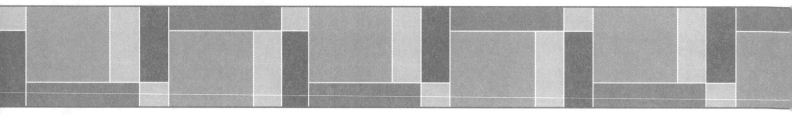

We extend a sincere thanks to our contributors, who generously gave their time, effort, and expertise to the development and writing of chapters and resources.

CONTRIBUTORS

Marlys Bohn, PhD, RN

Assistant Professor and Department Head,
Nursing Student Services
South Dakota State University
Brookings, South Dakota
Chapters 8–10

Nancy E. Joyner, RN, MS, APRN-CNS, ACHPN

Clinical Nurse Specialist-Palliative Care
Altru Health System – Altru Hospital
Grand Forks, North Dakota
Chapters 4–6 and portions of Chapters 1 and 11

NCLEX-STYLE QUESTIONS

Heather Lane Bradley, RN, MSN

University of Kentucky Hospital
Lexington, Kentucky
Chapters 8–11

Rhonda Hutton Gann, RN, MSN

State Fair Community College
Sedalia, Missouri
Chapters 4–7

Jane Walker, BBA, RN, MSN

Walters State Community College
Morristown, Tennessee
Chapters 1–3

REVIEWERS

We extend sincere thanks to our colleagues from schools of nursing throughout the country who gave their time generously to help create this textbook.

Mary J. Baukus, MS, MA, RN

Faculty Specialist II (Clinical Instructor)
WMU Bronson School of Nursing
College of Health and Human Services
Western Michigan University
Kalamazoo, Michigan

June M. Belt, MSN, APRN, BC (ANP, GNP, PCM)

Clinical Assistant Professor
School of Nursing
University of Kansas
Kansas City, Kansas

Marcia Bosek, DNSc, RN

Associate Professor
Rush University College of Nursing
Chicago, Illinois

Susan Breakwell, RNC, DNP

Assistant Professor
Rush University College of Nursing
Chicago, Illinois

Janet Witucki Brown, PhD, CNE

Associate Professor
The University of Tennessee,
Knoxville
Knoxville, Tennessee

Juliana Cartwright, RN, PhD

> Associate Professor
> School of Nursing
> Oregon Health & Science University
> Ashland, Oregon

Virginia Conley, PhD, ARNP

> Assistant Professor of Nursing
> Fay W. Whitney School of Nursing
> University of Wyoming
> Laramie, Wyoming

Karen K. Cox, MNSc, RN

> Assistant Professor
> Arkansas Tech University
> Russellville, Arkansas

Susan L. Fox, PHD, CNAA, BC

> Senior Associate Dean
> College of Nursing
> University of New Mexico
> Albuquerque, New Mexico

Polly Cameron Haigler, PhD, RN

> Clinical Associate Professor
> College of Nursing
> University of South Carolina
> Columbia, South Carolina

Roseann Kaminsky, RN, MSN, BSN, BSEd

> Associate Professor
> Lorain County Community College
> Allied Health and Nursing
> Elyria, Ohio

Mary E. McNair, MSN, RN, OCN

> Instructor
> School of Nursing
> University of Mississippi
> Jackson, Mississippi

Joseph Molinatti, EdD, RN

> Assistant Professor
> College of Mount Saint Vincent
> Bronx, New York

Stephanie Myers Schim, PhD, RN

> Associate Professor
> College of Nursing
> Wayne State University
> Detroit, Michigan

Craig R. Sellers, PhD(c), RN, ANP-BC

> Director, ANP Program
> University of Rochester School of Nursing
> Rochester, New York

M. Josephine Snider, EdD, RN

> Associate Professor
> College of Nursing
> University of Florida
> Gainesville, Florida

Diane Young, PhD, RN, CNE

> Professor
> Allen College
> Waterloo, Iowa

Preface

When I was a new nursing graduate, one of the most challenging aspects of caring for patients in an acute-care setting concerned patients at the end of life. Though I was fairly confident that my physical care for the patient was adequate, I often wondered how to better assure that I was also appropriately caring for additional aspects of their care, including their psychosocial, emotional, and spiritual needs and the many needs of their loved ones. I also felt that there were multiple aspects of the care of these very special patients for which I was not prepared. This lack of preparation motivated me to explore what was known about the care of patients at the end of life and began my journey to ensure that future nurses would have this knowledge and skills so that the patients these nurses encountered would receive the expert nursing care they so rightfully deserved. Over the years, my research and personal experience have slowly evolved to the extent that I feel very confident caring for patients at the end of life.

Thus, when I was offered the opportunity to create a text addressing the unique and multiple needs of terminally ill patients across the life span, written specifically for nursing students completing their basic programs of study or newly graduated, I was excited and eager to begin writing. My sincere hope and that of my co-authors is that this multifaceted text will adequately prepare newly employed nursing graduates about nursing care for patients at the end of life and their loved ones and instill in these nurses the beginning of life-long education in the field of nursing.

Using a proven modular, self-study approach, this text is designed so readers will understand each of the concepts prior to completing the chapters. Each chapter begins with an overview, learning objectives, and an NCLEX-style pretest that determines the base knowledge of the reader. Concepts are developed throughout the chapter, with outcome assessments following the individual concepts, so that the reader is assured that he or she has comprehended the concept before going on. For the sake of students in a prelicensure program, selected outcome assessments include questions written in the NCLEX format. Answers to the questions can be found in the appendix at the end of the book.

The book content explores all facets of care, beginning with a general overview of introductory concepts related to end-of-life nursing care, then exploring the ethical and the legal aspects of nursing care at the end of life. Physical care of the patient is divided into three separate chapters (Chapters 4–6). Recognizing that pain and pain relief is one of the more important aspects of these patients' care, this content has its own chapter. Other physical care measures are then presented, with symptoms ranging from less to more severe. The final physical care chapter (Chapter 6) outlines the issues involved in providing nutrition and hydration to patients at the end of life. Chapter 7 gives an overview of the care of the terminally ill patient, conceptualized on the stages of growth and development as developed by Erickson in the 1950s. Issues related to psychosocial, spiritual, and communications are explored in Chapters 8–10, and the concluding chapter (Chapter 11) explores care of the caregiver.

Chapter Features

Pretest: Each chapter begins with an NCLEX-style pretest that determines the reader's prior knowledge of the subject and alerts them to areas of knowledge that they should focus on.

Glossary: Important terms that will be introduced are presented at the beginning of the chapters.

Section Reviews: At the end of each section, the reader can complete an NCLEX-style review.

Case Studies: Throughout the chapters and concluding at the end of the chapter, the case studies allow the reader to put a human face on the chapter content.

Chapter Summaries: Core content from the chapter is summarized in bulleted format.

Chapter Reviews: All chapters conclude with a case study, incorporating the key concepts of the chapter.

Acknowledgments

I am deeply indebted to two nursing colleagues who wrote multiple chapters for their expertise and dedication in the writing of the text. Dr. Marlys Bohn has extensive clinical experience working with breast cancer patients in a major medical center. She has also worked in long-term, parish, and hospice nursing. Prior to entering the nursing profession, Dr. Bohn served in a chaplaincy role, which further enhanced her knowledge and understanding of spirituality and human emotions. In her current role as a faculty member at South Dakota State University, Dr. Bohn has a unique perspective regarding the understanding of nursing students in this content area. For this text, Dr. Bohn authored Chapters 8–10.

Ms. Nancy Joyner completed her master's degree in nursing in hospice and palliative care nursing and is certified as a Clinical Nurse Specialist in Hospice and Palliative Care Nursing. She is currently working as the Clinical Nurse Specialist in Palliative Care nurse at Altru Health System in Grand Forks, North Dakota. Prior to accepting this position, Ms. Joyner worked for several years in hospice nursing settings. She was also one of the first to complete the End of Life Nursing Consortium (ELNEC) program of study when the program premiered. Ms. Joyner's primary contributions to this text include Chapters 4–6 and selected aspects of Chapters 1 and 11.

For myself, I have continued to care for patients and their families at the end of life, with the greater confidence that I am truly incorporating all aspects of needed nursing care. I am now employed full-time in a university nursing program at Washington State University Vancouver. My expertise is primarily in the area of legal and ethical issues in nursing. I was the primary author for Chapters 2, 3, and 7 and selected aspects of Chapters 1 and 11.

Ginny Wacker Guido, JD, MSN, RN, FAAN

Contents

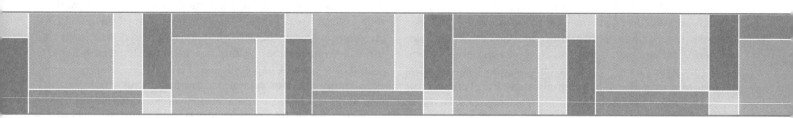

Nursing Care at the End of Life: Introductory Concepts

OBJECTIVES Following completion of this chapter, the learner will be able to:

1.1. Describe principle features of palliative care, focusing on the philosophy and principles of palliative care.

1.2. Discuss quality-of-life issues and implications for nursing care at the end of life.

1.3. Differentiate between palliative care assessment and interventions and curative assessment, treatment, and care.

1.4. Analyze the similarities and differences between hospice nursing care and palliative care.

1.5. Use a quality of life model to examine impact on palliative care needs.

1.6. Discuss unique changes patients manifest as their life comes to closure.

1.7. Identify opportunities for growth for all involved persons during the dying process.

1.8. Analyze the nurse's role as a member of the palliative care interdisciplinary health care team.

This chapter introduces multiple concepts and principles that are essential for nurses to understand and employ in assuring quality end-of-life care. The chapter begins with a description of the principle features of palliative care, incorporating the philosophy and principles upon which palliative care is based. Quality-of-life issues are explored, using a quality of life model to examine the impact of palliative care needs. Palliative care is contrasted with curative care and the similarities and differences between palliative care and hospice care are explored. The chapter concludes with a discussion of the unique changes patients undergo as they near death and identifies opportunities for growth for all persons involved during the dying process.

PRETEST

1. Which best defines palliative care?
   1. Curative therapies and interventions related to treatment of a disease or condition
   2. Care overcoming the underlying disease etiology and promoting recovery
   3. Aggressive treatment of presenting symptoms and provision of comfort care
   4. Care provided solely to terminally ill patients

2. Which statement most accurately represents the effect that advancements in health care have had on end-of-life care?
   1. Advancements in health care have allowed health care providers to enhance the provision of quality care for patients at the end of life.
   2. Advancements in health care have created fear that the only alternative to aggressive treatment is abandonment and suffering.
   3. Advancements in health care have created additional awareness in patients and families about treatment of pain and suffering.
   4. Advancements in health care have assisted health care providers in recognizing care that is considered medically futile.

3. Which statement most accurately describes the majority of elderly patients? They:
   1. Have special needs due to concomitant health problems and age-related changes in functioning.
   2. Have no difficulty expressing their health care needs.
   3. Are more frequently independent in their need for assistance.
   4. Exhibit the same cognitive, physical, and complex medical impairments as other adult patients exhibit.
4. Which statement correctly describes hospice care?
   1. Hospice care has been recognized only within the past 5 to 10 years.
   2. Hospice is synonymous with palliative care.
   3. Hospice allows for individual qualification guidelines within a geographic region.
   4. Hospice care has developed in direct response to patients living with life-threatening and life-limiting illnesses.
5. Palliative nursing care:
   1. Must address a single important health care need facing individuals and their families.
   2. Has the potential to increase patient burden and distress.
   3. Provides vigorous comfort care measures aimed at maintaining the best quality of life.
   4. Is provided in limited clinical and home settings.

GLOSSARY

curative treatment   Remedies, therapies, and interventions used in the cure of diseases; the intent of such treatment is to cure or restore the individual to a healthy state.

healing   To restore or return to health and soundness; to become whole and sound in mind and body; perfecting balance, harmony, and equilibrium.

hospice   The philosophic approach to providing comfort and care at life's end rather than providing heroic lifesaving measures; a program that provides special care for people who are near the end of life and for their families, usually during the last 6 months of life.

palliate   (from Latin *pallium*—to cloak, conceal) To reduce or relieve the symptoms of a disease or disorder, without curing the underlying disease.

palliative care   (also called comfort care, supportive care, or symptom management) The active, comprehensive care of patients whose diseases are not responsive to curative treatment, but are considered chronic or terminal. Control of pain and other symptoms with respect to physical, psychological, social, and spiritual problems is principal. The goal is to achieve the best possible quality of life for patients and their families (World Health Organization, 1990, 2007).

quality of life   The well-being of an individual, measured not by monetary issues, but by the individual's perception of his or her enjoyment and satisfaction with life; a standard of living that attempts to measure satisfaction rather than longevity; often described as health-related quality of life as opposed to a more global determination of the economic and social impact relating to standards of living.

SECTION ONE: Quality of Life and Palliative Care

Individuals have similar health care goals, whether they are acutely or chronically ill or whether they are at the end stages of their lives. These health care goals are to live life as fully as possible and to function optimally in all aspects of living, which can be defined as **quality of life**. In addition, quality of life includes being able to engage in roles that are important to the individual, such as attending the graduation or wedding of a grandchild, continuing to be able to work in one's garden and live at home, or merely being an active part of family conversations. Quality of life encompasses feelings of self-esteem, self-worth and love, feelings of independence, and a sense of well-being despite having limitations imposed by circumstances and illness. Perhaps the overarching demands of having quality of life are to cope effectively and continue to have hope during the final days of one's life.

Health care advances coupled with a better appreciation of what constitutes quality of life for a given individual are beginning to change the way in which society views end-of-life care. For example, in two states in the nation, patients now have the right to determine not only if they will accept or not accept life-sustaining procedures and systems, but to accept medications that will terminate their life using their time lines. At the opposite extreme, individuals have the ability to accept expert palliative measures and hospice care rather than continue on a previously selected course of more curative medical interventions.

One of the earliest research studies to attempt to explore the relationship between a patient's prognosis and his or her preferences at the end-of-life with health care providers' perceptions was the Study to Understand Prognosis and Preferences for Outcomes and Risks of Treatment (SUPPORT), published in 1995. The data collection time frame for the study was a four-year period. The study included more than 9,000 adult patients who were hospitalized with one or more life-threatening illnesses and who were expected to die within a six-month window.

The study revealed that health care providers were significantly deficient in their delivery of care for individuals at the end of life, particularly in the areas of discussing prognoses and assisting patients during their last 6 months of life in decision making. The study also noted that the majority of patients, during these last 6 months, continued to suffer moderate to severe pain.

Though the study's finding confirmed what many nurses who cared for this population had voiced, the results did document the need for changes in the management of care for the dying. Further, the study reinforced the need for health care providers to initiate steps to evaluate the concept of quality care, particularly at the end of life, and to use evaluation findings to implement a more effective and beneficial approach to quality care.

Palliative care is one concept that addresses quality-of-life issues. **Palliative care** is specialized care most often provided to individuals with a potentially life-limiting, life-threatening, or chronic, progressive illness, and their families. It is often called comfort care, supportive care, or symptom management. Box 1–1 depicts the World Health Organization's definition of palliative care.

The National Consensus Project (2004) describes eight domains of palliative care theory and practice. Box 1–2 outlines these eight domains.

Information in each of these domains addresses specifics for the interdisciplinary care team regarding composition of the team members and the provision of continuity of care across varied health care settings.

Palliative care is a philosophy of humanistic, individualized, total care for patients and families across the continuum of health care throughout the lifespan and in multiple health settings, who need comfort with or without curative treatment. **Curative treatment** involves remedies, therapies, and interventions intended to cure the individual undergoing the treatment and may be beneficial in preventing further pain or exasperation of physical symptoms. Whether curative care measures are incorporated or not, the emphasis of palliative care is on optimizing quality of life, represented by a holistic, interdisciplinary, patient-centered approach. The goals of care include relief of pain and suffering and, when necessary, provision of comfort (versus cure) care measures, offering support toward a peaceful dying process and death. Palliative care also includes psychosocial and spiritual needs of the patient and family, as well as physical, cultural, and emotional needs (Ferrell & Coyle, 2006).

The overall purpose, therefore, is to prevent or treat the symptoms of the disease and/or side effects caused by its treatment as early as possible and also to address related psychological, social, and spiritual problems. Palliative care is that which "**palliates**," or

BOX 1–1   Definition of Palliative Care
■ Embraces life and regards death as a normal process ■ Neither speeds up death nor delays it ■ Provides relief from pain and other distressing symptoms ■ Integrates the psychological and spiritual aspects of care ■ Offers a support system to help patients live as well as possible until death ■ Offers a support system to help families cope with their loved one's death and to help them cope afterward with their own bereavement

Source: World Health Organization, 2007

BOX 1–2   Eight Domains of Palliative Care
1. Structure and process of care 2. Physical aspects of care 3. Psychosocial and psychiatric aspects of care 4. Social aspects of care 5. Spiritual, religious, and existential aspects of care 6. Cultural aspects of care 7. Care of the imminently dying patient 8. Ethical and legal aspects of care

Source: National Consensus Project, 2004, p. 616

relieves, pain and distress. Implemented when treatment to cure is no longer effective, palliative care measures attempt to ease the sufferings that often accompany terminal illness, making the end-of-life experience as positive and pain-free as possible by providing care and compassion for the whole person. Palliative care also incorporates supporting the dying person's family and friends. Palliative care can be provided in any setting, including the home, skilled care facility, or hospital (Virani & Sofer, 2003).

Palliative care expands traditional disease-model treatments by helping patients and their families with support and decision making, and providing opportunities for personal growth. The interdisciplinary team is an integral part of palliative care, incorporating the professions of medicine, nursing, social work, chaplaincy, counseling, nutrition, rehabilitation, pharmacy, and physical therapists, among others in delivering quality care to patients and their families. Palliative care affirms life by supporting the patient's and family's goals for the future, including their hopes for cure or life-prolongation, as well as their hopes for peace and dignity throughout the course of an illness, the dying process, and death. Appropriate for all patients regardless of age, from the time of diagnosis with a life-threatening or debilitating condition through the course of their illness, palliative care provides for assessment and treatment of pain and other symptoms, helps with patient-centered communications and decision making, and coordinates care across the continuum of care settings (Center to Advance Palliative Care [CAPC], 2007; National Consensus Project, 2004).

SECTION ONE REVIEW

1. Which best describes palliative care?
   1. The nurse provides care to a patient with a terminal illness.
   2. The nurse provides care for patients in any setting or unit.
   3. Care provided follows a standard protocol and is not individualized.
   4. Care can be provided only by certified palliative care nurses.
2. A nursing student is studying the concepts of palliative care. The instructor knows more studying is needed if which statement is made? "The World Health Organization definition of palliative care states providers:
   1. May speed up death or delay death."
   2. Embrace life and regard death as a normal process."
   3. Provide relief from pain and other distressing symptoms."
   4. Integrate the psychological and spiritual aspects of care."
3. For which signs or symptoms as experienced by patients would palliative care be most useful? (Select all that apply.)
   1. Physical disabilities
   2. Changes in sensorium
   3. Psychological responses
   4. Emotional distress
4. Additional instruction is needed if a family member makes which statement? "Palliative care practice includes the:
   1. Structure and process of care."
   2. Psychosocial and psychiatric aspects of care."
   3. Spiritual, religious, and existential aspects of care."
   4. Community aspects of care."

SECTION TWO: Historical Perspectives

Until the late 1880s, health care providers lacked adequate technology, skills, and tools to manage the seriously ill. Most care was provided by immediate and extended family members and most patients died at home, usually within days of the onset of illness (End of Life Nursing Education Consortium [ELNEC], 2008, CAPC, 2007). Given the limitations of health care treatments and interventions, much of the early care of these dying patients was directed at comfort measures. During the 1900s, however, advances in health care extended life such that the average American's lifespan increased by approximately 30 years, and, as a result, the focus of health care shifted from primarily alleviating suffering to curing disease.

Impact of Medical and Technical Advances on Dying

During the past several decades, medical and technical advances have continued to change the way Americans die. The dying process has often been prolonged, in part, because medical treatments can manage such issues as pneumonia, infections, kidney failure, and other immediate causes of death. Though true **healing**, the restoration of a person to total health and soundness, is often not possible, patients may be able to enjoy enhanced longevity because of medical and technical advances.

Many deaths entail a difficult period of decision making between the patient's family and the clinical team concerning the application of aggressive treatment choices or their cessation. Because medical futility is often difficult to recognize, many patients experience burdensome procedures and/or therapies that can be exhausting, expensive, unsettling, and unsuccessful (Agency for Health Care Policy and Research [AHCPR], 1996).

Some of the more obvious reasons for these burdensome and costly experiences include a societal view that death is a failure and is to be avoided at all costs, a medical philosophy that sees death as a personal failure rather than a natural conclusion, and primary health care providers who request family members to make major medical decisions without the necessary explanations of realistic outcomes. Family members frequently fail to realize the limitations of therapies and medications, advocating for "doing everything that can be done," and not being apprised that even if everything is done, the outcome will still be death, but it will come more slowly. Additionally, the fear of potential lawsuits continues to make physicians reluctant to advise comfort rather than cure measures for countless patients.

Finally, there is widespread thought that the only alternative to aggressive treatment is abandonment and suffering. Since the American health care system is primarily oriented toward the cure of patients with acute medical conditions and injuries, it fails to recognize that the medical needs of the dying patient are fundamentally different and therefore require a multidisciplinary approach. One of the challenges of facing a shift in the kind of care given the dying is the coordination among interdisciplinary team members to avoid unnecessary transitions between medical care institutions.

Since the exact timing of death is not predictable, many patients may spend years as the illness advances and becomes terminal. As more technology is developed and recommended for these individuals, the patient's prognosis becomes more difficult to diagnose. Many patients have comorbidities, adding to the dilemma of predicting the future.

Accompanying these disease processes are multiple symptoms that create additional dilemmas when making choices and decisions. The physician may continue to offer treatment, but the interventions may become more futile and may not result in the quality of life the patient desires.

In response to these concerns, national initiatives are being developed to improve care of persons at the time of death. Significant efforts are being made to improve the education of health professionals and to encourage public awareness of the issues. One of the most promising efforts in this area is the End of Life Nursing Education Consortium (ELNEC) project developed in partnership with the American Association of Colleges of Nursing (AACN) and the City of Hope in California. The project provides comprehensive, nationally offered courses designed to educate nurses in end-of-life care issues. A sister project involves inclusion of end-of-life content in nursing textbooks so that this content may be incorporated into undergraduate nursing programs (ELNEC, 2000). Despite these efforts, important gaps continue to exist in the knowledge base that is the foundation for evidence-based care of the dying (Ellershaw & Wilkinson, 2003).

Aging and Chronic Conditions

Given the aging and growth of the population, significant increases in chronic illnesses are predicted. Age-adjusted death rates in the United States declined significantly during 2006; the age-adjusted death rate fell to 776.4 deaths per 100,000 from 799 deaths per 100,000 in 2005 (Centers for Disease Control

[CDC], 2008). Thus individuals are living longer and these more elderly patients often have special needs due to their frailty, including difficulty in communicating their health care needs. They may be unprepared to find themselves dependent on others. Moreover, they may be cognitively impaired or demented, and often have other complex medical problems, so that they are forced to deal with an increasingly intimidating health care system, often without adequate advocacy support.

Persons who are told they have a life-threatening disease or terminal illness often suffer in fear, and their families suffer with them. Tragically, in America today, these fears are well founded. People fear tangible things related to when and how they will eventually die, including being abandoned, becoming undignified in terms of what they do, how they look, or the way they smell. People are afraid of dying in pain and of dying alone. As one recent study noted, no patient should face death alone (Beckstrand, Callister, & Kirchhoff, 2006). This supports the findings of Dr. Ira Byock, a past president of the American Academy of Hospice and Palliative Care (1997).

Between the years 2010 and 2030, the number of people in the United States who are 65 years or older will increase more than 70%. The number of people over 85 will double to 10 million by 2030 (Administration on Aging, 2000; CAPC, 2007). These statistics, in addition to increased longevity, higher costs of health care, and a larger number of individuals living with chronic illness, will create a significant financial and human resource burden on health care services in the United States.

SECTION TWO REVIEW

1. The focus of health care in the 1900s shifted from:
   1. Alleviating suffering to curing disease.
   2. Dying in a hospital to dying at home.
   3. Perceiving deterioration and death as the failure of health care to seeing decline and death as the only options.
   4. Focusing on the needs of the individual to the needs of the community.
2. Which are reasons why patients, families, and team members experience difficult decision making in life-threatening and terminal illnesses? (Select all that apply.)
   1. Discussing after-death care and inheritances
   2. Understanding medical futility
   3. Experiencing and/or refusing burdensome procedures and/or therapies
   4. Ensuring the patient makes the correct decision
   5. Discussing medical and technical advances
3. What must the nurse take into consideration when a comorbidity exists in a patient with a terminal illness?
   1. Only abandonment and suffering exist as an alternative to aggressive treatment.

2. The comorbidity only adds to the unpredictability of determining life expectancy.
   3. The nurse recognizes that the medical needs of the dying patient are basically the same as for other patients.
   4. The nurse should limit choices to ease the decision-making process.
4. Fear in people who have a life-threatening disease or terminal illness:
   1. Is not justified; there are ways to alleviate suffering.
   2. Can often be related to how he or she might look to others or how the disease might change body odors.
   3. Is a tangible concern related to when and how they will eventually die.
   4. Has no connection to pain.
5. Which is the most likely effect of an aging population?
   1. Health care costs will decline.
   2. A smaller number of patients will be living with chronic illness.
   3. There will be a negative impact on health care services.
   4. Younger people will outnumber the aging population.

SECTION THREE: Importance of Palliative Care Measures

At some point, individuals with life-threatening or terminal conditions and their families may wish to know the trajectory of the disease process. They have a right to this information as well as the right to be kept comfortable, as free of pain as is possible, and have all other symptoms managed in a therapeutic manner. From the time a treatment is initiated, individuals and families need to know what course or direction their disease may take, alternatives that are possible, and the consequences of these possible alternatives. Primary health care providers, though they understand that patients need full information and honesty, often have difficulty with these discussions of "breaking the bad news."

Other issues further illustrate the need for quality palliative care. Patients may have decreased functional capacity, causing loss of independence and a sense of loss of control over their lives. It may also leave them unable to continue the activities that are meaningful and valuable to them. Family roles may shift, and patients may perceive the potential of being abandoned as change and tensions in their family and social relationships develop. Lack of socialization may contribute to loneliness as their illness progresses.

With this increased need for assistance for daily activities, a patient may fear being both a personal and a financial burden to their families. This may lead to psychological or spiritual conflict or loss. Ultimately, patients may experience the inability or unwillingness to cope with life-limiting illness and pending death.

Difficulty in making decisions about treatment choices that have not been clearly defined can be overwhelming. Perhaps their options are not clear with regard to expected outcome goals. Perhaps these options are overwhelming.

SECTION THREE REVIEW

1. Which most accurately describes the status of health care?
   1. Advancements in health care and the extension of life have made it easier for nurses to provide quality care for those who need it.
   2. The basics of human pain and suffering are being overlooked.
   3. Research and medical treatments are aimed at positively affecting a patient's quality of life.
   4. There are no discrepancies between patient desires and actual treatment.
2. Which statement most accurately describes the specific education a nurse working in palliative care should have? (Select all that apply.)
   1. The nurse should be familiar with the combined physiological changes, signs, and symptoms of the dying process and available treatment options.
   2. The United States is a death-defying society, focusing more on disease and cure than on comfort and palliation.
   3. Palliative care is provided by an interdisciplinary team approach.

4. Only nurses working with dying patients for many years are capable of working in palliative care arenas.
   5. The palliative care nurse must be able to think quickly and act alone in difficult situations.
3. In discussing care with a patient and family members, which is most important for the palliative care nurse to include?
   1. The current state and trajectory of the patient's disease process.
   2. All treatment options, even if they are all futile.
   3. The whole truth is to be avoided to maintain their hope.
   4. The nurse should tell the family that the health care team can best decide what the patient should be told.
4. A family member exhibits appropriate learning when which statement is made?
   1. "We can expect the same quality of life on a day-to-day basis."
   2. "We can expect him to feel a loss of control over his life as time goes by."
   3. "She will feel like she has gained some independence from us."
   4. "The role within the family will stay the same."

SECTION FOUR: The Interplay of Curative and Noncurative Measures

Caring for patients at the end of life does not necessitate doing "to patients" but more "doing for and being with patients" and their families. This requires exceptional caring, communication, knowledge, and skill (ELNEC, 2008).

The continuum of care as developed by Ferris and colleagues in 2001 (Figure 1–1) transcends from health and wellness through curative and palliative care. Patients and families have expectations and needs for care from presentation of disease to death and for the family after death. Health care providers need the capacity to offer a combination of disease-modifying and palliative therapies throughout their patients' illness experiences. The diagram in Figure 1–1 demonstrates this continuum. Palliative care extends

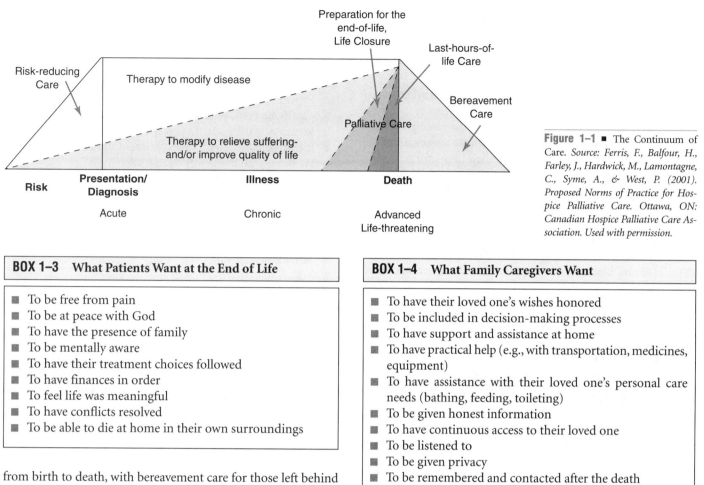

Figure 1–1 ■ The Continuum of Care. *Source: Ferris, F., Balfour, H., Farley, J., Hardwick, M., Lamontagne, C., Syme, A., & West, P. (2001). Proposed Norms of Practice for Hospice Palliative Care. Ottawa, ON: Canadian Hospice Palliative Care Association. Used with permission.*

BOX 1–3   What Patients Want at the End of Life
■ To be free from pain
■ To be at peace with God
■ To have the presence of family
■ To be mentally aware
■ To have their treatment choices followed
■ To have finances in order
■ To feel life was meaningful
■ To have conflicts resolved
■ To be able to die at home in their own surroundings

BOX 1–4   What Family Caregivers Want
■ To have their loved one's wishes honored
■ To be included in decision-making processes
■ To have support and assistance at home
■ To have practical help (e.g., with transportation, medicines, equipment)
■ To have assistance with their loved one's personal care needs (bathing, feeding, toileting)
■ To be given honest information
■ To have continuous access to their loved one
■ To be listened to
■ To be given privacy
■ To be remembered and contacted after the death

Source: McIlfatrick, 2006; Meier, 2003

from birth to death, with bereavement care for those left behind following the person's death. Essential in the model is the increasing implementation of palliative care interventions as the patient's illness progresses from acute to chronic and finally to a life-threatening stage. This increasing implementation of palliative care measures occurs as curative treatments are decreased. Equally important is that the patient approaching this final, life-threatening stage receives care designed to prepare him or her for life closure prior to the final hours of life.

Although similar to curative care, the assessment of palliative care needs focuses on the recognition of patient autonomy in choosing care or in working with family members if the patient is unable to make his or her wishes known. Palliative care recognizes that the patient must be presented with the choices available and the outcomes expected, and be assisted to understand that the options available may change as the patient's medical condition changes. When presented with these choices and assisted to understand outcomes and options, the person facing end-of-life decisions is given a sense of control over his or her life, often at times when he or she perceives that there is no control. These choices and options are parts of an ongoing process that continues from one care setting to another care setting.

Moving from just a curative approach, palliative care examines what patients themselves want. Seriously ill patients identified the topics displayed in Box 1–3 when asked what they would want as their condition progressed.

Studies of individuals with serious illness show they want the services that palliative care provides at the end of life. Overall, they want pain and other symptoms controlled. Patients want to avoid inappropriate prolongation of the dying process and to have a sense of control, good communication, and to be closely monitored so they need not feel abandoned. Patients do not want to be a burden on their family, but desire to strengthen relationships with their loved ones (Center to Advance Palliative Care [CAPC], 2007; Meier, 2003; National Quality Forum, 2006; SUPPORT, 1995).

Similarly, the result of two polls of bereaved family caregivers conducted in 2003 and repeated in 2006 found their needs to be those depicted in Box 1–4.

Palliative care is sometimes identified as the four Cs: comfort, communication, choices, and control, all of which focus on the patient and the family (ELNEC, 2008). These four Cs support ongoing reevaluation of goals of care and decision making, emphasizing therapeutic communication and remaining up to date on available choices. They also serve to augment transition management from curative to end-of-life care. All of these characteristics of palliative care help improve quality of life and increase patient and family satisfaction.

Palliative care is competent, compassionate care. In the course of illnesses, the time may come when patients may choose to forgo or not complete life-prolonging therapies. A palliative care specialist will honor and advocate for the patients' wishes and best interest.

The goals of palliative care fall in one of several categories as depicted in Box 1–5.

Palliative care affirms life by supporting the patient and family's goals for the future, which includes their hopes for cure or life prolongation, as appropriate, as well as their hopes for peace and dignity throughout the course of illness. Palliative care assists patients through the dying process and death with the intention to guide and assist the patient and family in making decisions that allow them to work toward their goals. The palliative care team collaborates with professional and informal caregivers to ensure coordination, communication, and continuity of care across institutional and home care settings. Palliative care is appropriate for all patients from the time of diagnosis with a life-threatening or debilitating condition, regardless of the patient's age.

BOX 1–5   Goals of Palliative Care

- Pain management
- Management of other symptoms
- Providing patient support
- Providing family support
- Clarifying goals of care
- Identifying the patient's perception of prognosis
- Identifying the family's perception of prognosis
- Working with the family dynamics
- Discussing Code Status—Cardiopulmonary Resuscitation/Do Not Resuscitate/Comfort Care only
- Establishing long-range health care directive plans
- Providing spiritual support
- Addressing health system issues
- Providing staff support
- Addressing discharge goals

SECTION FOUR REVIEW

1. Throughout life, options are given to promote health, from attempts to treat and cure disease, and finally to interventions of palliation. Which statement best confirms which beliefs are most important in the United States?
   1. Those working in health care are quick to recognize the need for palliative therapies.
   2. There are no deficiencies in current systems of care for patients and families at the end of life.
   3. Social and economic forces do not influence care at the end of life.
   4. The United States is a death-defying society focusing more on disease and cure than it does on comfort and palliation.
2. Which statement accurately describes the focus of palliative care?
   1. Increasing research monies spent looking for palliative interventions
   2. Caring for patients at the end of life—not doing "to" but more "doing for and being with"
   3. Stabilizing the many health conditions of the person
   4. Ensuring that the goals of care remain consistent
3. Which most appropriately describes the continuum of care? In palliative care, this continuum: (Select all that apply.)
   1. Begins at birth and does not end even after a patient's death.
   2. Does not include the presentation of disease.
   3. Delineates care between disease-modifying and palliative therapies throughout the patient's illness experience.
   4. Involves the primary care provider and the nurse assigned to the patient, as well as other team members as necessary.
   5. Includes all care for a patient until death occurs.
4. Seriously ill patients were asked what they would want at the end of their lives. The number one answer identified was:
   1. Dying in the hospital.
   2. Being alone.
   3. Avoiding inappropriate prolongation of the dying process.
   4. Allowing suffering to occur with little intervention.
5. Which statement by a family member best exemplifies the goals of palliative care? (Select all that apply.)
   1. "I know you are here to make things easier for us so we won't have to come here as often."
   2. "I want to make sure we all understand what changes in lifestyle my mother will need."
   3. "If I understand correctly, the goal is to make her comfortable and help her continue her life as she is able."
   4. "I know you will make sure my mother understands her disease process and what it will mean for her life expectancy."

SECTION FIVE: Principles of Hospice and Comparison to Palliative Care

Palliative care and hospice programs have grown rapidly due to the response in patients living with chronic, life-threatening, and life-limiting illness. Clinical interest has also grown to meet the needs of this population (National Consensus Project, 2004). In many ways, palliative care and hospice have similar characteristics. All of hospice care is palliative, but not all of palliative care involves hospice. Palliative care can often be the transition from treatment options to noncurative goals of care. Even today, though, not all health care providers, especially physicians and nurses, are either aware of or educated to manage end-of-life care that incorporates the philosophy of both hospice and palliative care options for their patients facing death, greatly limiting the referral process for patients who might benefit from these services.

Benefits of both palliative care and hospice can be found in the literature. Skilled nursing facilities with hospice care have cited the benefits shown in Box 1–6.

Palliative Care

Palliative care programs care for patients with life-threatening illnesses at any time during that life-threatening illness, even if life expectancies extend to years. These programs address the physical, psychosocial, emotional, and spiritual needs of patients as described in the previous section of this chapter. Palliative care can often serve as the bridge or transition from treatment options to noncurative and curative goals of care. Palliative care programs aim to serve patients throughout their illness experience, particularly, although not exclusively, in acute care hospitals and ambulatory outpatient settings. Palliative care may begin much earlier than the last 6 months of life, often while a patient continues to receive curative treatment for a disease. Patients may receive palliative care while in the hospital or in a home care program. Palliative care teams may consult with patients, families, and other health care team members to treat pain and other symptoms, help with discussion of goals and wishes, or provide extra support. Many patients may choose to transition to a hospice program at a later date. Table 1–1 shows the comparison of palliative care and hospice care components.

Hospice Care

In contrast, **hospice** is a philosophical approach to providing comfort and care at life's end that does not incorporate curative care, though may incorporate palliative care principles. Hospice care has specific guidelines under Medicare reimbursement. If a hospice program wishes to have services paid for under the Medicare Hospice Benefit, the hospice program must meet federal regulations. Most hospice programs and their patients

---

BOX 1–6   **Benefits of Hospice Care in Skilled Nursing Facilities**
■ Reduced number of hospitalizations
■ Decreased length of hospital stays
■ Decreased use of restraints
■ Decreased use of analgesics administered by injection
■ Reduced number of intravenous lines and feeding tubes
■ Increased likelihood that pain will be detected and treated

Source: National Hospice and Palliative Care Organization [HPCO], 2007, paragraph 6

and families rely on this payment option. The United States Medicare Hospice Benefit limits care to patients who:

1. Agree to therapy with a palliative intent;
2. Have a life expectancy of less than 6 months if the disease presents with its usual course in the judgment of the patient's attending physician and the hospice medical director; and
3. Elect the Medicare Hospice Benefit for coverage of all services related to their terminal condition.

There are four levels of hospice care under Medicare in the United States. Box 1–7 outlines these four levels.

When attempting to determine if a patient is a candidate for hospice care, a useful question to ask is, "Would you be surprised if this patient were to die within the next year?" This question yields a more accurate answer than, "Will this patient die in the next 6 months?" Determining prognosis can be difficult and needs to be addressed with each individual case. While no one knows how long anyone will live, there are certain signs that one's prognosis is very poor and that the time before death could be very limited.

Language is also important when discussing hospice with patients and families. Consider saying, "Because of the severity of your illness, you and your family are eligible for the assistance of hospice at home," rather than, "There is nothing more I can do for you. I am referring you to hospice." In the alternative, noting that "hospice is exceptionally good with pain and symptom control and will assist your loved one to remain comfortable" is another means of helping patients and their family members see the positive potential of hospice. Additional questions that may be asked in determining if hospice care would be a better alternative for an individual patient may be found in Box 1–8.

The philosophy of hospice is that every individual has the right to die as free of pain as possible, with dignity, knowing that his or her loved ones will receive the necessary support to allow this to occur. Hospice focuses on caring, not curing. In most cases, care is provided in the patient's home or where he or she resides (e.g., assisted living facility, skilled nursing facility, group home, etc.). Hospice care can also be provided in freestanding hospice centers and hospitals.

TABLE 1–1 Comparison of Palliative and Hospice Care Components

COMPONENT	PALLIATIVE CARE	HOSPICE CARE
Care recipient	Anyone who requires comfort measures for an illness or condition; is not dependent on life expectancy	Anyone who requires comfort care for an illness or condition; life expectancy is not expected to exceed 6 months
Type of care	Can continue to receive curative care measures while receiving palliative care measures	Care measures are aimed at relieving symptoms; curative measures are not continued
Length of care	Depends on the care needs; there is no maximum length that care can be received	The maximum length of care should be 6 months or less
Provider organizations	■ Acute care facilities ■ Long-term care ■ Skilled nursing ■ Health care clinics ■ Hospices	■ Hospices ■ Hospital-based hospice programs ■ Selected other organizations
Provider sites	■ Home ■ Assisted living facilities ■ Long-term care facilities ■ Skilled nursing facilities ■ Acute care facilities	■ Home ■ Assisted care facilities ■ Long-term care facilities ■ Skilled nursing facilities ■ Acute care facilities ■ Resident hospice facility
Providers of services	Usually done with an interdisciplinary team approach	Involves an interdisciplinary team approach
Experts in end-of-life care	Depends; may or may not be experts in this type of care	Yes
Insurance coverage	Medicaid, Medicare, and private insurance policies: some treatments and medications may be covered	Medicaid: In the majority of states, Medicaid pays all hospice charges Medicare: Pays all hospice charges Private insurance: Most insurance plans have a hospice benefit

---

BOX 1–7   The Four Levels of Hospice Care

1. Routine Home Care, the most frequently seen level of hospice care, is delivered on an intermittent basis wherever the patient resides.
2. Continuous Home Care consists of shifts of care, usually short term.
3. Inpatient Respite Care relieves the primary caregiver and provides care for the caregiver.
4. General Inpatient Care is delivered on a continuous basis in an acute or chronic care setting.

BOX 1–8   To Determine If the Patient Is a Candidate for Hospice Care, Question If the Patient:

■ Has more than one hospital admission for the same diagnosis in last 30 days.
■ Has a prolonged length of stay without evidence of progress.
■ Has a prolonged length of stay in the intensive care unit (ICU) or been transferred from the ICU without evidence of progress.
■ Is in an ICU with documented poor or futile prognosis.
■ Has family support needs or communication challenges.
■ Has a life-limiting illness and has chosen not to have life-prolonging therapy.
■ Has unacceptable pain for a period greater than 24 hours.
■ Has uncontrolled symptoms (e.g., nausea, vomiting).
■ Has unresolved psychosocial or spiritual issues.

Hospice services are available to patients of any age, religion, race, or medical condition/diagnosis. Hospice care, in contrast to many palliative care services, is covered under Medicare, Medicaid, most private insurance plans, and health maintenance organizations. Discharge from hospice can occur

SIX: Individualizing Palliative Care Assessment Using a Quality of Life Model

Grant (2008) described a quality of life model that es the physical, psychological, social, and spiritual s of a person (Figure 1–2). Throughout health and specifically during the dying experience, all dimen- ality of life can be impacted.

eaning of quality of life differs from person to per- ty of life can be defined only by the patient based on own life experience. It is important to try to examine of each dimension from the patient's and family's per- ne cannot just assume what "quality" means to pa- or family members. Dimensions are interrelated and considered from a holistic approach. The significance everal of the aspects within the dimensions may be af- ny change in individual circumstances.

s need to focus on both negative and positive con- o quality of life. This is similar to the "glass half full" r example, if nurses assessed and focused on only sing would be the opportunity to help patients and alize their hopes, which may have changed over time. f life is considered throughout the illness and dying This includes the time of death and the bereavement proving prognostication can affect quality of life by rategies of care for patients and their families (White, Patel, 2001).

The four dimensions that comprise this quality of life model are described briefly in the following text and in much greater depth in subsequent chapters. This more comprehensive understanding of each of these dimensions will assist nurses in developing and implementing care plans that encompass all four dimensions of the quality of life model.

Physical Well-Being

There are multiple physical symptoms due to disease progression and debility, including organic and metabolic changes that affect the physical well-being of the patient, including pain, fatigue, and dyspnea, to name but a few physical symptoms. Additionally, functional ability, appetite, and balancing sleep and rest have significant bearing on the patient's overall physical well-being.

Psychological Well-Being

Psychological well-being consists of a wide range of emotions and psychological issues/concerns that can occur at the end of life. Communication and support components are as important as the physical care. Addressing and working through unresolved issues may greatly assist the individual patient and family member to more positively address physical, social, and emotional aspects of dying.

The loss of privacy and dignity has a great impact on a patient's overall psychological well-being. Moving from independence to dependency often creates a feeling of being a burden to

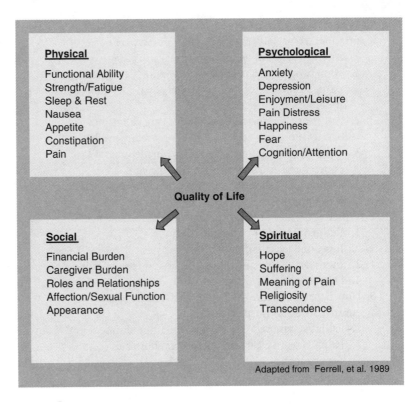

■ Quality of Life Dimensions. *Source: Ferrell, B. R. M., City of Hope Medical Center, 2008. Used with*

if prognosis improves or if a patient wishes to seek curative treatment. A patient may be readmitted at any time as long as the criteria for hospice are met.

Hospice has been referred to as the "gold standard" of palliative care in the United States (National Hospice and Palliative Care Organization [NHPCO], 2007). Hospice programs in the United States have focused on caring for the terminally ill in their own homes or in skilled nursing facilities. Hospice care is a family-centered approach that includes a health care team that works together, focusing on the dying patient's needs as a whole person. The goal is the same as in palliative care: to help keep the patient as pain-free as possible, with loved ones nearby until death. The hospice team develops a care plan that meets each patient's individual needs for pain management and symptom control. Box 1–9 depicts the more frequently encountered hospice team members.

It is important to identify the role of the patient's primary physician once the person begins receiving hospice care. Most often, a patient chooses to have his or her personal physician involved in the medical care. The patient's personal physician and the hospice medical director work together to coordinate the patient's medical care, especially when a patient's symptoms are difficult to manage. Regardless of the patient's choice for treatment options, the personal physician's involvement is important to ensure continuous quality hospice care for the individual patient. The hospice medical director is also available to answer

BOX 1–9   Hospice Team Memb

- Hospice physician (or medical
- The person's personal physicia
- Nurses
- Home health aides
- Social workers
- Clergy or other counselors
- Trained volunteers
- Speech, physical, and occupatio
- Music, art, and massage therapis

questions the individual or loved one
pice care.

Support that hospice provides to bers can include communication wit members, teaching caregiving skills, loved ones, including family member companionship, and help from volur death, bereavement support is offere 1 year. These services can take a vari telephone calls, visits, written materials port groups. Individual counseling ma pice, or the hospice may refer them to (NHPCO, 2007).

SECTION FIVE REVIEW

1. Which is the most likely reason that health care providers, especially physicians and nurses, are not knowledgable about end-of-life care?
   1. Both hospice and palliative care options are given to patients and their family members by other team members.
   2. Appropriate referrals to palliative care or hospice occur before physicians and nurses are involved.
   3. Medical and nursing schools have inadequate courses and education on end-of-life care.
   4. The benefits of both palliative care and hospice are well known.
2. Which is a benefit of both palliative care and hospice?
   1. Reduced number of hospitalizations
   2. Increased length of hospital stays
   3. Increased use of intravenous lines and feeding tubes
   4. Decreased time from diagnosis to death
3. How is palliative care the bridge between ongoing curative care and hospice care?
   1. Palliative care serves patients for a limited time.
   2. Patients receive care only in certain hospital departments.

   3. Patients are cared for only durin 6 months of life.
   4. Palliative care is provided to pati continue to receive treatment for
4. Why has hospice been referred to as standard" of palliative care in the Un
   1. It focuses on caring for only the te patient in his or her own home or nursing facility.
   2. Hospice develops a care plan meet individual needs for pain manager symptom control.
   3. Hospice care uses a medical model
   4. It ensures the patient gets only thos or she desires.
5. Which are included in the four levels of h Medicare in the United States? (Select all
   1. Inpatient respite care
   2. Outpatient respite care
   3. General inpatient care
   4. General outpatient care
   5. Routine or continuous home care

Ferrell a
encompa
dimensi
illness, a
sions of
The
son. Qu
his or he
all aspec
spective
tients ar
should
of one o
fected b
Nu
tributor
theory.
fears, n
families
Quality
trajecto
period.
guiding
Coyne,

Figur
and
perm

if prognosis improves or if a patient wishes to seek curative treatment. A patient may be readmitted at any time as long as the criteria for hospice are met.

Hospice has been referred to as the "gold standard" of palliative care in the United States (National Hospice and Palliative Care Organization [NHPCO], 2007). Hospice programs in the United States have focused on caring for the terminally ill in their own homes or in skilled nursing facilities. Hospice care is a family-centered approach that includes a health care team that works together, focusing on the dying patient's needs as a whole person. The goal is the same as in palliative care: to help keep the patient as pain-free as possible, with loved ones nearby until death. The hospice team develops a care plan that meets each patient's individual needs for pain management and symptom control. Box 1–9 depicts the more frequently encountered hospice team members.

It is important to identify the role of the patient's primary physician once the person begins receiving hospice care. Most often, a patient chooses to have his or her personal physician involved in the medical care. The patient's personal physician and the hospice medical director work together to coordinate the patient's medical care, especially when a patient's symptoms are difficult to manage. Regardless of the patient's choice for treatment options, the personal physician's involvement is important to ensure continuous quality hospice care for the individual patient. The hospice medical director is also available to answer

---

BOX 1–9   Hospice Team Members

- Hospice physician (or medical director)
- The person's personal physician, if desired
- Nurses
- Home health aides
- Social workers
- Clergy or other counselors
- Trained volunteers
- Speech, physical, and occupational therapists, if needed
- Music, art, and massage therapists as needed

---

questions the individual or loved ones may have regarding hospice care.

Support that hospice provides to patients and family members can include communication with the patient and family members, teaching caregiving skills, prayer, telephone calls to loved ones, including family members who live at a distance, companionship, and help from volunteers. After the person's death, bereavement support is offered to families for at least 1 year. These services can take a variety of forms, including telephone calls, visits, written materials about grieving, and support groups. Individual counseling may be offered by the hospice, or the hospice may refer them to a community resource (NHPCO, 2007).

SECTION FIVE REVIEW

1. Which is the most likely reason that health care providers, especially physicians and nurses, are not knowledgable about end-of-life care?
   1. Both hospice and palliative care options are given to patients and their family members by other team members.
   2. Appropriate referrals to palliative care or hospice occur before physicians and nurses are involved.
   3. Medical and nursing schools have inadequate courses and education on end-of-life care.
   4. The benefits of both palliative care and hospice are well known.

2. Which is a benefit of both palliative care and hospice?
   1. Reduced number of hospitalizations
   2. Increased length of hospital stays
   3. Increased use of intravenous lines and feeding tubes
   4. Decreased time from diagnosis to death

3. How is palliative care the bridge between ongoing curative care and hospice care?
   1. Palliative care serves patients for a limited time.
   2. Patients receive care only in certain hospital departments.
   3. Patients are cared for only during their last 6 months of life.
   4. Palliative care is provided to patients while they continue to receive treatment for a disease.

4. Why has hospice been referred to as the "gold standard" of palliative care in the United States?
   1. It focuses on caring for only the terminally ill patient in his or her own home or in a skilled nursing facility.
   2. Hospice develops a care plan meeting each patient's individual needs for pain management and symptom control.
   3. Hospice care uses a medical model approach.
   4. It ensures the patient gets only those treatments he or she desires.

5. Which are included in the four levels of hospice care under Medicare in the United States? (Select all that apply.)
   1. Inpatient respite care
   2. Outpatient respite care
   3. General inpatient care
   4. General outpatient care
   5. Routine or continuous home care

SECTION SIX: Individualizing Palliative Care Assessment Using a Quality of Life Model

Ferrell and Grant (2008) described a quality of life model that encompasses the physical, psychological, social, and spiritual dimensions of a person (Figure 1–2). Throughout health and illness, and specifically during the dying experience, all dimensions of quality of life can be impacted.

The meaning of quality of life differs from person to person. Quality of life can be defined only by the patient based on his or her own life experience. It is important to try to examine all aspects of each dimension from the patient's and family's perspective. One cannot just assume what "quality" means to patients and/or family members. Dimensions are interrelated and should be considered from a holistic approach. The significance of one or several of the aspects within the dimensions may be affected by any change in individual circumstances.

Nurses need to focus on both negative and positive contributors to quality of life. This is similar to the "glass half full" theory. For example, if nurses assessed and focused on only fears, missing would be the opportunity to help patients and families realize their hopes, which may have changed over time. Quality of life is considered throughout the illness and dying trajectory. This includes the time of death and the bereavement period. Improving prognostication can affect quality of life by guiding strategies of care for patients and their families (White, Coyne, & Patel, 2001).

The four dimensions that comprise this quality of life model are described briefly in the following text and in much greater depth in subsequent chapters. This more comprehensive understanding of each of these dimensions will assist nurses in developing and implementing care plans that encompass all four dimensions of the quality of life model.

Physical Well-Being

There are multiple physical symptoms due to disease progression and debility, including organic and metabolic changes that affect the physical well-being of the patient, including pain, fatigue, and dyspnea, to name but a few physical symptoms. Additionally, functional ability, appetite, and balancing sleep and rest have significant bearing on the patient's overall physical well-being.

Psychological Well-Being

Psychological well-being consists of a wide range of emotions and psychological issues/concerns that can occur at the end of life. Communication and support components are as important as the physical care. Addressing and working through unresolved issues may greatly assist the individual patient and family member to more positively address physical, social, and emotional aspects of dying.

The loss of privacy and dignity has a great impact on a patient's overall psychological well-being. Moving from independence to dependency often creates a feeling of being a burden to

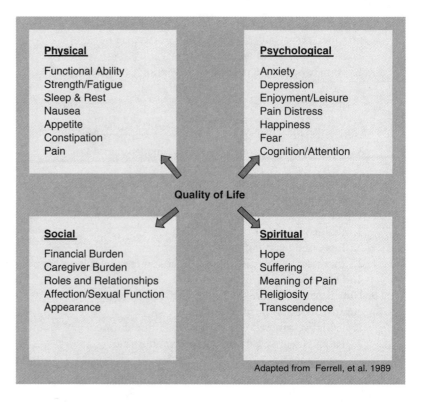

Figure 1–2 ■ Quality of Life Dimensions. *Source: Ferrell, B. R. and Grant, M., City of Hope Medical Center, 2008. Used with permission.*

Adapted from Ferrell, et al. 1989

others. Subsequent lowered self-esteem can intensify feelings of psychological and physical pain, aloneness, and depletion of energy. The feeling of helplessness often leads to hopelessness (ELNEC, 2008). This feeling of a loss of control can lead patients to try to control the little things around them. Additional methods of coping should be explored.

Social Well-Being

Social well-being must also be considered. The social structure and integrity of the family may be endangered. Relationships and roles are often disrupted, which may cause turmoil, dysfunction, and may need restructuring. Becoming dependent on one's family may be seen as a burden by the patient and is often a concern to the patient near the end of his or her life (McIlfatrick, 2006). Children may manifest their emotional concerns by isolating themselves or by acting out in a classroom or at home. Financial concerns may arise due to lost income from the patient and/or family members missing work because of caregiver responsibilities. All of these factors must be individualized and addressed in the plan of care.

As patients near death, it is common for them to withdraw from the people around them. Health care providers should explain this to the family and friends of the patient, so that they understand this is a natural part of the dying process (ELNEC, 2008).

Spiritual Well-Being

Religion and spirituality may have a great impact on a patient's overall well-being and may be a course of great comfort to the person and/or family members. These two terms are not synonymous; religion relates to a particular system of faith and worship, with specific rules, doctrines, customs, and practices, while spirituality is used to refer to matters of the soul apart from specific religious affiliation and aligned with inspiration, ultimate ends and values, and the search for existential meaning. Spiritual assessment and interventions in health care should be part of the plan of care and the interdisciplinary team members all assist in providing aspects of spiritual comfort to terminally ill patients.

SECTION SIX REVIEW

1. Quality-of-life dimensions encompass dimensions of the person: physical, psychological, social, and:
    1. Emotional.
    2. Human.
    3. Spiritual.
    4. Secular.
2. Which statement describes the significance of knowing that quality-of-life dimensions may be affected by any change in individual circumstances?
    1. Nurses need to focus on just the positive aspects.
    2. Quality of life should be considered throughout the illness and dying trajectory.
    3. Improved prognosis can decrease quality of life.
    4. Patients and families realize their hopes without hearing from health care providers.
3. Which two components of psychological well-being are as important as the physical care component?
    1. Communication and support
    2. Drug intervention and psychotherapy

3. Dependence and loss of control
    4. Anxiety and depression
4. In the United States, which describes the social structure and integrity of many families? They are:
    1. Healed.
    2. Without family input.
    3. Unrelated to the patient.
    4. Endangered.
5. What is the reason spiritual care is often a neglected component of quality of life?
    1. Interdisciplinary teams do not have time to devote to spirituality.
    2. The comfort level of the caregivers is not established with the health care providers.
    3. Health care providers may not realize the need for spiritual care.
    4. There is a lack of understanding of all religious practices.

SECTION SEVEN: Life Closure

Care of the dying patient is an intense interval for the patient, family, and health care team. Initiating discussion with the patient and family is the first step in establishing the individual plan of care for the dying patient. There is usually less anxiety and depression in the dying process if it has been clearly discussed. Removing the fear of the unknown can reduce this stress. Ongoing communication

with the family and the patient regarding the dying process and the goals of care is necessary (Berzoff & Silverman, 2004).

The stages and tasks as the patient approaches death vary and may occur at any time, not following this nonlinear pattern but involving all dimensions of quality of life. The first aspect is from a broader, more worldly, outer perspective. Callanan (2001) gave the visual example of a stone dropped in a puddle. At the beginning of life, the ripples are centralized, inward, and then moving outward. However at the end of life, it is in reverse, and the ripples diminish.

The goal, therefore, at the end of life is to gain a sense of completion about the meaning of one's individual life.

The second aspect or perspective is more sensitive and internal. These are the goals of relationship closure with families and friends, and accepting the finality of life brought on by impending death. Byock (1997) describes how patients may see a different self beyond the personal loss, as well as finding new meaning in life, as he or she approaches death. This becomes the ultimate acceptance, the "letting go."

The patient's transition to the dying phase should be consistently communicated by all members of the health care team. Mixed messages should be avoided, as they can lead to loss of trust, miscommunication, and poor care management (NQF, 2006). The National Consensus Project Clinical (2004) and the National Quality Forum (2006) endorse open communication with the patient, family, and care team regarding the dying phase and plan of care. Everyone involved in the patient's care should be supportive of the plan of care.

The plan of care for the dying patient and his or her family must be individually directed to meet their specific needs. This allows for clarification of prognosis, identification of end-of-life goals, and identification of care preferences, including the site of care and setting for death. Agreement between care team members that the patient is dying, and communicating this to the patient and family, improves satisfaction and fosters trust (Balaban, 2000). The treatment plan should include education for the patient and family about the signs and symptoms of imminent death. Understanding of and sensitivity to developmental, cultural, and religious needs are of critical importance. Attention to adequate symptom management allays fears and allows comfort during the dying process. The comprehensive treatment plan must be medically sound and concordant with the patient's wishes and values (Byock, 1997).

Diagnosing the dying process is a complex process due to multiple factors. Health care providers can sometimes narrow a prognosis to hours, days, or weeks, but are more frequently inaccurate about the length of time left to a patient before the patient dies. Health care providers are trained to cure and treat patients and will often continue aggressive, invasive procedures and treatments at the expense of making the patient comfortable. They are more doing "to" than "for" a person during that last phase of their lives. There is often a reluctance to make the diagnosis of dying if any hope of improvement exists and even more so if no definite diagnosis has been made. However, when recovery is uncertain, it is better to discuss this rather than giving false hope and offering ineffective treatment options to patients and their families.

Box 1–10 depicts some of the more common signs and symptoms that indicate death is approaching, though not all individuals will manifest all of these signs and symptoms.

BOX 1–10   Signs and Symptoms of Impending Death

One to three months prior to death:

- Social withdrawal from the world and some people
- Withdrawal from active participation in social activities
- More going inside of self
- Increased periods of sleep, lethargy
- Decreased intake of food and liquids
- Decreased communication

Weeks prior to death:

- Disorientation and delirium, often manifested by: increased restlessness, confusion, agitation, inability to stay content in one position and insisting on changing positions frequently
- Stating the need to "go" somewhere or "get out of bed" without physical need
- Picking at clothes, reaching in the air
- Talking with the unseen, but usually calmly
- Reports seeing people who have already died
- Patient states that he or she is dying.
- Patient requests family visit to settle unfinished business and reach closure, putting affairs in order.
- Complaints of body being extremely tired and/or heavy
- Significantly decreasing oral intake or ability to intake food and fluids
- Body temperature hot or cold
- Inability to heal or recover from wounds or infections
- Increased respiratory congestion or fluid buildup in the lungs; shortness of breath.
- Sleeping but not responding
- Decreasing blood pressure
- Pulse increasing or decreasing
- Diaphoretic (increased perspiration)
- Abnormal breathing patterns and irregular respirations

Days or hours before death:

- Intense surge of energy—often family confuses this with "getting better and stronger"
- Periods of (apnea) whether awake or sleeping
- Very rapid breathing or cyclic changes in the patterns of breathing (Cheyne-Stokes respirations)
- Increased edema (swelling) of either the extremities or the entire body
- Ability to arouse patient only with great effort, but patient quickly returns to unresponsive state (stupor or semi-coma)
- Severe agitation in patient, hallucinations, acting "crazy" and not in patient's normal manner or personality
- Inability to swallow any fluids at all; not taking food by mouth; vomiting
- Patient breathing through wide-open mouth continuously and no longer able to speak, if awake
- Urinary or bowel incontinence in a patient who was not incontinent before
- Marked decrease in urinary output and darkening color of urine or very abnormal color of urine such as red or brown
- Blood pressure dropping dramatically from patient's normal blood pressure range (more than a 20–30 point drop)
- Systolic blood pressure below 70; diastolic blood pressure below 50
- Patient's extremities feel very cold to the touch.
- Fever
- Patient complains that his or her legs/feet are numb and cannot be felt at all.
- Cyanosis or mottling (a blue or purple coloring to the patient's arms, legs, hands, knees, and feet)
- Patient's body is held in a rigid unchanging position.
- No tactile response when eyelashes touched
- No radial pulse

Minutes before death:

- Open-mouthed, gasping respirations
- Unresponsive (inability to arouse patient at all)
- Mouth open, unable to shut
- Eyes partially open

Source: Ellershaw & Ward, 2003; ELNEC, 2008

SECTION SEVEN REVIEW

1. When the nurse is establishing the individual plan of care for the dying patient, which is the priority action?
   1. Initiating discussion with the patient and family members
   2. Alleviating any fears that the patient and family members may have
   3. Asking questions of the patient and family members
   4. Taking notes with the patient and family members
2. A family member is learning about the expected events of a family member completing life. Appropriate learning has taken place when which statement is made?
   1. "I know the outer perspective includes the process of 'letting go' ."
   2. "Closure with family and friends is the first task of completing life."
   3. "The last task is seeing a different self beyond the personal loss."
   4. "Completing community affairs is part of the outer perspective of completing life."

3. Which is an early sign of the dying process?
   1. Mottling
   2. Social withdrawal
   3. Changes in respiratory status
   4. Decreased heart rate
4. Weeks prior to death, signs may include:
   1. Periods of apnea.
   2. Unresponsiveness.
   3. Hallucinating.
   4. Intense surge of energy.
5. Which would be the most appropriate statement for the nurse to assist the family to understand death is moments away?
   1. "Her eyes may stay open but she isn't really seeing anything."
   2. "She may talk until death occurs."
   3. "Her breathing will become more regular in rate and intensity."
   4. "Her skin color will look more normal."

SECTION EIGHT: Opportunities for Growth at the End of Life

Patients and families have often described the personal growth that takes place at the end of life even during struggles to overcome physical, emotional, and spiritual distress, and at times, denying the dying process as well. Death can profoundly affect those who are intimately involved with the patient. This includes the health care providers, who find their own personal growth related to caring for individuals facing life-threatening illnesses. This growth often comes about from assisting a patient to experience a good, or peaceful death, and from coming to understand what is meant by dying well (Byock, 2004). All the dimensions of quality of life model provide opportunity for growth and healing even when facing or witnessing the death. Patients and families are often able to find meaning through life review, working toward personal goals and closure, and exploring their relationship with others and God at this point.

The meaning of hope shifts from that of cure and limited or measured time to one in which individuals strive to reach personal end-of-life closure goals. Despite the reality that the patient will die and the potential for suffering, many people do find new ways to hope. Patients can maintain hope as they die, and families regain hope even as they experience loss (Ersek, 2006; Byock, 2004). Family members often recognize that the care they give to their dying family member is a final gift of love. Many who die from a more progressive illness are able to rise above suffering to feel a sense of well-being, even as they are dying. Patients who die from sudden or traumatic deaths and their families may miss these opportunities for growth (Byock, 1996).

For the health care professional, accepting death and the dying process as a natural part of the life cycle is one of the first steps in growth. Such caregivers take comfort in learning that dying well—a patient's good death, marked by controlled pain, resolved life issues, not dying alone, and reaching other goals he or she established—can be viewed as successful care for those reasons. Having emotions emerge when caring for, and from assessing the suffering of others during the dying process opens nurses to the opportunity of dispelling personal fears and of providing heartfelt therapeutic presence and compassionate end-of-life care. Personal satisfaction develops through processing and sharing stories about patients and families facing death (Byock, 1997). Often nurses feel that they receive much more than they give from these experiences. Additionally, facing one's own mortality can usually initiate the need for a deeper examination of personal priorities, beliefs, and values.

SECTION EIGHT REVIEW

1. Dying well and a good death may depend on which consideration?
   1. Denying that the dying process is an inevitable part of life
   2. Recognizing growth and well-being can emerge from relieving symptoms caused by treatments
   3. Knowing that life review is not a component of end-of-life care
   4. Experiencing decreasing spiritual awareness as death approaches
2. At the end of life, which option indicates how hope shifts?
   1. From cure to quality
   2. From life's meaning to afterlife
   3. From suffering to realization
   4. From loss to success
3. The nurse should ensure that family members recognize that the care they give:
   1. Instills hope.
   2. Provides nutrients.
   3. Shows love.
   4. Encourages a cure.
4. For the nurse, accepting death and the dying process as a natural part of the life cycle serves which purpose?
   1. Promotes that care should only be given to gain knowledge and experience
   2. Encourages the acceptance of depression instead of fighting the experience
   3. Encourages the admission of personal dissatisfaction
   4. Dispels personal fears and allows the nurse to provide therapeutic presence
5. Which type of patient is more likely to rise above suffering and emerge with a sense of well-being even as he or she is dying? The patient who dies from: (Select all that apply.)
   1. A myocardial infarction.
   2. Terminal cancer.
   3. A motor vehicle collision.
   4. Chronic obstructive pulmonary disease.
   5. Alzheimer's disease.

SECTION NINE: Role of the Nurse Providing End-of-Life Care Across All Clinical Settings

Nurses spend more time with patients and patient's families than any other health care professional, placing them in a unique position to be advocates for patients and families as the patient approaches the end of life. Additionally, nurses often assume a lead role in the health care team and frequently act as not only the primary care provider, but as a consultant and educator, assisting patients and family members to address the multitude of needs that accompany an approaching death. Expert nursing care has the potential to reduce the burden and distress greatly. Indeed, nurses have the ability to offer support for the many diverse needs of patients, families, and caregivers.

The palliative care team works closely with the primary physician to deliver well-coordinated and communicated care, and to provide guidance and counseling about complex treatment choices to the patient and family members. The team provides the highest quality of care by building the necessary systems to treat the growing number of people with serious, advanced, and complex illnesses. Beckstrand et al. (2006) confirm that incorporation of the entire team when treating patients in their final days of life gives family members the support they need to make difficult decisions when withholding and withdrawing life-sustaining systems and interventions.

Nurses, working as part of the interdisciplinary team, may be required to provide palliative care in a variety of different settings, which requires nurses to have a knowledge base in palliative care.

These locations include all areas of the acute care facility, in nursing homes, home care, assisted living facilities, outpatient, and numerous other settings.

One of the means through which nurses and other members of the interdisciplinary team provide palliative care effectively is therapeutic presence. This strategy is a way of expressing compassionate caring without having to "do" anything and is not treatment or intervention by standard definitions. To be present with dying patients and their families allows the nurse or another team member to enter into another person's circumstances and personal world while responding with compassion and care. Presence is often the greatest gift we can give to dying patients and their families.

Although the goal is for comfort, not all deaths are peaceful or without suffering. There are times when symptoms cannot be adequately controlled or there is unfinished business that can impact a peaceful death. At times, nurses may feel guilty or responsible for situations that may or may not have been under their control. It is important to value the efforts taken and review what could be done in future situations.

Dignity and respect are hallmarks of palliative nursing. Interventions needed to meet these characteristics include effective, therapeutic communication, awareness of choices, providing comfort, and giving as much control to the patient and family as possible. Even when faced with overwhelming losses of autonomy and independence, patients and families can ideally retain the freedom to choose, regarding their perceptions. Nurses, individually, and collectively as a profession, play a vital role in improving care at the end of life. A patient or family member may not remember what was done, but will remember how he or she was made to feel.

SECTION NINE REVIEW

1. Which describes nurses' first responsibility in end-of-life care?
   1. Decrease the time we spend with patients and families.
   2. Educate patients and families on questions to discuss with other health care professionals.
   3. Remember that patients and their families are similar.
   4. Limit support for the physical, psychological, social, emotional, as well as spiritual needs of patients, families, and caregivers.

2. How might a nurse assist in relieving a family member's distress?
   1. Encourage frequent rest periods.
   2. Discourage asking for assistance from other places.
   3. Discourage distressed family members from assisting in care.
   4. Encourage brief conversations with the patient.

3. Which are included in roles nurses can undertake since nurses spend more time with patients and patient's families than any other health care professional? (Select all that apply.)
   1. Advocate
   2. Consultant and educator
   3. Support
   4. Cheerleader
   5. Errand runner

4. Which indicates the outcome of palliative care nursing?
   1. Limited treatment of the pain, symptoms, and stress of serious illness
   2. Focus only on long-term needs and activities
   3. Well-coordinated and communicated care
   4. Separation from the physician and team to practice independently

5. Which are obstacles to providing quality palliative care? (Select all that apply.)
   1. Patients refusing care
   2. Continuity of care
   3. Multiple health care providers with different views
   4. Adequate staffing needs and time
   5. Multiple family members asking many questions

CHAPTER SUMMARY

- Quality of life has multiple meanings for individual persons, but generally encompasses feelings of self-esteem, self-worth and love, independence, a sense of well-being despite having limitations imposed by circumstances and illness, and the ability to cope effectively and retain hope during one's final days.
- Palliative care, provided to individuals with a potentially life-limiting, life-threatening illness, has a core goal of providing quality of life to individuals through a holistic, interdisciplinary, patient-centered approach.
- Historically, care at the end of life was centered on comfort care measures, delivered to patients in their home settings; palliative care allows health care providers to incorporate comfort and curative measures when caring for individuals at the end of life.
- National initiatives, including the End of Life Nursing Education Consortium (ELNEC), have been created to assist health care providers provide quality, competent care to individuals at the end of life.
- Caring for patients at the end of life does not necessitate doing "to patients" but more "doing for and being with patients" and their families. This requires exceptional caring, communication, knowledge, and skill.

- Palliative care is sometimes identified as the four "Cs": comfort, communication, choices, and control, all equally important in the provision of quality care.
- All of hospice care is palliative, but not all of palliative care involves hospice.
- The philosophy of hospice is that every individual has the right to die as free of pain as possible, with dignity, knowing that their loved ones will receive the necessary support to allow this to occur. Hospice focuses on caring, not curing.
- The quality of life model encompasses four spheres: physical, psychological, social, and spiritual.
- Personal growth occurs for those involved in end-of-life care, accepting death and the dying process as a natural part of the life cycle, and understanding that the four spheres of the quality of life model are equally important in resolving closure issues.

CHAPTER REVIEW

MRS. JONES

CHIEF COMPLAINT(S). Chest wall and abdominal pain, constipation.

HISTORY OF PRESENT ILLNESS. The patient is a 75-year-old female admitted to an acute care hospital from the cancer center. She has a known history of metastatic breast cancer. Her breast cancer was first diagnosed some years ago, and metastases were diagnosed 5 years ago with one area of metastasis to the bone. Over the past week, she has had increasing pain in her sternal area, which is also causing more shortness of breath. Her fentanyl patch was increased from 150 mcg/hr to 200 mcg/hr 2 weeks ago. She has also developed increasing constipation and has not been compliant with routine bowel regimen.

PAST SPECIFIC SYMPTOM HISTORY. Loss of appetite, weakness and fatigue, insomnia, anxiety, upper chest pain, abdominal pain, constipation, shortness of breath

MEDICATIONS/IVs.

1. Timolol ophthalmic drops daily
2. Ambien 10 mg at bedtime
3. Hydromorphone 1–3 tablets every 3 hours as needed for pain
4. Lorazepam 1 mg four times a day as needed
5. Milk of magnesia as needed
6. MiraLax 17 g daily as needed
7. Fentanyl 200 mcg/h patch topically, change every 72 hours

ALLERGIES. No known allergies

PAST MEDICAL/SURGICAL HISTORY.

1. Metastatic breast cancer
2. Hypertension
3. Gastroesophageal reflux disease
4. Hypercholesterolemia
5. History of anxiety
6. History of chronic headache
7. Insomnia
8. Left foot drop secondary to Taxol
9. History of shingles

SOCIAL HISTORY. The patient has been widowed for 17 years. She lives in an apartment and has two adult sons and an adult daughter. One of her sons lives in the same town as Mrs. Jones. Another son lives out of state, and her daughter about 75 miles away. She has two grandsons. She enjoys her kitten. Mrs. Jones also enjoys watching TV. She did smoke, but quit 12 years ago and does not drink alcohol or use illicit drugs.

ADVANCE DIRECTIVE. She has a valid living will, and desires only comfort care if she is terminal and unable to make her own decisions. Her surrogate decision maker is aware of these desires.

CODE STATUS. DNR (do not resuscitate)

SPIRITUAL SOURCES OF STRENGTH. Mrs. Jones is a Lutheran and an active member of her church. She has requested that her church include her on their prayer list.

REVIEW OF SYSTEMS. GENERAL: She is alert and answers questions appropriately. EYES: History of glaucoma. Has eyedrops. Uses glasses for reading. ENT: Denies sore mouth, dry mouth, or hearing difficulties. CV: Denies angina or palpitations. RESPIRATORY: Mild shortness of breath caused by the increased pain. Denies cough or hiccups. GI: Reports poor appetite. Eats small quarter-portions. Fluid intake decreased. Ongoing problem with constipation. GU: Denies bladder pain or spasms. MUSCULOSKELETAL: Mild weakness and fatigue. Wears brace on her left leg when she is ambulatory. SKIN: Denies rash, pain, masses, or decubitus. PSYCH: Uses Ambien routinely for insomnia. Denies any depression. ENDOCRINE: Reports weight loss of 6 pounds in the past month and 1 pound in the past week. No edema. HEME/LYMPH: Denies fever, chills, or night sweats. Appreciates a cool environment, but likes her feet wrapped for warmth. NEUROLOGIC: Reports intermittent use of lorazepam for anxiety once every day or 2, denies any confusion or dizziness.

PAIN ISSUES. Upper chest and abdomen reports pain at a 7–8 level intensity on a 10-point scale; the lowest her pain level reaches is 2 on the 10-point scale. Often describes her pain as a constant ache. Not relieved except with medications, though she does note some relief or worsening of her pain with positioning. Does not radiate, but does have sharp, episodic increase in her chest pain at times. Denies any headache.

OVERALL WELL-BEING. Described by the patient as Fair

PATIENT'S/FAMILY'S AREA(S) OF GREATEST CONCERN. Pain control

PHYSICAL EXAMINATION. VITAL SIGNS: Temperature 36.6 degrees; heart rate 108; respiratory rate 20; blood pressure 151/50; O2 saturation 97% in room air. LAST BOWEL MOVEMENT: 3 days ago. CURRENT IV ACCESS: Port-A-Cath. GENERAL: Alert, sociable, but in moderate pain. HEENT: Mucous membranes moist, pink. CHEST/RESPIRATORY: Regular rate and rhythm. CARDIOVASCULAR: Heart sounds tachycardic, but regular rate and rhythm. ABDOMEN/GI: Mildly distended, soft, slightly tender to palpation. Bowel sounds slightly diminished, but present. EXTREMITIES: No edema. SKIN: Pale, warm, and dry. MUSCULOSKELETAL: Mild weakness, able to move extremities by herself. NEUROLOGICAL: Alert and sociable; oriented, appropriate affect and mood for situation.

PERTINENT LABS/DIAGNOSTIC TESTS. No pertinent labs or diagnostic tests

PALLIATIVE PERFORMANCE LEVEL. 40% (100% = fully ambulatory, normal activity, no evidence of disease, fully self-care, normal intake, and full LOC; and 0% = death)

ASSESSMENT. Mrs. Jones's pain is currently being managed with fentanyl patch 200 mcg/hr, breakthrough hydromorphone (not started at home yet), bed rest, positioning, medical equipment, and staff support. Her shortness of breath is being managed with bed rest and positioning. Her appetite is being managed with diet of choice. Her weakness and fatigue are being managed with bed rest and positioning. Mrs. Jones's insomnia is being managed with Ambien, pain control, bed rest, and support. Her anxiety is being managed with lorazepam and staff support. The patient's psychosocial and spiritual needs are being adequately managed with family and staff support.

Question

You are the nurse caring for Mrs. Jones. What are some of the indications for palliative care and related nursing management?

Suggested Responses

Areas that should be considered in addressing this question include:

- Pain Control: Treat symptoms, identify underlying cause(s)
- Treatment of other symptoms: Anxiety, breathlessness, weakness, fatigue, insomnia, constipation, mobility, and loss of appetite
- Psychosocial—patient support/needs: Diversion, life review, self-disclosure, and self-esteem
- Spiritual support: Incorporate chaplain or home pastor/priest, rabbi as appropriate.
- Family support: Consider a family conference.
- Clarifying goals of care: Consider whether this patient can return to her apartment after discharge or to an alternate setting.
- Patient's perception of prognosis: Consider what she knows and how realistic this perception is based on her disease etiology.
- Family's perception of prognosis: Consider what they know and how realistic their perceptions are.
- Level of care: Is she terminal at this stage and would hospice care be the most appropriate care at this stage of her illness?
- Consider if a pet visit could help.
- Are there additional interventions/considerations that might be addressed?

REFERENCES

Administration on Aging. (2000). *Older population by age: 1900 to 2050.* Retrieved from http://www.aoa.gov./prof/statistics/online_stat_data/popage2050.xls

Agency for Health Care Policy and Research Clinical Practice. (1996). In M. Field & C. Cassel, editors. *Approaching death: Improving care at the end of life.* Washington, DC: National Academy Press.

Balaban, R. (2000). A physician's guide to talking about end-of-life care. *Journal of General Internal Medicine, 15,* 195–200.

Beckstrand, R., Callister, L., & Kirchhoff, K. (2006). Providing a "good death": Critical care nurses' suggestions for improving end-of-life care. *American Journal of Critical Care 15*(1), 38–45.

Berzoff, J., & Silverman, P. (2004). *Living with dying: A handbook for end-of-life healthcare practitioners.* New York: Columbia University Press.

Byock, I. (1996). The nature of suffering and the nature of opportunity at the end of life. *Clinics in Geriatric Medicine, 12*(2), 237–251.

Byock, I. (1997). *Dying well: The prospect for growth at the end of life.* New York: Riverhead Books.

Byock I. (2004). *The four things that matter most: A book about living.* New York: Free Press.

Callanan, M. (2001). Journeying Home. Video series, Hospice of the Red River Valley, Grand Forks, ND.

Centers for Disease Control. (2008). U.S. mortality drops sharply in 2006. *National Vital Statistics Report, 56*(16), 1–56.

Center to Advance Palliative Care. (2007). Defining palliative care. Retrieved from http://www.capc.org/building-a-hospital-based-palliative-care-program/case/ definingpc

Ellershaw, J., & Ward, C. (2003). Care of the dying patient: Last hours or days of life. *British Medical Journal, 326*, 30–34.

Ellershaw, J., & Wilkinson, S, eds. (2003). *Care of the dying: A pathway to excellence*. New York: Oxford University Press.

End of Life Nursing Education Consortium. (2000). *Advancing end-of-life nursing care*. Washington, DC: American Association of Colleges of Nursing.

End of Life Nursing Education Consortium (ELNEC). (2008). *Advanced end of life nursing care: ELNEC supercore training program 2008. Washington, DC: American Association of Colleges of Nursing.*

Ersek, M. (2006). The Meaning of Hope in the Dying. In B. R. Ferrell, & N. Coyle (Eds.) *Textbook of palliative nursing*. New York, NY: Oxford University Press.

Ferrell, B. R., & Coyle, P. (2006). Understanding the moral distress of nurses witnessing medically futile care. *Oncology Nursing Forum, 33*(5), 922–930.

Ferrell, B. R., and Grant, M. (2008). ACE Project Curriculum. Retrieved from http://www.cityofhope.org/education/health-professional-education/nursing-education/ACE-project/Pages/ACE-project-curriculum.aspx

Ferris, F., Balfour, H., Farley, J., Hardwick, M., Lamontagne, C., Syme, A., et al. (2001). *Proposed norms of practice for hospice palliative care*. Ottawa, ON: Canadian Hospice Palliative Care Association.

McIlfatrick, S. (2006). Assessing palliative care needs: Views of patients, informal careers and healthcare professionals. *Journal of Advancing Nursing, 57*(1), 77–86.

Meier, D. (2003). Palliative care: Making the case. Center to Advance Palliative Care, Training Seminar, October 2003, San Diego, CA.

National Consensus Project. (2004). National Consensus Project for Quality Palliative Care: Clinical Practice Guidelines for Quality Palliative Care, Executive Summary. *Journal of Palliative Medicine, 7*(5), 611–627.

National Hospice and Palliative Care Organization. (2007). Hospice Information. Retrieved from http://www.caringinfo.org/LivingWithAnIllness/Hospice/TheHospiceTeam.htm

National Quality Forum. (2006). *A national framework and preferred practices for palliative and hospice care quality*. Washington, DC: Author.

SUPPORT Study. (1995). A controlled trial to improve care for seriously ill hospitalized patients. The study to understand prognoses and preference for outcomes and risks of treatments. *Journal of the American Medical Association, 274*(20), 1591–1598.

Virani, R., & Sofer, D. (2003). Improving the quality of end-of-life care: Making changes at every level. *American Journal of Nursing, 103*(5), 52–60.

White, K., Coyne, P., & Patel, U. (2001). Are nurses adequately prepared for end of life care? *Journal of Nursing Scholarship, 33*, 147–151.

World Health Organization. (1990). Cancer pain relief and palliative care. Geneva: WHO Technical Report Series 804.

World Health Organization. (2007). World Health Organization's Definition of Palliative Care. Retrieved from http://www.who.int/cancer/palliative/definition/en/

Ethics and Ethical Issues in End-of-Life Nursing Care

2.1 Differentiate law from ethics.

2.2 Discuss the utility of various ethical theories when determining the nurse's approach to nursing care at the end of life.

2.3 Explore key ethical principles that can be applied by health care providers at the end of life.

2.4 Define the principle of double effect and its application to end-of-life nursing care.

2.5 Analyze the role of therapeutic jurisprudence as a tool to guide nurses in the implementation of ethical decision making during end-of-life care.

2.6 Analyze the role of advocacy from an ethical perspective.

2.7 Discuss the important role that ethics committees play in caring for this population.

2.8 Apply the respectful death model in end-of-life care.

This chapter compares and contrasts legal and ethical issues as well as introduces and discusses ethical theories and key ethical principles that guide nursing practice. The role of therapeutic jurisprudence and the importance of the nurse as a patient advocate at the end of life are presented. The value of ethics committees when presented with ethical dilemmas have been shown to be critical to the resolution and delivery of quality and sensitive nursing care. The chapter concludes with an overview of the respectful death model and its application for end-of-life nursing care.

PRETEST

1. Ethics as a discipline differs from law in that ethics concerns:
   1. Society as a whole and may be enforced through statutes.
   2. Individual decisions rather than society as a whole.
   3. A person's actions rather than the reasons for the actions.
   4. Attitudes and beliefs and is enforced through the judiciary.

2. Ethical theories deriving norms and rules from the duties human beings owe to each other fall under the broad classification of:
   1. Teleological theories.
   2. Deontological theories.
   3. Utilitarian theories.
   4. Situational ethics.

3. The patient benefit model in ethics committee structures:
    1. Facilitates decision making for the competent patient.
    2. Facilitates substituted judgment and facilitates decision making for the incompetent patient.
    3. Considers broad social issues and is accountable to the institution.
    4. Facilitates decision making by health care providers.
4. Therapeutic jurisprudence has developed over the past several years to address:
    1. The impact of legal and ethical decisions on the psychological well-being of the patient involved.
    2. Nurses' ability to determine the decisional capacity of patients who have moments of competency and moments of incompetency.
    3. How the patient can more fully express his or her autonomy rights when there are choices in therapeutic management of the patient.

4. The belief that concerns patients and their families have about legal issues should be considered above ethical issues in determining the care that the patient will receive.
5. The values-based decision making approach to advocacy is predicated upon:
    1. The inherent human dignity that is deserving of respect.
    2. Sharing information and assisting the individual to become empowered to speak or defend his or her right to choices made.
    3. The autonomy rights of the patient.
    4. The principle of maleficence.

GLOSSARY

act deontology   Based on the personal moral values of the person making the ethical decision.

act utilitarianism   Attempts to determine, in a given situation, which course of action will bring about the greatest happiness, or the least harm and suffering, to a given individual.

autonomy   Personal freedom to make choices or decisions.

autonomy model   In hospital ethics committees, this model facilitates decisions for the competent individual.

beneficence   The ethical duty to do good.

best interest standard   An objective test that looks at personal preferences made while the now-incompetent patient was rational and capable of stating what he or she would want in the event of a catastrophic happening; frequently relied on in the incompetent person's right-to-die issues.

bioethics   This term describes the application of ethics to the human person.

deontological theories   In ethics, these theories derive norms and rules from the duties human beings owe one another by virtue of commitments that are made and roles that are assumed.

ethical committees   In health care settings, such groups of persons provide structure and guidelines for potential problems, serve as an open forum for discussion, and function as true patient advocates.

ethics   Discipline relating to moral actions and moral values; rules of conduct recognized in respect to a particular class of human actions.

ethics of caring   The harmonious relations and holistic nature of treatment and therapies; "care for, emotional commitment to, and willingness and act on behalf of persons with

whom one has a significant relationship" (Beauchamp & Childress, 2001, p. 369).

fidelity   In ethics, keeping one's promises or commitments.

justice   In ethics, states that people should be treated fairly and equally.

law   Law is the sum total of rules and regulations by which a society is governed.

nonmaleficence   The duty to do no harm.

nonnormative ethics   Also referred to as metaethics, attempt to analyze the meaning, justification, and inferences of moral concepts and statements; a branch of ethics that is not used in everyday clinical situations.

normative ethics   Are universally applicable, involve questions and dilemmas requiring a choice of actions, and entail conflicts of rights and obligations on the part of the nurse decision maker.

paternalism   In ethics, allows one to make decisions for another; also known as parentalism.

patient benefit model   In ethics committees, this model uses substituted judgment and facilitates decision making for the incompetent patient.

principle of double effect   Used as an argument for allowing nonmaleficence in selected situations, such as when the nurse administers a morphine drip to a patient in respiratory distress.

principalism   An emerging theory in ethics, this theory incorporates the various ethical principles in attempting to resolve conflicts in clinical settings.

respect for others   In ethics, the highest principle as it incorporates all the other principles; transcends cultural differences, gender issues, religious differences, and racial concerns.

rule deontology   In ethics, is based on the belief that certain standards for ethical decisions transcend the individual's moral values, such as the belief that all human life has value.

rule utilitarianism   In ethics, seeks the greatest happiness for the greatest number.

self-determination   Mandates that patients are informed about advance directives when admitted to health care settings and given the opportunity to enact such directives.

situation ethics   A branch of deontological ethics, this theory takes into account the unique characteristics of each person and seeks the most humanistic course of action given the circumstances.

social justice model   In ethics committees, this model considers broad social issues that affect the entire health care institution.

substituted judgment   A subjective determination of whether persons, were they capable of making their opinions and wishes known, would have chosen to either accept or refuse medical therapy; frequently relied on in the incompetent person's right-to-die issues.

teleological theories   In ethics, these theories derive norms or rules for conduct from the consequences of actions.

therapeutic jurisprudence   The impact of legal and ethical decisions are considered from the perspective of their effect on the psychological well-being of the person.

utilitarianism   Ethical theory that allows decisions to be made based on their utility.

values   Personal beliefs about the truths and worth of thoughts, objects, or behavior; motives and attitudes and the relationship of these motives and attitudes to the good of the individual.

veracity   In ethics, truth-telling.

SECTION ONE: Law and Ethics Defined

Providing quality nursing and medical care for patients at the end of their lives has become a major concern in the United States today (Beckstrand, Callister, & Kirchoff, 2006). Some decisions when providing quality nursing and medical care pivot on doing what is "right" for the person and family from an ethical and legal consideration. Though these two concepts are often interwoven, there are major differences.

Law is most frequently defined as the sum total of rules and regulations by which a society is governed. Law includes the rules and regulations established and enforced by custom within a given community, state, or nation. Thus law is created by people and exists to regulate people. Law reflects ever-changing needs and expectations of a given society and is therefore dynamic and fluid. Though not an exact science, law is an ongoing and organized system of change in response to current conditions and public expectations (Guido, 2006).

Ethics is the science relating to moral actions and values. Derived from the Greek word "ethos" meaning character, customs, or habitual uses, ethics encompass principles of appropriate/ acceptable conduct. A broader conceptual definition is that ethics is concerned with motives and attitudes and the relationship of these attitudes to the individual. "Ethics has to do with actions we wish people would take, not actions they must take" (Hall, 1990, p. 37). Many people envision ethics as dealing solely with principles of morality—that which is good or desirable as opposed to that which is bad or undesirable. This ability to discern right from wrong and propriety from impropriety is but one aspect of ethics. The second aspect of ethics is best described as a "system or philosophy of conduct and principles" (Barrocas, Yarbrough, Becnel, & Nelson, 2003, p. 37). This latter aspect provides the structure for placing conduct into action, for ethics involves a commitment to do what is right or proper. Thus ethics is an action concept rather than merely a thought concept (Reamer, 2006).

When using a broader conceptual definition of ethics, values are interwoven with ethics. **Values** are personal beliefs about the truths and worth of thoughts, objects, or behavior. Videbeck (2004), describes values as "abstract standards that give a person a sense of what is right and wrong and establish a code of conduct for living" (p. 93). Such abstract standards include honesty, truthfulness, and appropriateness. Values are usually derived from societal norms, family orientation, and religion; as one matures, values often change. Values may be subdivided into personal, professional, and societal value systems. Ultimately, one's values help determine the actions that one takes in his or her everyday life. Values clarification, a process aimed at understanding the nature of one's own value system and its vast impact on the individual, has emerged as a means of beginning to define what these values mean to the individual person.

Ethics, like values, is individualistic to the person. One's values and ethics are fashioned, as noted above, by previous experiences, quality and quantity of educational experiences, and the person's surrounding environment. It is essential to remember that nurses' ethics and values are just as individualist as patients' ethics and values. Ethics generally become more defined as the individual matures and/or encounters new environments and cultures. However, understanding how one's value system influences one's ethical decision making is the first step in understanding and respecting the ethics and values of others (Guido, 2006). This perspective will promote the delivery of appropriate nursing care, especially as is needed when caring for persons at the end of their lives.

Similarly, health care values may change over time and will therefore impact ethical decision making. For example, during the late 1960s the concept of resuscitation for all hospitalized individuals became a standard. The slogan, "A heart too good to die," was often cited as the reason that all hospitalized individuals, should they suffer a cardiac or respiratory arrest, had resuscitation efforts initiated rather than allowing the person to die without such heroics. As societal values changed, including allowing individuals to determine for themselves what they would want at the end of life, the approach to resuscitation began to more accurately reflect the individual's value system as well as the value system of individual practitioners (Harkness & Wanklyn, 2006).

The legal system is founded on rules and regulations that guide society in a formal and binding manner. Although made by individuals and capable of being changed, the legal system is a general foundation that gives continuing guidance to health care providers, regardless of their personal views and value system. For example, the law recognizes the competent patient's right to refuse therapy, whether at the end of life or for less terminal conditions. The patient retains this right whether health care deliverers agree or disagree with the choice (Guido, 2006).

This right, however, is not absolute. If there are overriding state or legal interests, treatment may be mandated against an individual's wishes. Examples of overriding state interests include legal cases concerning mandatory immunization statutes and epidemic outbreaks that threaten the lives of large numbers of people.

Ethics are subject to philosophical, moral, and individual interpretations. Health care providers and health care recipients have systems of rights and values. Most health care providers have difficulty in areas that transect both the law and ethics, such as the issues of death and dying, euthanasia, genetics, abuse of others, and futility of health care. Table 2–1 shows the distinction between ethics and law.

To truly appreciate the interaction between these two areas, one must first understand ethics and ethical decision making. To further analyze the interaction between these two areas, a scenario is presented in the following section review.

TABLE 2–1 Distinction Between Law and Ethics

CONCEPTS	LAW	ETHICS
Source	External to oneself; rules and regulations of society	Internal to oneself; values, beliefs, and individual interpretations
Concerns	Conduct and actions; what a person did or failed to do	Motives, attitudes, and culture; why one acted as one did
Interests	Society as a whole as opposed to the individual	Good of the individual within society
Enforcement	Courts, statutes, and boards of nursing	Ethics committees, Professional organizations

Source: Adapted from Guido, G. W. (1988). Legal Issues in Nursing: A Sourcebook for Practice. Norwalk, CT: Appleton and Lange.

SECTION ONE REVIEW

1. _____ is concerned with motives and attitudes and the relationship of these attitudes to the individual.
2. If the nurse discovers a patient has been asking other patients for their narcotic pain medications, what is the nurse's priority action?
   1. Notify the nursing supervisor as this is against the law.
   2. Keep the patient away from the other patients.
   3. Present the discovery to the ethics committee as this is an ethical problem.
   4. Make sure the other patients know to take their own medications.
3. Which are examples of values? (Select all that apply.)
   1. Honesty
   2. Veracity
   3. Maleficence
   4. Justice
   5. The Golden Rule
4. The nurse is caring for a patient who has differing values than the nurse's. The nurse needs further instruction about the possible reasons for the differences when which statement is made?
   1. "I know values can be different because of a person's familial background."
   2. "Religious background can affect a person's values."
   3. "Values are different because of the person's race."
   4. "The patient's values may be different from mine because I am older."

Case Study 1 (Part 1)

Juan, aged 19, has been diagnosed with a rare carcinoma for the past 12 years. He has endured multiple hospitalizations, chemotherapy regimes, sessions of radiation, and surgeries. He now states that he has made his peace with God and wants to be allowed to die without further treatment and hospitalization. Juan is adamantly refusing inpatient hospitalization at this point. His parents, who are devout in their faith and cannot imagine life without their only child, feel that Juan must continue to pursue whatever medical and/or surgical treatments are available to him. They insist that he be hospitalized and request that additional specialists consult about further treatment for Juan.

Question

What are the ethical concerns that permeate this scenario and what are the legal issues that must be considered in caring for this patient and his parents?

Suggested Response

An important legal question concerns the patient's competency and age; at 19, he has the right of informed consent and it appears from the facts that he is competent and able to make his own medical determinations. His right to refuse care does not violate public safety; that is, his disease will not present a risk for exposure if he is allowed to refuse medical care. His actions in refusing further medical care, though personal, represent what many would like to see for all society, not just this individual. If the health care personnel dismiss Juan's wishes, he does have recourse within the legal system to enforce his preferences.

His parents' behavior represents ethical dilemmas that often complicate death and dying situations. They epitomize the beliefs and attitudes that arise, such as the need to preserve life at all costs despite the futility of further care efforts, the values they hold for their only child, and what they consider the "good" of the individual within their society. The situation also reflects the lack of ethical enforcement from the care providers that is so often seen in these types of cases. One role of health care personnel is to be present, to listen, and to serve as sounding boards. How one begins to resolve this very complex situation is with extreme tact and extended therapeutic communications.

SECTION TWO: Ethical Theories

A variety of different ethical theories have evolved over the course of history. The most basic distinction in ethical theories concerns nonnormative and normative ethics. **Nonnormative ethics**, sometimes referred to as metaethics, attempt to analyze the meaning, justification, and inferences of moral concepts and statements. Metaethical professionals may seek to understand why one should be good, or how one distinguishes the concept of "good." Generally, only true philosophers, or those dedicating their lives to the understanding of such meanings and inferences, concern themselves with nonnormative ethics (Fieser, 1999).

Normative ethics concerns norms or standards of behavior and value and the ultimate application of these norms or standards to everyday life. Normative theories are universally applicable, involve questions and dilemmas requiring a choice of action, and entail a conflict of rights and obligations on the part of the decision makers. When these ethics concern the human person, they are called **bioethics**. Most normative approaches to ethics fall into two broad categories, although a third category has slowly evolved.

One category, **deontological** (from the Greek *deon*, or "duty") **theories** derive norms and rules from the duties human beings owe one another by virtue of commitments that are made and roles that are assumed. Generally, deontologists hold that a sense of duty consists of rational respect for the fulfilling of one's obligations to other human beings. The greatest strength of deontological theory is its emphasis on the dignity of human beings (Fieser, 1999). Though not to be confused with moral aspects, this sense of duty often follows the religious thought that one must do certain things such as praise God, keep holy one day a week dedicated to God, and refrain from certain actions such as murder, theft, and telling falsehoods.

Deontological ethics look not to the consequences of an action, but to the intention of the action. It is one's good intentions that ultimately determine the praiseworthiness of the action (Volbrecht, 2002). A subset of deontological ethics is commonly referred to as **situation ethics**, wherein the decision maker takes into account the unique characteristics of each individual, the caring relationship between the person and the caregiver, and the most humanistic course of action given the circumstances. Situation ethics are frequently relied on when the nurse has cared for a particular patient over a long time frame. Sometimes situation ethics are referred to as love ethics, conveying the deep respect for the human person.

An example of this subset of deontological theory is illustrated throughout many long-term care facilities today. As the nurses who care for these residents over extended periods of time learn more and more about their fears and expectations, nursing interventions become more individualized. Dr. Chris Tanner (personal conversation, September 18, 2008) related the story of an elderly woman in such a facility who became more and more fearful of dying alone. First the nurses moved the resident to a room that was closer to the nursing station, checking on her frequently during the night. When the resident began spending all night in a chair in the nursing station, the nurses moved her mattress and bedding to the nursing station so that she could rest more comfortably and actually sleep at night during the final days of her life.

Deontological theories can also be subdivided into act and rule deontology. **Act deontology** is based on the personal moral values of the person making the ethical decision, whereas **rule deontology** is based on the belief that certain standards for ethical decisions transcend the individual's moral values (Fieser, 1999). Examples of such a universal rule could be "all human life has value and should be preserved at all costs" and "one should always tell the truth."

A second major division, **teleological** (from the Greek telos or "end") **theories** derive norms or rules for conduct from the consequences of actions. Right or preferable conduct consists of actions that have good consequences, and wrong or undesirable conduct consists of actions that have bad consequences. Teleologists disagree, though, about how to determine the rightness/preferability or wrongness/undesirableness of an action (Volbrecht, 2002).

This theory is often referred to as **utilitarianism**; what makes an action right or wrong is its utility, with useful actions bringing about the greatest good for the greatest number of people. An alternate way of viewing this theory is that the usefulness of an action is determined by the amount of happiness it brings.

Utilitarian ethics can then be subdivided into rule and act utilitarianism. **Rule utilitarianism** seeks the greatest happiness for all. It appeals to public agreement as a basis for objective judgment about the nature of happiness. **Act utilitarianism** attempts to determine, in a given situation, which course of action will bring about the greatest happiness, or the least harm and suffering, to a single individual. As such, utilitarianism makes happiness subjective (Butts & Rich, 2005).

Examples of nursing application of utilitarian ethics can be seen in multiple health care settings. Deciding which patients should be given priority in emergency situations, deciding which patients are most deserving of hospitalization when facilities are full to capacity, or deciding how to distribute needed vaccines should there be a major epidemic influenza outbreak may all be examples of utilitarian thought.

A more recent emerging theory, **principalism**, incorporates various existing ethical principles embodied in these concepts (e.g., autonomy, beneficence, and justice) and attempts to resolve conflicts by applying one or more of these principles (Guido, 2006). Ethical principles are much more easily used to guide professional decision making than application of ethical theories. Principles encompass basic premises from which rules can be developed and provide a framework for moral norms for practice in health care settings.

SECTION TWO REVIEW

1. Which correctly describes normative ethics?
    1. They are the standards of behavior applying to everyday life.
    2. They are personal beliefs about the truths of everyday life.
    3. They are the beliefs one has about conflicts in clinical settings.
    4. They are the subset of ethics that enables a person to make decisions for others.
2. The nurse is trying to decide between two actions and bases the final decision on the duty owed to the patient. Of which ethical theory is this an example?
    1. Teleology
    2. Deontology
    3. Utilitarianism
    4. Nonnormative ethics

3. If a family member is trying to make the most ethical decision for a dying family member and uses act utilitarianism to decide, which is the most ethical action?
    1. Ask the physician to write an order for tube feedings to give the patient nourishment.
    2. Insist the nurses leave the dying family member completely alone.
    3. Discontinue the services of the hospice team to allow the patient rest.
    4. Allow the physician to discontinue the use of the ventilator.
4. The ethical theory most often used by health care professionals, especially nurses is _____ or _____ .

Case Study 1 (Part 2)

Reconsider Juan's case as described in the first section review. Before Juan completed the process of refusing therapy in the hospital scenario, he suffered a severe seizure that left him incompetent to either give or refuse consent for further treatment. The health care workers, who are well aware that Juan would refuse care if he were able to do so, want to give comfort care and assist Juan through the dying process. His parents, desperate to keep their son alive, sign full consent forms for additional consultants and both medical and surgical interventions.

Question

Which ethical theory, deontological or teleological, could you argue that his parents are portraying in overriding Juan's wishes?

Suggested Response

The parents appear to be applying the theory of teleological ethics in their determination to keep their son from dying. They are certainly doing what seems best to bring them the most happiness, at least temporarily; this could also be described as act utilitarianism or bringing about the greatest good for an individual rather than **rule utilitarianism**, which is seen as bringing about the greatest good for society. An alternate evaluation of the situation can be considered and reasoned. Given the very devout faith of these parents, it could be that they are following the tenets of deontological theory in that one must not kill another or that all human life has value. If there is value, then there is a duty to preserve that life.

SECTION THREE: Ethical Principles and Their Application

Nurses apply a variety of ethical principles in everyday clinical practice, some to a greater degree than others. There are eight principles commonly incorporated into nursing care at the end of life. Each principle is discussed separately in the following text.

Autonomy

Autonomy addresses personal freedom and **self-determination**—the right to choose what will happen to one's own person. The legal doctrine of informed consent is the direct complement of this principle. Autonomy involves health care deliverers' and family members' respect for patients' rights to make decisions affecting care and treatment, even if health care deliverers and family members do not agree with the decisions made. Every patient plan of care must address the overall issue of autonomy and incorporate the patient's wishes and desires, if possible (Cimino, 2003). Because autonomy is not an absolute right, restrictions may be placed on a person's right to endanger others, as in the case of communicable diseases (Guido, 2006).

The principle of autonomy is often one of the more difficult principles in end-of-life decision making, if not the most difficult principle to enforce. For patients to make decisions about what therapies they will or will not accept there must be truthful disclosure regarding the diagnosis, prognosis, and therapies that are available to the patient. Sometimes these disclosures are limited as they involve facts about diagnoses or prognoses that are not fully known, especially when new therapies or new medications are experimental. There may be reluctance on the part of the family members or members of the health care team to impart the full extent of the illness and prognosis to their loved ones. While withholding information may be perceived as "kind" or

"in the patient's best interest," not fully informing the competent patient about all aspects of his or her care prevents the person from making informed decisions, thus denying them the ethical principle of autonomy.

A separate issue arises when health care providers and family members, pleading that they are doing what is best for an incompetent person, select to disregard advance directives that protect the autonomy of the person (Burt, 2005). Health care providers and family members need to be reminded that the very purpose of self-determination directives is to protect the autonomy rights of the person at times when the person is unable to speak for himself or herself. Though the patient's written desires are not necessarily what the nurse would determine as the "better" solution, the second statement in the *Code of Ethics for Nurses* (American Nurses Association, 2001) reinforces this directive: "The nurse's primary commitment is to the patient, whether an individual, family, group, or community."

Autonomy may also be problematic when the health care team and the patient or patient's family disagree about proposed therapies and realistic expectations. Health care providers may believe that previous experiences working with patients who had similar diagnoses and prognoses allow the health care providers to have a more realistic perspective of the type of care that should be offered or delivered to a given patient. Remember, there can be disagreements as each individual involved in a given situation expresses his or her own feelings and perspectives. The final decision, though, rests with the competent patient or the surrogate decision maker who has the legal capacity to speak for the incompetent patient.

Beneficence

Beneficence states that the actions one takes should promote good. This principle incorporates the prevention of harm and promotion of good and is most closely associated with utilitarian principles (Beauchamp & Childress, 2001). In caring for patients, good can be defined in a variety of ways, including allowing a patient to die without advance life support interventions. Good can also prompt nurses to encourage a person to undergo multiple treatment procedures if these procedures will increase the quality of the patient's life and provide additional comfort for the patient. Nurses frequently consider this principle when viewing the long- and short-term outcomes of invasive and noninvasive procedures. The complexity of this principle, though, is in defining the individual's interpretation of "good."

Nursing care at the end of life presents opportunities for nurses and interdisciplinary health care members to truly listen and communicate with the dying individual. Persons in this stage of their lives are frequently experiencing one of the five stages of grieving. Therefore, there is a need for the patient to freely express personal thoughts and feelings to supportive, caring health care professionals. Neuberger (2004) noted that in order to provide quality care, health professionals must have some emotional involvement with patients and be "prepared to support them and encourage them to express their emotions" (p. 134). This is true for all stages of the grieving process: denial, anger, depression, bargaining, and acceptance. To "do good" is to allow patients and their loved ones to express themselves, knowing that the health care provider understands and accepts the person's need to express his or her emotions.

Some of the ways that nurses may be able to "do good" in caring for the terminally ill patient and considering the needs of the patient's family members is in being respectful of the time that the person and family members require in coming to terms with the realization that death is imminent. Being available if and when the person is ready to verbalize thoughts about dying and bringing closure to relationships is one way that health care providers understand that patients are unique and will not necessarily react or respond as other dying persons may respond. Sometimes just sitting quietly with a patient is sufficient, as one's presence can be the source of comfort that a person most desires.

Nonmaleficence

The complement of beneficence, **nonmaleficence** states that one should do no harm, including nonintentional infliction of pain and/or suffering. Health care providers frequently employ the concept of a detriment-benefit analysis when the issue of nonmaleficence is raised. Using this approach, the focus of the projected treatment or procedure is on the consequences of the benefits to the patient and not on the harm that occurs at the time of the intervention. An example is when a nurse gives a patient an injection for the relief of pain. Even though the injection imposes some degree of discomfort and suffering at the moment the injection is administered, the overall benefit is less suffering from the pain.

A second way to support interventions that may have harmful effects is through application of the **principle of double effect**. Four conditions must be present for this principle to occur. One, the action itself must be "good" or at least morally neutral in itself. Two, the practitioner must intend only the good effect. The fact that there will also be an undesirable effect is secondary to the primary goal of beneficence. Three, the undesired effect must not be the means of attaining the good effect. Four, there is a proportional or favorable balance between the desirable and the undesirable effects of the action (Quill, 1997). Applying this concept, one could be justified in administering a morphine drip in a terminally ill patient with pulmonary edema to ease breathing and control further anxiety and suffering, yet be sensitive to the potential risk of respiratory depression as a side effect of the morphine. Such actions are in direct compliance with the *Code of Ethics for Nurses*, interpretive statement 1 (American Nurses Association, 2001).

Nurses may encounter struggles with the principles of beneficence and nonmaleficence in caring for terminally ill patients who have opted for life-sustaining treatments during the final stages of their lives. Often these treatments increase pain and potentially mental suffering by the very nature of their effects on the person, particularly in the case where intubation and prolonged mechanical ventilation are involved. The circumstances surrounding the final stages of Terri Schiavo's life vividly portray what can occur when family members disagree with an incompetent patient's care (Guido, 2007).

Veracity

Veracity concerns truth telling and incorporates the concept that individuals should always tell the truth. This principle also dictates that the whole truth be told. Most patients who are diagnosed with a terminal illness want to know the truth about their condition so that they can best plan for their remaining time (Vivian, 2006). Secondarily, without veracity, the principle of autonomy cannot fully be experienced. The principle of veracity is evident when one completely answers patients' questions, giving as much information as the patient and/or family can understand, and telling the patient when information is not available or known. Arguments against using veracity center on the issue that patients might forgo appropriate and necessary medical care if they knew the entire truth.

Self-determination cannot happen if one does not know the truth about his or her condition, diagnosis, and prognosis. When caring for persons at the end of their lives, it is important that health care members use language that the persons can understand and that one takes the needed time to assure that the person understands as fully as possible what has been said. Remember, without full disclosure in terms that the person can comprehend, informed and valid decision making cannot occur.

Equally important, though, is that health care providers honor the patient's wishes not to be told too much or to be told information over multiple time intervals so as not to receive information faster than the patient can process the information. In order to know how much or what to tell patients, it is important that the care deliverer listen to the cues that patients deliver. Generally, patients and/or patients' family members will use subtle hints regarding the relating of health care information. An example could be the patient who quickly verbalizes a different conversational topic whenever the issue of hospice care is discussed.

Conversely, the health care provider can initiate the information-giving process to determine if limited information is desired over full information. Questions by the health care provider such as "Would you like to know about your prognosis?" or "I understand that you are considering moving to a hospice unit" can assist the health care provider in making a determination about disclosure. Regardless of the amount of disclosure, all information provided should be reinforced at timed intervals so that patient processing of diagnosis, prognosis, and course of care delivery results in clear understanding.

Fidelity

Fidelity is keeping one's promises or commitments. Staff members know not to promise patients what they cannot deliver or what they do not control, such as when the patient asks that heroic measures not be implemented. With the advent of hospice care, this has become less of an issue. Perhaps the more difficult aspect is to respect and adhere to the patient's request when family members demand that more heroic measures and invasive measures be taken. It is difficult for family members to watch as their loved one no longer is able or refuses to take any type of nourishment. For example, when the patient is no longer consuming food and/or water, it can be very traumatic and difficult for the care provider to convince the family that the patient's inability or refusal of oral nourishment does not cause undue distress and pain. Teaching and continued communication with these family members are critical in continuing to respect the patient's wishes.

Paternalism/Parentalism

Paternalism allows one to make decisions for another and has been frequently viewed as an undesirable principle. By definition, paternalism allows no collaboration in the decision-making process, but totally removes the decision from the patient or patient's family members. Because parents of younger children also make decisions for the entire family, the principle has also been known as *parentalism.*

Called the **best interest standard** by many ethics professors, this principle is a quality-of-life assessment that is used to determine the highest net benefit among available options and

is most often employed when preferences are not known (Butts & Rich, 2005). Though most patients are competent to express their wishes in general terms, this principle allows health care personnel to assist in decision making when patients lack the full data to make decisions or are unable to fully comprehend the significance of the decision. For example, patients and/or family members may express their need for assistance in making decisions when they ask health care providers "If it was your decision, what would you do?" or "If it were your father, what type of treatment would you recommend?" Such queries indicate that the person is either not ready to make a decision or is unable to make a decision. Health care providers can then proceed to clarify options or give additional information.

Justice

Justice states that people should be treated fairly and equally, with access to health care services in order to maximize the welfare of the person. Social justice embodies the concept that there is a fair distribution of community resources, essentially assuring that all persons are treated with equality (Harris, 2003). Thus, justice attempts to examine ethics from the perspective of all persons rather than more narrowly addressing the individual. How does one, though, begin to "cherish" life and address the issues of whether withholding or withdrawing artificial feeding is allowable when multiple numbers of poorer individuals in this country lack appropriate nutrition and are denied the means to live their lives?

The principle of justice, which demands the fair and equitable treatment of all persons, must be tempered with the **ethics of caring**, which involves the harmonious relations and holistic nature of treatments and therapies (Botes, 2000). This ethics of caring is best described as "care for, emotional commitment to, and willingness to act on behalf of persons with whom one has a significant relationship" (Beauchamp & Childress, 2001, p. 369).

Viewing justice and the ethics of caring as polar opposites, Botes (2000) wrote:

> The ethics of justice is characterized by fairness and equality, rational decision-making based on universal rules and principles, an autonomous, impartial, and objective decision-making. At the other pole, the ethics of care is characterized by caring, involvement, and the maintenance of harmonious relationships from a need-centered, holistic, and contextual point of view. (p. 1074)

However, an argument can be made concerning the need for health care providers to consider both aspects in the delivery of competent, quality end-of-life care. Thus justice, which demands the fair and equitable treatment of all persons, must be tempered with the ethics of caring, which involves the harmonious relations and holistic nature of treatments and therapies.

Respect for Others

Respect for others is considered by many as the overriding principle that undergirds all of the principles. Respect for others acknowledges the right of individuals to make decisions and to live or die based on those decisions. Respect for others transcends cultural differences, gender issues, religious differences, and racial concerns. This principle is a major core value underlying the Americans with Disabilities Act and several discrimination statutes. It is also the first principle enumerated in the American Nurses Association's *Code of Ethics for Nurses* (2001). Nurses positively reinforce this principle daily in assuring that all patients receive quality, competent nursing care.

Implementing Ethical Principles

Health care providers seldom rely on a single ethical principle when caring for patients. Therefore, ethical principles that practitioners employ every day in practice settings frequently come into conflict with each other. For example, envision the scenario of a patient who is dying, who also cherishes his independence and ability to remain at home. As a caregiver, one must balance the need to preserve this independence (autonomy) while discussing with him and his family alternative care measures such as home hospice care, specific care that is essential to maintaining his comfort and safety, and factors that will herald the need for more continual care (beneficence).

One way to resolve potential conflicts is through a systematic, ethical decision-making approach. One framework for resolution involves reflection on the questions that appear in Box 2–1.

When making ethical decisions, health care providers should consider all the elements using an orderly, systematic, and objective method. Ethical decision-making models assist toward this end.

Though there are multiple models for ethical decision making, one of the easiest to remember is the MORAL model because the letters of the acronym remind nurses of the subsequent steps of the model, and thus the model can easily be used in all patient care settings. The steps of this model may be found in Box 2–2.

BOX 2–1   Questions to Consider in Resolving Ethical Conflicts

1. Who should make the choice?
2. What are the possible courses of action?
3. What are the available options or alternatives?
4. What are the consequences, both positive and negative, of these possible options?
5. Which rules and values should direct choices?
6. What are the desired goals and outcomes for all parties involved in the ethical issue?

Source: Guido, 2006, p. 8

BOX 2–2   Steps in the Moral Model

M	Massage the dilemma. Identify and define issues in the dilemma. Consider the opinions of the major players—patients, family members, nurses, physicians, clergy, and other interdisciplinary health care members—as well as their value systems.
O	Outline the options. Examine all options fully, including the less realistic and conflicting ones. Make two lists, identifying the pros and cons of all the options identified. This step in the model is designed to fully explore options and alternatives available, not to make a final decision. Remember, some of the options may be more realistic than others, but all can be enumerated and examined.
R	Resolve the dilemma. Review the issues and options, applying basic ethical principles to each option. Decide the best option based on the views of all those concerned in the dilemma.
A	Act by applying the chosen option. This step is usually the most difficult because it requires actual implementation, whereas the previous steps had allowed for dialogue and discussion. This step also mandates that all involved in the person's care understand and implement the chosen option.
L	Look back and evaluate the entire process, including the implementation. No process is complete without a thorough evaluation. Ensure that all those involved are able to follow through on the final option. If not, a second decision may be required and the process must start again at the initial step.

Source: Thiroux, 1977, refined for nursing by Halloran, 1982

SECTION THREE REVIEW

1. In planning a discussion about a patient's prognosis with the patient and family member, which ethical principles apply to the nurse's actions? (Select all that apply.)
   1. Veracity
   2. Paternalism
   3. Nonmaleficence
   4. Beneficence
   5. Fidelity
2. Which is an example of the principle of double effect?
   1. The doctor orders a pain medication for a terminally ill patient and the nurse administers it.
   2. The nurse administers a pain medication to a patient in severe pain experiencing difficulty breathing.
   3. The patient's family requests pain medication for their comatose family member who is moaning.
   4. The patient requests pain medication more frequently than necessary to ensure that double the pain relief is achieved.

3. The nurse is providing end-of-life care for a young adult patient who has alternating periods of lucidity and confusion. Which principle is most likely to be in conflict for the nurse?
   1. Nonmaleficence
   2. Beneficence
   3. Veracity
   4. Autonomy
4. For the nurse working in end-of-life care, which indicate questions to assist in resolving an ethical issue? (Select all that apply.)
   1. How can I best make this decision?
   2. What are the available options from which to choose?
   3. Who should make the decision or assist in the decision making?
   4. When should the decision be made?
   5. What are the consequences of each option?

SECTION FOUR: Therapeutic Jurisprudence and Patient Advocacy

Therapeutic Jurisprudence

The concept of **therapeutic jurisprudence** has evolved over the past 25 years, focusing the impact of legal and ethical decisions on the psychological well-being of a person. Therapeutic jurisprudence was first applied in discussions regarding mental health law and recognized that legal and ethical decisions could have both therapeutic and anti-therapeutic consequences (Wexler & Winick, 2005). These authors of therapeutic jurisprudence desired that professionals be aware of these two opposite outcomes and work to ensure that the beneficial aspects of legal and ethical decisions be recognized and implemented. Parameters of nursing care may be developed through the guidance of therapeutic jurisprudence so that thoughtful, compassionate care is delivered to all patients, especially those patients whose diagnoses and prognoses dictate a more complex integration of ethics and law (Beauchamp & Childress, 2001).

Many practitioners find it difficult to care for persons at the end of life from both an ethical and legal perspective, as the two disciplines may appear to represent the opposite ends of a pendulum. Respecting and adhering to legal demands within the framework of ethics is a challenge for nursing, and no case better portrays this type of difficult decision making than does the recent case of Theresa Marie (Terri) Schiavo. Perhaps no case

also demands that one employ therapeutic jurisdiction more than does that of Terri Schiavo.

Ms. Schiavo suffered a cardiac arrest in February 1990, and was without oxygen for approximately 11 minutes, which is 5 to 7 minutes longer than most medical experts believe is possible without suffering severe and permanent brain damage. She was resuscitated and, at the insistence of her husband, intubated and placed on a ventilator. When it became apparent that she would require long-term ventilator support, she had a tracheotomy. It was hypothesized that the cause of her cardiac arrest was a severe electrolyte imbalance caused by an eating disorder, based on the fact that in the six years preceding the cardiac event, Ms. Schiavo had lost approximately 140 pounds, going from 250 to 110 pounds.

During the first two months after her cardiac arrest, Ms. Schiavo was in a coma. She then regained some wakefulness and was eventually diagnosed as being in a persistent vegetative state (PVS). She was successfully weaned from the ventilator and was able to swallow her saliva, both reflexive behaviors (breathing and swallowing). She was not, though, able to eat food or drink liquids, which is characteristic of PVS. A permanent feeding tube was placed so that she could receive nutrition and hydration.

Throughout the early years of her PVS, there was no challenge to the diagnosis or to the appointment of her husband as her legal guardian. Four years after her cardiac arrest, a successful lawsuit was filed against the fertility physician who had failed to detect her electrolyte imbalance. A judgment of $300,000 went to her husband for loss of companionship and $700,000 was placed in a court-managed trust fund to maintain and provide continuing medical and nursing care for Ms. Schiavo.

Sometime after this successful lawsuit, the close family relationship between Ms. Schiavo's husband and her parents began to erode. As her family continued to fight for who should have custody of Ms. Schiavo, her plight became public. As her court appointed guardian noted:

> Thereafter, what is for millions of Americans a profoundly private matter catapulted a close, loving family into an internationally watched blood feud. The end product was a most public death for a very private individual.... Theresa was by all accounts a very shy, fun loving, and sweet woman who loved her husband and her parents very much. The family breach and public circus would have been anathema to her. (Wolfson, 2005, p. 17)

The continual and seemingly unending court battles regarding the removal or retention of her feeding tube also began about this time frame. At these court hearings, adequate medical and legal evidence were presented to show that Ms. Schiavo had been correctly diagnosed and that she would not have wanted to be kept alive by artificial means. Laws in the state of Florida, where Ms. Schiavo was a patient, allowed the removal of tubal nutrition and hydration in patients with PVS. The feeding tube was removed and later reinstated following a court order.

In October 2003, there was a second removal of the feeding tube after a higher court overturned the lower court decision that had caused the feeding tube to be reinserted. With this second removal, the Florida legislature passed what has become to be known as Terri's Law. This law gave the Florida governor the right to demand the feeding tube be reinserted and also appoint a special guardian ad litem to review the entire case. The special guardian ad litem was appointed in October 2003. Terri's Law was later declared unconstitutional by the Florida Supreme Court, and the U.S. Supreme Court refused to overrule their decision (Wolfson, 2005).

In early 2005, during the last weeks of Ms. Schiavo's life, the U.S. Congress attempted to move the issue to the federal rather than Florida state court system. The legal challenges ended with the federal district court in Florida and the 11th Circuit Court of Appeals ruling that there was insufficient evidence to create a new trial, and the U.S. Supreme Court refused to review the findings of these two lower courts (Wolfson, 2005). Ms. Schiavo died on March 31, 2005; she was 41 years of age.

Whichever side of the case one supported, the plight of Terri Schiavo created numerous ethical concerns for the nurses and health care providers caring for her. Issues that created these conflicts were multiple and varied and included working with feuding family members, attempting to prevent media personnel from invading the privacy of this individual through continuous media coverage, working with the masses of people lined at the borders of the hospice center insisting that Terri be fed and given hydration, and the individual emotions centering on the appropriateness of either keeping or removing the feeding tube.

One thing, though, remained clear. The nurse managers and nurses caring for the patient had a legal obligation to either remove or reinsert the feeding tube based on the prevailing court decision or legislative act. Their individual reflections about the right action to take or justice of such court decrees were secondary to the prevailing court orders. For the nurses and family members whose ethical values differed from the court orders, though, there must be some way to ensure that there are opportunities for these individuals to voice their concerns and feelings, and/or time for quiet reflections. While practice limits deviations from one's legal obligation, nurses must ensure that the emotional and psychological well-being of those persons for whom he or she cares are respected and acknowledged. Acknowledging and appreciating that such discord can occur and allowing positive means to express this concern may be the best solution in handling these difficult legal and ethical patient situations (Guido, 2007).

Patient Advocacy

Advocacy concerns the active support of a cause or issue that has importance to persons directly involved in the cause or issue. Advocates are those who defend and speak for such a cause or issue. In nursing, one frequently addresses the role of the nurse in advocating for the legal rights of patients; equally important, though, is that nurses advocate for the ethical concerns of patients and peers.

Nursing has identified three models of advocacy that are employed in clinical practice settings. The *rights protection model* is perhaps the best known model of advocacy. In this model, nurses advocate for the legal and ethical rights of the patient (Guido, 2006). Often seen as an extension of autonomy, nurses assist patients in asserting their autonomy rights, for example, in assisting an individual patient in successfully convincing health care providers that he or she does not desire surgical intervention, but rather desires solely palliative care. The third principle in the American Nurses Association *Code of Ethics for Nurses* (2001) reinforces this mandate: "The nurse promotes, advocates for, and strives to protect the health, safety, and rights of the patient."

A second approach to advocacy is the *values-based decision model*. Using this approach, the nurse assists the patient by discussing his or her needs and desires and helps the patient make choices that are most consistent with the patient's values, lifestyle, and desires (Guido, 2006). This model is predicated on the honest and truthful sharing of information and assisting the individual through the development of a strong nurse-patient relationship to become empowered to speak on his or her own behalf rather than relying on the nurse to speak or defend these rights. Using this approach, the patient is assisted to exert his or her right to autonomy and self-determination.

The third model is the *respect for persons model*, sometimes known as the patient-advocate model. Though not as fully developed as the two previous models, this approach centers on the inherent human dignity of a person who is deserving of respect. The respect for persons model is a direct application of the principle of respect for others (Guido, 2006). In this model, the nurse, always valuing the human person who is involved, acts to protect the rights, dignity, and choices of the patient. If the patient is not able to assist in making decisions about his or her care and treatments, the nurse advocates for the best

interests of the patient. The ultimate goal of this model is to promote the autonomy and individual uniqueness of the patient.

Each of these models may be used as a tool in caring for patients at the end of their lives. All of the models build on the ethical principles of autonomy, beneficence, justice, veracity, fidelity, and respect for others.

SECTION FOUR REVIEW

1. Which patient advocacy model specifically promotes the dignity of the patient as a person by requiring the nurse act to protect the rights, dignity, and choices of the patient? (Select all that apply.)
   1. The rights protection model
   2. The respect for persons model
   3. The values-based decision model
   4. The patient advocate model
   5. The interdisciplinary patient protection model
2. Which patient advocacy model is in use by a nurse who advocates for the patient even though the nurse does

not approve of the patient's lifestyle and disagrees with the patient's decision?
   1. The rights protection model
   2. The respect for persons model
   3. The values-based model
   4. The interdisciplinary patient protection model
3. Which ethical principles do the patient advocacy models rely upon? (Select all that apply.)
   1. Nonmaleficence
   2. Beneficence
   3. Justice
   4. Veracity
   5. Paternalism

SECTION FIVE: Hospital Ethics Committees

With the increasing numbers of ethical dilemmas in patient situations today, health care providers, patients, and patients' families are requesting guidance with decision making, and in particular decision making with end-of-life issues. Perhaps one of the best solutions for both long-term and short-term issues has been the creation and use of an institution ethics committee. **Ethical committees** can (1) provide structure and guidelines for potential problems, (2) serve as an open forum for discussion, and (3) function as a true patient advocate by placing the patient at the core of the committee discussions (Guido, 2006).

To form such a group, if one does not already exist, the proposed committee should first begin as a bioethical study group so that ethical principles and theories as well as common health care issues can be explored by members of the group. The committee should be composed of nurses, physicians, clergy, clinical social workers, nutritional experts, pharmacists, administrative personnel, and legal experts. Once the committee has become active, individual patients or patients' family members may also be invited to the committee deliberations. Ideally, the committee serves a variety of health care entities in the community, including acute care institutions, long-term care agencies, clinical settings, hospice, and community health agencies.

Ethics committees generally follow one of three distinct structures, though some ethics committees blend the three structures. Box 2–3 displays these three structures for ethics committees. Other committees may differ in their approach depending on the individual case.

BOX 2–3   Ethics Committee Structures

- **Autonomy model:** Facilitates decision making for the competent patient and family members.
- **Patient benefit model:** Uses **substituted judgment** and facilitates decision making for the incompetent patient.
- **Social justice model:** Considers broad social issues, including issues of organizational ethics, and is accountable directly to the institution.

Each of these models serves to advance the quality of care at the end of life. For example, in the case of Juan as described at the beginning of this chapter, the ethics committee would have used the **autonomy model.** Hopefully, the committee would have considered his perspectives and desires and assisted in intervening with his parent's desire to keep him alive, regardless of his desire to end his life with dignity and comfort. The advantage of the ethics committee is that it would have served as an open forum for the parents by allowing them to vent their frustrations and concerns and for Juan by allowing him to better describe his feelings and ultimate desires. Additionally, such an open discussion would have prevented the health care providers from being placed in the middle of the dispute.

The **patient benefit model** is most often relied upon to assist family members in determining what is best for the patient who is incompetent and cannot speak for himself or herself. This model combines preferences and desires that the patient may have expressed while competent, including oral and written statements, with families' goals and values, health care providers' goals and values, and existing laws and ethical standards. An example is the case of Terri Schiavo, as previously described in this chapter.

The **social justice model** is one that often involves better education of health care providers as well as patients and their families. Many of the disagreements that arise with patients at the end of life can be described as misinformation about the role of advance directives, benefits of palliative versus curative care, pain associated with voluntary stoppage of fluids and nutrition, and the withdrawal versus withholding of life-sustaining therapies. Opposing perceptions concerning care can also be at the core of issues that present to ethics committees, particularly perceptions that differ between health care providers who are involved in the care of patients at the end of life.

A study by Oberle and Hughes (2001) examined physicians' and nurses' perceptions of ethical problems regarding end-of-life decisions. The researchers concluded that while both professions felt an obligation to reduce the suffering in terminally ill patients, there was uncertainty about the best courses of action for these patients. Competing values, scarce resources, and communications as well as differences in the physicians' and nurses' professional roles impact end-of-life care. Ethics committees, through education and open discussions, could begin to help generate creative strategies for working toward optimal patient outcomes.

The utility of the social justice model was also supported in a study that examined the meaning and enactment of ethical nursing practice in three groups of nurses, including those in direct patient care positions, nursing students, and nurses in advanced practice positions (Doane, Pauly, Brown, & McPherson, 2004). Results from this study highlighted the need for further education across all three groups of nurses regarding how to develop the knowledge base that will assist nurses in ethical decision making. The study suggested that this educational process can occur

through the attendance of nurses at ethics committee hearings and ethical grand rounds. A second approach or format could be to develop educational programs on ethical decision-making that are sponsored and led by ethics committee members.

In most settings, ethics committees are a reality, in part because of the complex issues that are common to health care. In 1992, the Joint Commission for the Accreditation of Healthcare Organizations (JCAHO) first mandated ethics committees or, in the alternative, other credible vehicles for addressing ethical concerns. Included in the commission's manual was a chapter on patient rights, further supporting the important role of ethics committees.

These initial standards have been expanded to include the patient's participation in health care decisions, the creation of advance directives, and the enactment of do-not-resuscitate orders and policies (JCAHO [now known solely as the Joint Commission], 2007). The commission's premise is that the hospital supports the rights of each patient and that the hospital's policies and procedures describe the means by which those rights are protected and exercised. The hospital policies must also include a means for resolving conflicts in decision making and a description of the respective roles of physicians, nurses, and family members in decisions involving do-not-resuscitate orders or the withholding of treatment.

In many medical centers, the Joint Commission (JC) mandates are met by having ethical rounds, which are conducted on a weekly or monthly schedule. These ethical rounds allow staff members to be exposed to the decision-making process using common ethical dilemmas in preparation for the possibility of actually being in the position of contributing to a committee decision. These ethical rounds may also serve as an alternative to actual ethics committees. Another alternative to meet the requirements of the JC is to employ a bioethics consultant or pastoral staff care member rather than having the more traditional ethics committee.

SECTION FIVE REVIEW

1. The nurse and other members of the interdisciplinary team for an incompetent patient are meeting to discuss an ethical issue based on the beliefs of the patient. This is an example of:
   1. The social justice model.
   2. Nonnormative ethics.
   3. Deontological ethics.
   4. The patient benefit model.
2. What purpose do ethical rounds serve? They:
   1. Facilitate ethical decision making by staff members.
   2. Assist family members in understanding how to assist their loved one in making decisions at the end of life.
   3. Assure decisions reached by ethics committees are implemented.
   4. Begin to educate physicians and nurses about ethical principles so that they can become

comfortable with ethical issues arising in clinical practice settings.
3. The nurse is orienting a new graduate nurse and is discussing committees within the institution. The new nurse shows understanding of ethics committees when which statement is made? "The purpose of the ethics committee is to:
   1. Provide structure and guidelines for resolving ethical issues as they arise."
   2. Serve as an open forum for discussion among institution personnel."
   3. Function as a true patient advocate by placing the patient's concerns at the core of the discussion."
   4. Provide a solution for ethical dilemmas when health care providers cannot agree on the best solution for selected patients."

SECTION SIX: Respectful Death Model

The respectful death model (RDM) has been developed in recent years to support terminally ill patients, their family members, and professionals at the end of life. The model is a research-based, holistic model first described by Farber and colleagues (2004) and more fully developed for nursing by Wasserman (2008). Recognizing that the attitudes toward death have not significantly altered in the past 40 years, the RDM was developed as a process method that begins with the development of a therapeutic relationship with the terminally ill patient and members of his or her family and enables this relationship to continue until death. The communication that is established at all steps in the process assists in clarifying end-of-life issues and helps to provide solutions that reduce conflict, misunderstanding, and suffering (Farber & Farber, 2006). Steps in the process incorporate the ethical principles of autonomy, beneficence, veracity, fidelity, and respect for others.

Steps in the model begin with the establishment of a therapeutic relationship between the nurse and other members of the health care team with the patient and family members. Two possible steps flow once the therapeutic relationship is established: the need for end-of-life care is acknowledged or the patient and family talk about their concerns, enabling the health care team to incorporate these concerns into the care plan while providing realistic solutions to conflicts that may arise. Nurses and members of the health care team carefully listen to the patient and family concerns so that these potential conflicts can be addressed early in the care of the patient and future conflicts can be prevented.

The next step involves frank discussions about death and dying, clarifying knowledge of the underlying illness and knowledge of the dying process. Family members' fears and hopes are elicited and acknowledged as are concerns that the terminally ill person may have about desires and hopes for his or her family members, termed as patient beliefs about the future by Wasserman (2008). Also addressed are questions and concerns about who will assume the role of caregiver in the days and months ahead.

Essential to the entire model is the "mindful listening" (Farber & Farber, 2006, p. 223) that must occur between all parties to the discussions and the open and honest discussions that ensue. Members of the family as well as the terminally ill individual must be willing to express what he or she believes and is feeling while other members of the family and the terminally ill individual listen. Farber and Farber (2006) noted

that establishing these relationships and mindfully listening are established through "commitment, connection, and consciousness" (p. 223). Commitment denotes the fact that the health care providers will continue to support the patient and family through all stages of the dying process, including the final stages. Connection means that all individuals discuss all topics of importance openly and honestly, receiving responses from members of the health care team in the same open and honest manner. Consciousness refers to experiences and life meanings as shared by the terminally ill individual and family members (Farber, Egnew, & Farber, 2004). Underlying all of these concepts and conversations is that the professionals involved have first clarified their own values and beliefs concerning death and dying before entering into the RDM.

Farber and Farber (2006) identified benefits of the model as the formation of the therapeutic relationship, the extensive understanding of both the terminally ill individual and the family about their knowledge of death and dying, and possible solutions that decrease the conflict and suffering of the patient and family members. Wasserman (2008) further identified benefits as the potential for growth and learning for the patient, family, and health professionals as well as the ability of the person to achieve a respectful death and come to closure through death. Because the focus of the RDM is on the patient and family, their values and preferences support the respectful death of the terminally ill person.

Barriers to implementing the model in clinical settings include the continuing culture of many health care providers that does not value allowing adequate time for conversations with patients and families and resolution of their conflicts, and lack of adequate knowledge concerning death and dying. A second barrier is that health care professionals must become "guides, collaborators, and consultants" (Farber et al., 2004, p. 115) in allowing the patient and family to control the process and make decisions that affect the family relationship.

The RDM allows nurses to use skills and talents that well exemplify some of nursing's finest qualities, including the ability to effectively listen as patients and family members tell their stories and to help them to define what they want and desire at the end of life for their loved one. Nurses, educated to give holistic and comprehensive care that includes all aspects of physical, emotional, psychosocial, and spiritual care, are well positioned to ensure that the family develops the therapeutic relationships they need to achieve in order to fully support both the patient and the family at all aspects of end-of-life care and a respectful death.

SECTION SIX REVIEW

1. Which statement indicates a need for further instruction when a nurse describes why it is important for health care professionals involved in caring for patients at the end of their lives to understand patients' perceptions?
   1. "Many of the ideas that have been expounded for years about dying patients may be unfounded."
   2. "Appropriate plans of care can only be developed and implemented when health care providers try to understand the dying process from the view of the dying person."
   3. "Family members need guidance in understanding what to expect as they care for their dying loved ones."
   4. "Each person during the dying process undergoes the same thoughts and emotions, and health care workers must elicit those thoughts to obtain closure."

2. When using the respectful death model, which is the most important aspect for the patient, family, and health care professionals?
   1. Open communication
   2. Respite care for family
   3. Confidentiality
   4. Decreasing discomfort

3. Before entering into a situation in which the respectful death model is in use, which action is most important for the nurse to do?
   1. Discuss his or her feelings about the dying process with the family
   2. Ensure the dying person is of the same religion as the nurse
   3. Spend time reflecting on his/her own values and beliefs about dying
   4. Allow time to pass between meeting the patient and family and entering into the situation

CHAPTER SUMMARY

- Law is the sum total of rules and regulations by which a society is governed; ethics encompasses principles of appropriate/acceptable conduct and is generally concerned with motives, attitudes, and values.
- There are three major ethical theories that are applicable to health care settings:
  - Deontological, or "duty" theories
  - Teleological, or "consequential" theories
  - Principalism, or application of ethical principle theories.
- Ethical principles include:
  - Autonomy, or personal freedom and self-determination
  - Beneficence, or the duty to do "good"
  - Nonmaleficence, or the duty to avoid harm
  - Veracity, or truth telling
  - Fidelity, or keeping one's promises
  - Paternalism/parentalism, or making decisions for another
  - Justice, or the duty to treat others fairly and equally
  - Respect for others that is the overriding principle.
- The ethics of caring involves the harmonious relations and holistic nature of treatments and therapies.
- The MORAL model is one ethical decision-making model that can be easily used in nursing settings and that assists nurses in ethical decision making.

- Therapeutic jurisprudence focuses on the impact that ethical and legal decisions have on the psychological well-being of a person and seeks to ensure that the beneficial aspects of these decisions are recognized and implemented.
- Patient advocacy concerns the active support of a cause or issue that has importance to persons directly involved in the cause or issue.
- There are three models of advocacy employed in clinical practice settings:
  - Rights protection model
  - Values-based decision model
  - Respect for persons model.
- Hospital ethics committees provide structure and guidelines for resolving ethical dilemmas in a variety of health care settings.
- There are three models for ethics committees:
  - Autonomy model
  - Patient benefit model
  - Social justice model.
- The respectful death model guides the interdisciplinary health care team in assisting terminally ill persons and their family members develop the necessary therapeutic relationship that leads to a successful closure at the end of life.

CHAPTER REVIEW

Gladys Kwan, an 84-year-old retired nurse, recently moved to an assisted living center. She has been widowed for the past 20 years and has four adult children and multiple grandchildren and great-grandchildren, none of whom live within 50 miles of the living center. She has always been independent and has repeatedly said that if she were to suffer a major cardiac event or a stroke she would want no "heroics." Four months ago she was diagnosed with acute lymphocyte leukemia (ALL) and is being treated nonaggressively with prophylactic antibiotics, blood transfusions, and symptomatic management. Despite this fact, Mrs. Kwan has not signed any form of self-determination document nor has she indicated which child she would have named as her surrogate decision maker if she had signed such self-determination documents.

She recently fell while in the assisted living center, was hospitalized for hip-replacement surgery, and moved to a rehabilitation center. While at the rehabilitation center, she suffered a major stroke and was admitted to an acute care facility. Completely paralyzed on her right side, she is unable to vocalize her wishes, but adamantly refuses to cooperate with the nursing and medical staff; she is now fully restrained as she continues to disconnect and infiltrate her intravenous therapy and discontinue her feeding tube. When approached by staff or family members, she pulls the covers over her head and turns as far away from them as she can. Her family is divided between further therapy or allowing her to be admitted to a hospice center.

Question

You are the primary nurse for Mrs. Kwan. What are your ethical obligations to the patient?

Suggested Response

While she was fully competent, Mrs. Kwan was very assertive in her demand that she be allowed to die without "heroics." There should be no dispute about what her wishes entail as she has now experienced a devastating stroke and previously had been diagnosed with a terminal illness for which she is receiving palliative care. Mrs. Kwan's behavior also demonstrates her autonomy needs; she had disconnected any invasive lines that she perceives as keeping her alive and actively turns away from health care providers and family members. Her autonomy rights are to be allowed to die as naturally as possible with no further treatments or therapies. Beneficence, to do good, entails giving comfort care and assuring Mrs. Kwan that she will be kept comfortable in the dying process. Doing "good" for this particular person also entails assuring her that you will keep any promise (fidelity) you might have made before she had her stroke, such as ensuring that someone will be at her bedside for support and comfort and that you will continue to tell her truthfully about her condition (veracity). The standard of best interest does not enter into this patient care scenario, as Mrs. Kwan was able to fully communicate her preferences for care prior to having the stroke. She also indirectly communicated the level of care she desired when she elected to have palliative care for the leukemia as opposed to more aggressive therapy.

Perhaps the biggest challenge for the nurse working with this patient's family members is their desire for more aggressive care. They need to understand why her preferences supersede their needs and desires and how to "let Mrs. Kwan go." Hopefully, they will be able to accept that the ultimate decision rests with Mrs. Kwan and cherish the final moments they have with her.

The eldest daughter of Mrs. Kwan, Judy Nobles, has requested that the court appoint her as a guardian for her mother. Judy believes that her mother could benefit from further inpatient hospitalization and petitions the health care providers to sedate her mother and begin rehabilitative care.

Questions

How would providing such inpatient care complement or contradict the concept of therapeutic jurisprudence? How would you, as the primary nursing provider for Mrs. Kwan, begin to advocate for the patient, and which model of advocacy would you employ?

Suggested Response

Therapeutic jurisprudence basically states that one use the principles of law and ethics in the most caring and compassionate means possible. What Judy Nobles is proposing is in direct violation of what her mother desires and has already rejected. Mrs. Kwan had the opportunity to be more aggressive in health care therapies when she was first diagnosed with leukemia, yet she chose the more conservative manner of care. She also adamantly declared that she wanted no heroics, should that course of action ever present itself. Secondly, her actions in the acute care setting following the stroke (discontinuing peripheral lines and invasive catheters as well as turning away from health care providers) presents a clear picture that she does not want continuing and life-prolonging care. Therapeutic jurisprudence seeks to provide compassion, integrity, and conscientiousness in its application; the direct opposite of what Judy is requesting.

One could argue that the rights protection model of advocacy is the model most likely to be employed in this instance. The nurse would be using previous statements of the patient as well as the patient's behaviors to determine what the patient would have desired and then advocate for the person. Mrs. Kwan is, through her actions, advocating for her right to reject further therapies and treatments. One could also use the respect for persons model as the advocacy model to be implemented with Mrs. Kwan for much of the same reasons.

REFERENCES

American Nurses Association. (2001). *Code of Ethics for Nurses.* Washington, DC: Author.

Barrocas, A., Yarbrough, G., Becnel, P., & Nelson, J. E. (2003). Ethical and legal issues in nutrition support of the geriatric patient: The can, should, and must of nutritional support. *Nutrition in Clinical Practice, 18*(1), 37–47.

Beauchamp, T. L., & Childress, J. F. (2001). *Principles of biomedical ethics.* Oxford: Oxford University Press.

Beckstrand, R. L., Callister, L. C., & Kirchoff, K. T. (2006). Providing a "good death": Critical care nurses' suggestions for improving end-of-life care. *American Journal of Critical Care, 15*(1), 38–45.

Botes, A. (2000). A comparison between the ethics of justice and the ethics of caring. *Journal of Advanced Nursing, 32*(5), 1071–1075.

Burt, R. A. (2005). The end of autonomy. Improving end of life care: Why has it been so difficult? *Hastings Center Report Special Report, 35*(6), S9–S13.

Butts, J. B., & Rich, K. (2005). Nursing ethics: Across the curriculum and into practice. Boston: Jones and Bartlett Publishers.

Cimino, J. E. (2003). A clinician's understanding of ethics in palliative care: An American perspective. *Clinical Reviews in Oncology/Hematology, 46*(1), 17–24.

Doane, G., Pauly, B., Brown, H., & McPherson, G. (2004). Exploring the heart of ethical nursing practice: Implications for ethics education. *Nursing Ethics, 11*(3), 240–253.

Farber, A., & Farber, S. (2006). The respectful death model: Difficult conversations at the end of life. In R. S. Katz and T. A. Johnson, eds. *When professionals weep.* (pp. 221–236). New York: Routledge.

Farber, S., Egnew, T., & Farber, A. (2004). What is respectful death? In J. Berzoff and P. R. Silverman, eds. *Living with dying.* (pp. 102–127). New York: Columbia University Press.

Fieser, J. (1999). *Metaethics, normative ethics, and applied ethics: Contemporary and historical readings.* London: Cengage Learning.

Guido, G. W. (2006). Legal and ethical issues in nursing. (4th ed.). Upper Saddle River, NJ: Pearson Prentice Hall.

Guido, G. W. (2007). Legal and ethical issues. In P. S. Yoder-Wise, *Leading and managing in nursing.* (4th ed., pp. 59–90). St. Louis: Mosby Elsevier.

Hall, J. K. (1990). Understanding the fine line between law and ethics. *Nursing 90, 20*(10), 37.

Halloran, M. C. (1982). Rational ethical judgments using a decision-making tool. *Heart and Lung, 11*(6), 566–570.

Harkness, M., & Wanklyn, P. (2006). Cardiopulmonary resuscitation: Capacity, discussion, and documentation. *QJM: An International Journal of Medicine, 99*(10), 683–690.

Harris, D. M. (2003). *Contemporary issues in healthcare law and ethics.* (2nd ed.). Washington, DC: Foundation of the American College of Healthcare Executives.

Joint Commission for Accreditation of Healthcare Organizations. (2007). *Accreditation manual for hospitals.* Oakbrook Terrace, IL: Author.

Neuberger, J. (2004). *Dying well: A guide to enabling a good death.* (2nd ed.). San Francisco: Radcliffe.

Oberle, K., & Hughes, D. (2001). Doctors' and nurses' perceptions of ethical problems in end-of-life decisions. *Journal of Advanced Nursing, 33*(6), 707–715.

Quill, T. E. (1997). Rule of double effect: A critique of its role in end-of-life decision making. *New England Journal of Medicine, 337,* 1768–1771.

Reamer, F. G. (2006). *Social work values and ethics.* (3rd ed.). New York: Columbia University Press.

Thiroux, J. (1977). *Ethics: Theory and practice.* Philadelphia: Macmillan.

Videbeck, S. L. (2004). *Psychiatric mental health nursing.* (2nd ed.). Philadelphia: Lippincott, Williams, and Wilkins.

Vivian, R. (2006). Truth telling in palliative care nursing: The dilemmas of collusion. *International Journal of Palliative Nursing, 12*(7), 341–348.

Volbrecht, R. M. (2002). *Nursing ethics: Communities in dialogue.* Upper Saddle River, NJ: Prentice Hall.

Wasserman, L. S. (2008). Respectful death: A model for end-of-life care. *Clinical Journal of Oncology Nursing, 12*(4), 621–626.

Wexler, D. B., & Winick, B. J. (2005). *Judging for the 21st Century: A problem solving approach.* Ottawa, ON: National Judicial Institute Press.

Wolfson, J. (2005). Erring on the side of Theresa Schiavo: Reflections of the special guardian ad litem. *The Hastings Center Report, 35*(3), 16–19.

Legal Issues in End-of-Life Nursing Care

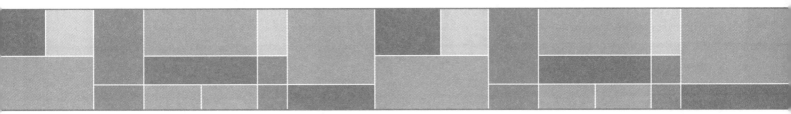

Following completion of this chapter, the learner will be able to:

3.1. Describe the historical roots of end-of-life legal issues.

3.2. Describe advance directives, including living wills, natural death acts, and durable powers of attorney for health care.

3.3. Compare and contrast alternatives to advance directives, including Respecting Choices, and the Physicians Orders for Life-Sustaining Treatment form. Describe informed consent and its importance in end-of-life issues.

3.4. Examine decision-making capacity in end-of-life issues.

3.5. Discuss physician-assisted suicide from a legal and professional practice perspective.

3.6. Enumerate the American Association of Colleges of Nursing's end-of-life nursing competencies.

This chapter examines legal issues as they relate to nursing care at the end of life. Individuals have the right of informed consent if they are competent and can make their wishes known to family members and health care providers. There are multiple legal doctrines that assist individuals to ensure that their wishes are known when and if they become incompetent to express their desires at a specific time. Physician-assisted suicide and its legal requirements are discussed in depth. The chapter concludes with an examination of end-of-life competencies that all nurses practicing in this arena should possess.

PRETEST

1. When did the issue of informed consent to treatment first arise in the context of end-of-life care?
   1. An attorney first coined the term during a hearing about a patient's rights.
   2. A patient gave the physician consent to receive treatment and then retracted the consent.
   3. People concerned about resuscitation efforts against their wishes allowed courts to decide.
   4. Physicians refused to resuscitate some people, and families sued.

2. Which document allows the patient to choose a surrogate decision maker in the event he or she becomes incompetent? (Select all that apply.)
   1. The natural death act
   2. A durable power of attorney for health care

   3. The Death with Dignity Act
   4. The Physician Orders for Life-Sustaining Treatment form

3. In which state(s) is physician-assisted suicide legal? (Select all that apply.)
   1. Washington
   2. California
   3. Oregon
   4. All states in the United States of America

4. Which statement is most accurate about consent given by a competent patient? Consent:
   1. May be revoked at any time prior to the initiation of the treatment or procedure.
   2. May be revoked only in writing if the original consent was written.

3. May not be revoked.
4. May be revoked only if a second procedure supersedes the procedure or treatment for which the original consent was given.
5. What does it mean when an adult patient enacts a valid natural death act?
   1. The document takes precedent over his or her expressed wishes that may be in direct conflict with the executed document.
   2. The document is legally binding and all health care providers must abide by its provisions or face legal liability.
   3. It can be revoked only if the person signs a subsequent natural death act that expressly revokes the original document.
   4. It prevents health care providers who abide by its provisions from being charged with criminal negligence.

GLOSSARY

best interest standard   An objective test that looks at personal preferences made while the now-incompetent patient was rational and capable of stating what he or she would want in the event of a catastrophic happening; frequently relied on in the incompetent person's right-to-die issues.

clinically designated surrogate decision maker   One or more health care providers who consult with available family members when the patient lacks decision-making capacity.

consent   A voluntary action by which one agrees to allow someone else to do something; may be oral, written, or implied based upon the selected circumstances.

decision-making capacity   Ability of an adult individual to determine what he or she will allow in terms of medical treatments/procedures; the ability of the individual to understand and appreciate the proposed treatment, potential complications, benefits and risks, as well as alternative interventions.

do-not-resuscitate directives   Executed by patients on admission to health care facilities, these directives allow patients to determine, while still competent, to what extent they will allow resuscitative measures, should such measures become necessary.

durable power of attorney for health care   Statutory directive that allows competent persons to appoint a surrogate or proxy to make health care decisions for them in the event that they are incompetent to do so.

futility standard   Decisions are based on goals in which the primary outcomes are the patient's safety and comfort rather than the vain attempt to delay the patient's ultimate death; acknowledges the fact that there are instances where further treatment is futile.

informed consent   The voluntary authorization by a patient or the patient's legal representative to do something to or for the patient; based on patient comprehension.

judicially designated surrogate decision maker   One whose authority to give or deny consent for another is established through a court appointment as part of a hearing during which it is determined that an individual lacks decision-making capacity.

legal guardian or representative   A person legally responsible for giving or refusing consent for the incompetent patient; appointed through the court system for incompetent persons.

living will   A directive from competent individuals to medical personnel and family members regarding the treatment that individuals wish to receive if they can no longer make decisions for themselves; has no legal enforcement as such.

medical durable power of attorney   Synonymous with the durable power of attorney for health care.

natural death act   Legally recognized living will; a directive of a competent person that allows the person to die without the use of extraordinary life-support systems; protects the health care provider from civil or criminal liability for following the directive.

patient-designated surrogate decision maker   Individual with capacity to give or deny informed consent whose authority is established via a valid natural death act or durable power of attorney for health care.

patient self-determination   Enacted into law in November 1991, the statute mandates that patients are informed about advance directives when admitted to health care settings and given the opportunity to enact such directives.

physician-assisted suicide   Aiding another person to end his or her life; in the health care arena, the act of prescribing or giving medications that will hasten a person's death.

statutorily designated decision-making capacity   Established when legislative law exists recognizing the right of family consent and designating which family members are authorized to act on behalf of the patient lacking decision-making capacity.

substituted judgment standard   Allows a surrogate to determine what the patient would have wanted were he or she capable of making such a determination; a subjective test of what the surrogate believes the patient would have wanted.

SECTION ONE: Historical Roots of End-of-Life Legal Issues

Legal concerns about a person's right to make end-of-life decisions continue to come to the forefront when caring for patients in all health care settings. These concerns take on greater relevance when the individual nearing the end of life is not able to make decisions for himself or herself, and family members struggle to determine their next actions as the health care team endeavors to provide quality and compassionate care in an environment that teems with newer technologies and medical advances.

These technologies and medical advances have greatly altered the manner in which death and dying have come to be viewed by health care providers, patients, and families. The advent of complex surgical procedures, institution of specialty intensive care units, and continuing development of new medications have all contributed to increased health and longer life for the majority of Americans. During the 1960s, the advent of cardiopulmonary resuscitation changed the way in which acute care hospitals approached death, mandating that performance of cardiopulmonary resuscitation was the new standard of care for patients who experienced cardiac arrest and cessation of respirations (Harkness & Wanklyn, 2006).

As cardiopulmonary resuscitation and life support became more prevalent, patients began to express concerns and doubts about whether they would want such treatment should there be a need to institute such measures. These concerns and doubts lead to questions about their rights to refuse care that was designed to preserve life. Legal experts, when approached on such issues, concluded that a competent adult did have the right to refuse medical treatment, even if the refusal was certain to cause death. But these early legal conclusions involved patients who had not yet been resuscitated or placed on life support systems. It was not until the mid-1970s that individuals and their families wishing to forgo life-sustaining medical treatment came to rely on the judicial system to solve the issues that undoubtedly might have been better resolved outside the court system.

Perhaps it was inevitable that the courts were designated to address these early cases. The first court case to challenge the judiciary in this respect was *In re Quinlan* (1976). Karen Ann Quinlan was in her late teens when she suffered a respiratory arrest and was not resuscitated in time to prevent permanent brain injury. Following successful resuscitation, she was placed on a ventilator. When it became apparent that she would remain in a vegetative state and that she would not be the lively person that she had always been, her family requested that the ventilator be discontinued and she be allowed to die. This seemed a logical conclusion, for her life, as her parents and friends had known it, was over. Two choices were open to them: accept what was an affront to their values, beliefs, and dignity, or fight against it. The parents chose to fight and filed a lawsuit so that Karen could die (Meisel, 2005).

In a lengthy decision, the New Jersey Supreme Court held that although patients generally have the right to refuse therapy, guardians for the incompetent usually do not. The court, though, did finally reach the conclusion that guardians should have this right as they stand in the place of the patient. The court then allowed the father of Karen Quinlan to authorize the withdrawal of life support systems for Karen. The decision was a difficult one to reach because Karen did not meet the Harvard criteria for brain death. Though she was ventilator-dependent at the time of the court case, she did have some brain activity on the electroencephalogram (EEG) and some reflex movements. The decision was also difficult because it conflicted significantly with a precedent-setting New Jersey case that held that one should always save a life, even if the patient's objection to life-saving procedures was based on religious beliefs (*John F. Kennedy Memorial Hospital v. Heston*, 1971).

Additionally the court, to assist the father in his decision making, mandated that an ethics committee be developed, as the court said this was too serious a decision for one person to make by himself. Such a committee, said the court, should be instituted to assist, as the decision to remove the ventilator rested solely with Karen's father.

Further lawsuits followed, primarily to further define the rights of the family or surrogate decision maker in deciding to withdraw life-sustaining measures. In these subsequent cases, the courts wavered on the need for ethics committees, addressed the issue of terminally ill individuals versus those in a persistent vegetative state, and slowly developed the **substituted judgement standard**. This standard is a subjective determination of how persons, were they capable of making their opinions and wishes known, would have chosen to exercise their right to accept or refuse therapy.

Cruzan v. Director, Missouri Department of Health (1990), appeared to be one of the final cases in a long string of such cases. In *Cruzan*, the court was faced with discontinuing a feeding tube, and that court made explicit that right-to-die issues would be decided on a state-to-state basis. They also decreed that "clear and convincing evidence" was required to uphold the right to discontinue life-sustaining procedures and measures. This imposed a standard of evidence that is a medium standard of proof, mandating that the individual convince the court that it is substantially more likely that a fact is true. In this particular case, this meant that the parents who brought this lawsuit had to convince the court that Nancy Cruzan would not have wanted to live in a permanent vegetative state and that she had made such statements during her lifetime to family and friends. Following the Cruzan decision, cases generally allowed more latitude to family members, and courts struggled to find instances in which patients had made some expression, however fleeting, about their desires for sustaining life with artificial or life-support measures (Guido, 2006).

Fifteen years after Cruzan was settled, Terri Schiavo's plight again brought forward litigation regarding end-of-life decision making. It is to be hoped that the legacy of Terri Schiavo's multiple court decisions is the final decision from a litigation perspective. In Schiavo, multiple courts heard the same arguments debated by a variety of attorneys, over the course of which her feeding tube was discontinued and reinserted multiple times. (Reread Chapter 2 for a more complete description and analysis of this case.)

These multiple lawsuits and court hearings have verified the limitations of litigation in such cases. Litigation in end-of-life cases has shown itself to be a piecemeal way of attacking an issue, as the litigation applies solely to the facts of a specific case and a specific person. Newer cases will have facts that are somewhat different, as the "evidence" in support of the person's request not to be kept alive on life-support systems will differ from facts or circumstances of previous cases, or the "evidence" in support of the medical tests used to verify a permanent vegetative state will be slightly different from the case before it.

Though even the Schiavo case probably will not prevent future lawsuits, there are some lessons to be learned from that case. Undoubtedly, there are some measures that could be implemented to assist other patients and families who find themselves at this stage of their lives. The first would be additional state statutes that begin to bring consensus to the right of competent patients to forgo medical treatment and the right of incompetent patients to have close family members make those decisions for them. Currently about half of the states address these issues with significant clarity and without multiple exceptions (Meisel, 2005).

A second consideration seems to be for the courts to further clarify some of the more ambiguous language used in the cases settled to date. For example, *Cruzan* revolved around the issue of "clear and convincing evidence," which is a legal standard and does not give guidance to surrogate decision makers. These surrogate decision makers should understand that what is required is evidence that the person now incapacitated would not have desired to be kept alive in such circumstances and burdened by such life-sustaining measures. What that evidence will encompass will vary according to the person, his or her values, and perhaps his or her culture (Meisel, 2005).

Finally, the interests of family members or those persons closest to the patient should be the ones that come to the forefront. These interests should be defined more in terms of a social connection rather than a formal relationship, as the social connection would allow for the interests of those closest to the patient to be a vital part of the decision-making process. In some family groups, those individuals who are closest to the terminally ill person may not have a direct family lineage. Acknowledging the wishes of these individuals who have the closest relationship to the person may ultimately prevent the conditions that created and perpetuated the conflict in the Terri Schiavo case.

SECTION ONE REVIEW

1. For which patient was a lawsuit filed for the first time bringing a person's right to die to the judicial system?
   1. Karen Quinlan
   2. Nancy Cruzan
   3. Terri Schiavo
   4. Jack Kevorkian
2. Which statement correctly describes the purpose of the doctrine of substituted judgment?
   1. It describes the method by which physicians are to choose the person or persons who can make decisions for an incompetent patient.
   2. It describes how decisions must be made for incompetent patients in the manner in which the patient would have accepted or refused treatments/procedures for themselves.

3. It assists the judicial system in making decisions for those incompetent patients who cannot decide for themselves.
   4. Ethics committees use the doctrine to determine how decisions should be made for an incompetent patient.
3. Following the Schiavo case and her subsequent death, which statement most accurately describes the consequences resulting from the court decision?
   1. New regulations were passed allowing family members to make right-to-die decisions for their relations.
   2. More complex decisions must now automatically go before the Supreme Court.
   3. Only spouses and children of patients are allowed to make decisions for patients.
   4. State statutes are becoming less ambiguous to make family rights more understandable.

SECTION TWO: Patient Self-Determination Act and Its Ramifications

The Patient Self-Determination Act (PSDA) was passed on November 5, 1990, as an amendment to the Omnibus Budget Reconciliation Act of 1990, becoming effective December 1, 1991. The PSDA was a direct response to the Cruzan case and was introduced by Senators Danforth of Missouri and Patrick

Moynihan of New York. They proposed the legislation so that all patients would be aware of their rights to refuse treatment and prevent another Cruzan-type case.

The PSDA requires Medicare and Medicaid providers (hospitals, nursing homes, hospice programs, home health agencies, and health maintenance organizations) to give adult individuals, at the time of inpatient admission or enrollment, information about their rights under applicable state laws governing advanced directives. Specifically, this information includes: (1) the right to participate in and direct their own health care decisions; (2) the right to accept or refuse medical or surgical treatment; (3) the right to prepare an advance directive; and (4) information on the provider's policies that govern the utilization of these rights. The act allows the person to enact **do-not-resuscitate directives**. The act also prohibits institutions from discriminating against a patient who does not have an advance directive. A separate aspect of the PSDA requires institutions to document patient information, comply with state laws concerning advance directives, and provide ongoing community education on advance directives.

Patient self-determination involves the right of individuals to decide what will or will not happen to them as well as documentation describing these wishes. Today, the right of self-determination most often concerns issues surrounding death and dying, with the term generally describing advance directives. These directives are discussed separately in the following text.

Living Wills

Living wills, first seen in the late 1960s, gained popularity following the Quinlan case. **Living wills** are directives from competent individuals to medical personnel and family members regarding the treatment they wish to receive when they can no longer make the decision for themselves. The living will is not necessary if the patient is competent and capable of making his or her wishes known. It becomes important when the previously competent person becomes unable to give informed consent regarding health care.

Usually the language of a living will is broad and vague, providing little direction to the health care practitioner concerning the circumstances and actual time the individual wishes the living will to be honored. There is typically no legal enforcement of the living will, and health care practitioners may choose to abide by the patient's wishes or to ignore them as they see fit. There is also no protection for the practitioner against criminal or civil liability, and many primary health care providers have been afraid to proceed under a living will's direction for fear that family members or the state will file charges of wrongful death.

Natural Death Acts

To protect health care practitioners from potential civil and criminal lawsuits and to ensure that patients' wishes are followed when they are no longer able to make their wishes known, the natural death act was enacted into state laws. **Natural death acts** are, in actuality, legally recognized living wills in that they serve the same function as living wills but with statutory enforcement, and virtually all states have enacted some form of natural death legislation. Recognizing that for a variety of reasons health care providers may be unwilling to follow the directive, several of these state laws require a reasonable effort on the part of the primary health care provider to transfer the patient's care to a provider who will honor these wishes.

Statutory provisions for natural death acts vary from state to state. Generally, persons over 18 years may sign a natural death act. Such persons must be of sound mind and capable of understanding the purpose of the document that they sign. The natural death act document is usually a declaration that withholds or withdraws life-sustaining treatment from the patient should he or she ever be in a terminal state. The natural death act ideally is in written form, signed by the patient, and witnessed by two persons, each of whom is 18 years or older. Recognizing that patients may not be physically capable of written enactments, a newer trend is to allow oral enactment of natural death acts. Most states also now allow the individual drafting the form to name a surrogate in the written document so that health care providers can obtain consent from an individual who is the most knowledgeable about the drafter's wishes.

To prevent any person from benefiting by the death of another, state laws also disallow certain individuals from serving as witnesses to a natural death act document. Box 3–1 lists persons who may not serve as witnesses for a valid document.

Other states incorporate some, but not all, of the previously enumerated restrictions.

The form of the natural death act also varies from state to state. Some states provide no suggestion as to the contents of the document, whereas other states have a mandatory form that must be completed. Still other states suggest a form but provide that additional directions may be added if they are not inconsistent with the statutory requirements. For states that have no set form, private organizations have suggested formats for these special living wills. Some states also have a clause stating that the person must have discussed these issues with his or her designated surrogate.

Once signed and witnessed, most natural death acts are effective until revoked, although some states require that they must be re-executed every 5 or 10 years. In some states, pregnancy invalidates the document. It may be advisable for individuals to review, re-date, and re-sign the natural death act every year or so. This assures family members and health care providers that the directions contained in the natural death act reflect the current wishes of the patient. If the individual wishes to revoke

---

BOX 3–1   Persons Who May Not Serve as Witnesses to a Valid Natural Death Act Document:

- Individuals related to the patient by blood or marriage
- Individuals who are entitled to any portion of the estate of the patient
- Individuals who have direct financial responsibility for the patient's medical care
- An attending physician, the institution's administrative personnel, or any employee of the facility in which the individual is a patient
- A person who, at the request of the patient, signed the declaration because the patient was unable to sign for himself or herself

- Physical destruction of the document
- Defacement of the document
- Written revocation that the person wishes to revoke the document
- Oral revocation that the person wishes to revoke the document

the document, there are a variety of means to revoke the document. Box 3–2 lists some of these possible means for revocation.

Some states have restrictions on revocation, such as the revocation may take place without regard to the mental condition of the patient and/or that the revocation is ineffective until the attending physician is notified of the revocation.

Once a valid natural death act exists, it is effective only when the person becomes qualified; that is, the person is diagnosed to have a terminal condition and the removal or withholding of life-support systems would merely prolong the patient's process of dying. Most states require that two physicians certify in writing that any procedures and treatments will not prevent the ultimate death of the patient but will serve only to postpone death in a patient with no chance of recovery. Medications and procedures used merely to prevent the patient's suffering and to provide comfort are excluded from this definition. A sample Natural Death Act form may be found in Figure 3–1.

Durable Power of Attorney for Health Care

The **durable power of attorney for health care** (DPAHC) or the **medical durable power of attorney** (MDPA) allows competent patients to appoint a surrogate or proxy to make health care decisions for them in the event that they are incompetent to do so. These legislative enactments were the next logical step following the limitations surrounding living wills and natural death acts. With DPAHCs, there is no need to guess if this is the time that the patient would have wanted the living will to be followed, as a surrogate decision maker has been named under the provisions of the DPAHC. This named surrogate has the same status as a **legal guardian or representative**, with full authority to either accept or refuse care and to speak for the patient.

Under the DPAHC statutes, individuals designate a surrogate to make medical decisions for them when they are unable to make such decisions. The power includes the right to ask questions, select and remove physicians from the patient's care, assess risks and complications, and select treatments and procedures from a variety of therapeutic options. The power also includes the right to refuse care and/or life-sustaining procedures. Health care providers are protected from liability if they abide, in good faith, with the surrogate's decisions. Additionally, surrogates have the authority to enforce the patient's treatment plans by filing lawsuits or legal actions as needed.

Patients are cautioned to appoint persons as their surrogates who understand what they desire for themselves and who are ca-

pable of making hard decisions. Friends, relatives, or spouses are generally the individuals appointed to serve as surrogates. As with natural death acts, some states mandate that the patient and the surrogate have discussed potential health care needs and options, at least superficially. Most states allow the patient or potential patient to appoint subsequent surrogates. In the event the first named person cannot serve or is unwilling to serve in this capacity, then a second or third person has the principal's authority. Without this latter provision, patients' wishes might still not be honored. Once appointed by the principal, surrogate decision makers have the ability to act as the now incompetent person would have acted if he or she were able to communicate with health care providers.

Limitations of Advance Directives

Though it was envisioned that advance directives would ensure that patient preferences would be honored, studies have shown that this may not be true. The most frequent reason for not honoring the patient's request is due to physician noncompliance (Lynch, Mathes, & Sawicki, 2008). Additionally, these same authors estimated that less than 30% of individuals in the United States have completed any form of an advance directive.

There are several reasons that individuals have not completed advance directives. Perhaps the primary reason is that the instructions given in the directives are too vague for the majority of people or too medically specific to be helpful. Consider, for example, the statements in several state advance directives that read "if I am close to death," "if death is imminent regardless of treatment," or "if I am in a persistent vegetative state." Often these vague instructions are at the heart of equally vague conversations with health care personnel or family members, resulting in patients making requests such as "do not keep me alive with machines" or "let me die if I am a vegetable" (Hickman, Hammes, Moss, & Tolle, 2005).

Other reasons that individuals may not complete advance directives include that health care personnel fail to assist these individuals to understand how the directives can help them achieve their values and goals for health care at the end of life, and that once the advance directive is complete, planning for end-of-life care is considered to be finished. The patient may be asked if he or she has an advance directive but not how he or she might envision health care interventions changing as the patient declines in health. Additionally, traditional advance directives are seen as the person's right, with little thought about incorporating the advance directive into clinical care.

Finally, the advance directives seen today are based on the ethical value of autonomy as the primary mode of decision making for individuals. However, many individuals, especially those from other than Western cultures, have a much broader social context for decision making rather than merely viewing the wishes and desires of an individual. Patients may choose that family members or a specific family member make decisions for them and thus will defer any discussions about prognosis and interventions for cultural or other reasons (Hickman et al., 2005).

Natural Death Act

Health Care Directive

Directive made this . . . . day of . . . . . . (month, year).

I . . . . . ., having the capacity to make health care decisions, willfully, and voluntarily make known my desire that my dying shall not be artificially prolonged under the circumstances set forth below, and do hereby declare that:

(a) If at any time I should be diagnosed in writing to be in a terminal condition by the attending physician, or in a permanent unconscious condition by two physicians, and where the application of life-sustaining treatment would serve only to artificially prolong the process of my dying, I direct that such treatment be withheld or withdrawn, and that I be permitted to die naturally. I understand by using this form that a terminal condition means an incurable and irreversible condition caused by injury, disease, or illness, that would within reasonable medical judgment cause death within a reasonable period of time in accordance with accepted medical standards, and where the application of life-sustaining treatment would serve only to prolong the process of dying. I further understand in using this form that a permanent unconscious condition means an incurable and irreversible condition in which I am medically assessed within reasonable medical judgment as having no reasonable probability of recovery from an irreversible coma or a persistent vegetative state.

(b) In the absence of my ability to give directions regarding the use of such life-sustaining treatment, it is my intention that this directive shall be honored by my family and physician(s) as the final expression of my legal right to refuse medical or surgical treatment and I accept the consequences of such refusal. If another person is appointed to make these decisions for me, whether through a durable power of attorney or otherwise, I request that the person be guided by this directive and any other clear expressions of my desires.

(c) If I am diagnosed to be in a terminal condition or in a permanent unconscious condition (check one):

I DO want to have artificially provided nutrition and hydration.

I DO NOT want to have artificially provided nutrition and hydration.

(d) If I have been diagnosed as pregnant and that diagnosis is known to my physician, this directive shall have no force or effect during the course of my pregnancy.

(e) I understand the full import of this directive and I am emotionally and mentally capable to make the health care decisions contained in this directive.

(f) I understand that before I sign this directive, I can add to or delete from or otherwise change the wording of this directive and that I may add to or delete from this directive at any time and that any changes shall be consistent with Washington state law or federal constitutional law to be legally valid.

(g) It is my wish that every part of this directive be fully implemented. If for any reason any part is held invalid it is my wish that the remainder of my directive be implemented.

Signed . . . .

City, County, and State of Residence

The declarer has been personally known to me and I believe him or her to be capable of making health care decisions.

Witness . . . .

Witness . . . .

(2) Prior to withholding or withdrawing life-sustaining treatment, the diagnosis of a terminal condition by the attending physician or the diagnosis of a permanent unconscious state by two physicians shall be entered in writing and made a permanent part of the patient's medical records.

(3) A directive executed in another political jurisdiction is valid to the extent permitted by Washington state law and federal constitutional law.

Figure 3–1 ■ Natural Death Act. *Washington State Legislature, 1992 c 98 § 3; 1979 c 112 § 4*

SECTION TWO REVIEW

1. Which advance medical directive is taking precedence over all other advance directives?
   1. The state natural death act
   2. The durable power of attorney for health care
   3. The do-not-resuscitate order signed by the attending physician
   4. No document, as all advance directives have equal weight
2. Once an adult patient has executed a valid natural death act, which illustrates the consequences?
   1. The document takes precedent over his or her expressed wishes that may be in direct conflict to the document.
   2. It is legally binding and all health care providers must abide by its provisions or face malpractice charges.
   3. It can be revoked only if the patient signs a subsequent living will revoking the first document.
   4. It prevents health care providers who abide by its provisions from being charged with criminal negligence.
3. Which statement indicates the need for further teaching when a family member is discussing the purpose behind having a durable power of attorney for health care?

1. "Individuals wanted a means to assure their final wishes would be respected should they not be able to express those wishes."
2. "Written living wills, handwritten and presented at the time of admission to hospitals, were followed by health care providers."
3. "Family disputes often prevented the patients' final wishes from being respected."
4. "Physicians and other health care providers frequently disregarded the final requests of patients who were competent and vocal about their requests."
4. Which describes the reason the durable power of attorney for health care is preferred over living wills/natural death acts? The durable power of attorney for health care: (Select all that apply.)
   1. Names the individual or individuals to approach for a valid consent.
   2. Provides a better understanding of what the patient would have wanted if he or she were still able to orally express his or her wishes.
   3. Represents a means of creating a document that is deemed as legal in all states without the need to have state-specific documents.
   4. Increases the patient's ability to better refuse unwanted therapies and procedures.

SECTION THREE: Alternatives to Advance Directives

Because of the limitations noted in the previous sections, other programs were initiated in the various states. The alternatives to advance directives have as their main mission the concept of advanced care planning. Advanced care planning refers to "the process by which patients, together with their families and health care practitioners, consider their values and goals and articulate their preferences for future care" (Tulsky, 2005, p. 360). More than a signature on a document, advanced care planning is a form of communication.

Respecting Choices

In La Crosse, Wisconsin, the Respecting Choices program began in 1991 as a community-wide effort to develop institutional policies in selected health care systems to ensure that written advance directives were always available when needed. Components of the program included: staff education about the program and advanced care planning; clearly defined roles and expectations of primary health care providers; educational training for advanced

care planning facilitators; routine public and patient engagement in advanced care planning; clinically relevant advance directives incorporated into clinical care; and written protocols so that emergency personnel could follow physician orders that reflected patient preferences (Hammes & Rooney, 1998).

An evaluation of the Respecting Choices program was done at 11 months. This evaluation showed that 85% of all decedents in that time frame had some type of written advance directive at the time of their death and that treatment decisions made in the last weeks of life were consistent with written instructions in 98% of the deaths where an advance directive existed (Hammes & Rooney, 1998). This program is now being implemented in multiple communities in the United States, primarily through religious organizations, including the Lutheran and Catholic churches.

Physician Orders for Life-Sustaining Treatment

A Physician Orders for Life-Sustaining Treatment (POLST) form, previously known as an Emergency Medical Service No Cardiopulmonary Resuscitation (EMS-No CPR) form, is intended for use by any person 18 years of age or older who has serious health conditions. The form contains information about the person's end-of-life directives, including cardiopulmonary resuscitation, medical interventions, antibiotics, and artificially administered nutrition. It is not an advance directive, but rather a physician's or other primary health care provider's orders regarding treatment that the person will accept or refuse to accept.

The program began in Oregon in 1991. Initially developed for use by emergency medical service (EMS) personnel, the main purpose of the POLST was to provide these initial responders with written physician orders that gave specific instructions concerning medical interventions that the EMS personnel were to implement. These mandatory orders allowed the EMS personnel to honor the person's end-of-life treatment preferences either to have or to limit treatment, even when the person was transferred from one care setting to another. This latter provision accomplishes a secondary purpose of the form in that it is portable and may be used from one setting to another.

The need for such a readily accessible form arose because advance health care directives do not give guidance to EMS personnel, as they are not physician's orders and because no state forces a physician or other primary health care provider to comply with an advance directive. The POLST form is easy to complete, requiring only that the physician or other primary health care provider sign the form, and there is no witness to the signature or notarization of the form required. The POLST form is generally brightly colored so that it is easily recognizable by both the patient and the health care provider.

Persons who complete the POLST are advised to also complete an advance directive. The POLST merely outlines the person's preferences for end-of-life care and does not give guidance regarding who the person would select to have as his or her surrogate decision maker or guidance about issues outside the four categories on the form itself. A POLST may be the initial orders that accompany the patient who is newly admitted to a health care facility, and the advance directive gives more detailed information about the patient's long-term care.

Currently, the POLST is an endorsed program in a few states, including Oregon, Washington, Pennsylvania, West Virginia, and New York and in some communities in Wisconsin. Another 20 states are developing programs, either for the entire state or for communities within the state (POLST State Programs, 2008).

Section Summary

Advance directives and the POLST have some similarities. They are designed to assist persons with making their final wishes known so that these wishes and desires can be followed even if the person cannot speak for himself or herself. They encourage open and frank conversations with health care providers and among family and close friends. They also encourage this communication to take place at a time when the patient is competent to understand the ramifications of alternative options and can execute advance directives and POLSTs.

To make these advance directives and POLSTs as effective as possible, health care providers must themselves understand their provisions and how to answer patients' and families' questions. One of the most challenging aspects of the process of preparing these documents is assisting patients to identify their preferences for treatment. Some individuals have clear opinions, while other patients are more comfortable trusting future choices to family members without articulating specific wishes. It is also important for health care providers and patients to remember that preferences change over time and that the willingness to undergo aggressive treatment is in large part dependent on perception of the likely outcome of that treatment.

Patients and families inevitably ask questions concerning initiating curative and palliative care measures, particularly when the benefits of those measures may mean that the person will live longer, but not necessarily with the same quality of life. Additional questions then arise concerning the discontinuance of such treatments and therapies, especially when any benefits from a treatment or therapy are shown to be nonexistent and the treatment futile. Many families find it more acceptable not to initiate therapy rather than to begin and then withdraw the therapy. Having a patient's desires and last wishes known, either through advance directives and/or POLSTs, often helps family members make these hard decisions.

SECTION THREE REVIEW

1. Which are considered alternatives to advance directives? (Select all that apply.)
   1. Respecting Choices
   2. Peaceful Death
   3. Physician Orders for Life-Sustaining Treatment (POLST)
   4. Death without Issues

2. Which represents the main difference between Respecting Choices, Physician Orders for Life-Sustaining Treatment (POLST), and advance directives?
   1. Respecting Choices and POLST are information-only documents.
   2. The Respecting Choices and POLST documents are less complex and easier to implement than advance directives.

3. Respecting Choices and POLST apply only to emergency medical services.
4. Advance directives require a physician signature, whereas Respecting Choices and the POLST documents do not.
3. Educational programming has been effective if a person makes which statement?
   1. "As an advance directive, the Physician Orders for Life-Sustaining Treatment assists emergency personnel in understanding the patient's wishes."
   2. "A patient cannot have both advanced care planning documents and advance directive documents, because they override each other."
   3. "Nurses do not have a role in assisting patients prepare advanced care planning documents, because they are for use outside the hospital environment."
   4. "Advanced care planning makes others aware of the values and goals of the person while communicating preferences for future care."

SECTION FOUR: Informed Consent and Decision-Making Capacity

Before one can discuss the patient's right to die or to forgo life-sustaining procedures, one must consider the issue of informed consent. Competent adults have long been recognized as having the right to refuse medical treatment. Competent adults may decide which treatments they will receive and which medical procedures they will refuse (Guido, 2006). As noted in Section Two of this chapter, any decision to forgo medical treatment will need to survive a period in which the health care receiver is incompetent.

Informed Consent

The health care provider's right to treat a person is based on a contractual relationship that arises through the mutual consent of parties to the relationship. **Informed consent** is the voluntary authorization by a patient or the patient's legal representative to do something to or for the patient. Informed consent is based on the mutual consent of the parties involved, and the key to true and valid consent is patient comprehension.

Consent, technically, is an easy yes or no: "Yes, I will allow the medical intervention" or "No, I want only comfort measures." With consent, patients and their family members may not fully understand or may understand only vaguely what is being allowed. The law concerning consent in health care situations is based on informed consent, which mandates to health care providers the separate legal duty to disclose needed material facts in terms that patients can reasonably understand so that these patients can make informed choices. There should also be a description of the available alternatives to the proposed treatment and the risks and dangers involved in each alternative. While failure to disclose needed facts in understandable terms does not negate the consent, it does place potential liability on the health care provider for negligence (Guido, 2006). Box 3–3 outlines the information that the patient or representatives must receive to be fully informed.

Equally important to giving patients all material facts needed on which to base an informed choice is that the correct

---

BOX 3–3   Information Required for Informed Consent

- A brief but complete explanation of the treatment or procedure to be performed
- The name and qualifications of the person to perform the procedure and, if others will assist, the names of qualifications of those assistants
- An explanation of any serious harm that may occur during the procedure, including death if that is a realistic outcome. Pain and discomforting side effects both during the procedure and following the procedure should also be discussed.
- An explanation of alternative therapies to the procedure of treatment, including the risk of doing nothing at all
- An explanation that the patient can refuse the therapy or procedure without having palliative care or support discontinued
- The fact that patients can still refuse, even after the procedure or therapy has begun

---

person(s) consent to the procedure or therapy. Generally, if the patient is an adult according to state law and is competent, he or she is the correct person to give or deny consent. The individual's competency is usually made based on an assessment of the person by a physician or other member of the health care profession. This assessment focuses on the person's understanding of the nature of the particular action in question and its significance.

If the person is incompetent to make decisions regarding his or her health care, a guardian or representative can give or deny consent for the person. Many individuals appoint their representative through a living will or a DPAHC document and guardians are generally appointed through the court system. In selected states, there may also be a family doctrine that allows family members to make health care decisions for loved ones. For example, a debilitating terminal illness may render the patient incapable of making decisions and giving consent, and the physician will frequently ask the family about medical matters for the noncompetent patient. The order of selection using this doctrine is generally (1) spouse, (2) adult children or grandchildren, (3) parents, (4) grandparents or adult brothers and sisters, and (5) adult nieces and nephews.

Decision-Making Capacity

Although the law clearly prescribes that treatment decisions for competent patients, whether at the end of life or not, are to be made based on informed consent, health care providers also work with patients who lack this ability to either give or deny consent. Decision making for those patients who are incompetent is far from simple and begins with the goal that health care providers, family members, and surrogate decision makers are attempting to implement the patient's values and desires.

In the American legal system, patients are presumed to have **decision-making capacity** unless some factor exists to question this presumption. In other words, there must be a triggering factor that causes the health care provider to question the patient's capacity for decision making. An obvious factor could be that the patient is unconscious and thus cannot make any determination for himself or herself. Often, though, individuals who may lack decisional capacity are those with mental disabilities (mental retardation, periods of dementia, and mental illness), those patients whose decisional capacity is compromised by illness (renal or hepatic insufficiency or severe respiratory diseases), or those patients whose decisional capacity is limited due to treatment for existing illnesses and conditions (drug toxicity or medications that compromise mental acuity). The degree of inability to make decisions is highly variable and may be either temporary or permanent (Meisel & Cerminara, 2004).

Standards for determining decision-making capacity, while not entirely clear, are beginning to emerge. Decisional capacity is now seen as "decision specific," in that a person may be able to make certain types of decisions, but not other types of decisions. For example, the person who lacks capacity to make financial decisions may be fully capable of making health care decisions and know exactly what he or she desires in terminal states. Secondly, the ability to understand remains at the core of decision-making capacity. In order to obtain valid informed consent, the person must be able to appreciate the proposed treatment, potential complications, benefits and risks, as well as possible alternatives. Additionally, the person must appreciate this from a cognitive perspective and how it will relate to his or her situation and not just in general terms (Meisel & Cerminara, 2004).

When an individual is unable to make decisions for himself or herself, a surrogate decision maker is generally consulted. Box 3–4 lists the four types of surrogate decision makers.

Standards for these surrogate decision makers vary, though legal experts agree that the first objective should be to promote the desires that the patient would have expressed if he or she were capable of such expression (Guido, 2006). Where there still exists some disagreement is the degree of

---

BOX 3–4   Surrogate Decision Makers

- **Patient-designated** as occurs with valid natural death acts and durable power of attorney for health care provisions
- **Judicially designated** and appointed by a court of law as part of a hearing during which the person is determined to lack decision-making capacity
- **Clinically designated** as occurs when health care providers consult readily available family members when the patient lacks decision-making capacity
- **Statutorily designated** when legislative law exists recognizing the right of family consent and designating which family members are authorized to give or deny informed consent for a person lacking decision-making capacity

Source: Meisel & Cerminara, 2004

---

certainty with which the surrogate must know the patient's wishes. Three standards have emerged to assist health care providers in determining the patient's wishes: the substituted judgment standard, the best interest standard, and the futility standard.

The **substituted judgment standard** essentially allows the surrogate to determine what the patient would have wanted were he or she capable of making a determination. Essentially this is seen as a subjective test, because the decision maker is attempting to determine what another individual would have wanted had he or she been able to make these wishes known. The standard is implemented when the patient has not previously made his or her wishes known or where the individual was never capable of making his or her wishes known, as in the case of a mentally retarded person with a cognitive capacity of a 1- or 2-year old. The caveat is that the decision maker must make the determination using good faith and truly do what he or she determines the person would have wanted for himself or herself.

The **best interest standard** allows the decision maker to actually implement what the patient would have wanted if the patient were capable of making his or her wishes known. This standard is an objective test that relies on what the person indicated as his or her preference while he or she was competent and able to verbalize future care needs.

Some legal experts now acknowledge that there is also a **futility standard** and that there are instances where further treatment is futile. Using this standard, decisions must be made based on goals that have as their primary outcomes the patient's comfort and safety rather than a vain attempt to prolong the patient's ultimate death. This standard has evoked the most controversy and initiated ethics committee hearings to assist with determining when care becomes futile rather than assistive (Meisel & Cerminara, 2004). Additional information regarding ethics committees may be found in the preceding chapter.

SECTION FOUR REVIEW

1. In discussing obtaining consent for a procedure, which statement correctly identifies the main reason informed consent is necessary?
   1. "Health care deliverers want to ensure that they will not be sued if there is an adverse outcome."
   2. "Individuals have the right to say what will or will not happen to them."
   3. "Patients may have the right to sue the practitioner if informed consent is lacking."
   4. "The Patient Bill of Rights demands that patients are informed of their rights if the patient so requests."
2. Which represents the goal of decision-making for incompetent patients?
   1. Family members try to implement the patient's wishes.
   2. Health care professionals try to implement the patient and family's wishes.
   3. Health care professionals and surrogate decision makers try to implement the patient's wishes.
   4. Family members discuss the options and choose the best one for the patient.
3. Which standard is becoming clearer in deciding patients' decision-making capacity?
   1. Decisional capacity is "decision specific."
   2. Decisional capacity is determined by the substituted judgment standard.
   3. The best interest standard assists in making good faith decisions.
   4. The futility standard can be used when the primary outcome should be the comfort and safety of the patient.
4. Who can be surrogate decision makers for incompetent patients?
   1. Distant family members
   2. Court-appointed persons
   3. Those responsible for medical care
   4. A stranger
5. For valid informed consent to exist, which must the patient receive, in terms he or she can understand? (Select all that apply.)
   1. A brief explanation of the proposed therapy or procedure.
   2. The names and qualifications of those who will be performing the procedure or treatment.
   3. An explanation of all possible complications or risks involved in the therapy or procedure.
   4. The fact the patient may not refuse the therapy or procedure once it has been initiated.
   5. The patient can refuse the procedure or treatment and palliative care will continue to be delivered.

Case Study 1

Jason, a healthy 55-year-old oil executive, was playing in the yard with his two grandchildren when he was stung by a bee. He immediately experienced signs of respiratory distress. His children, rather than waiting for an ambulance to respond to a 911 emergency, immediately helped him into their car and drove him to the local hospital, which was about a 15 minute drive from his home. On admission, Jason was pulseless, apneic, and cyanotic. His daughter stated that she had tried to begin cardiopulmonary resuscitation en route to the hospital and that he had become unconscious about 10 minutes ago.

Jason was intubated, given several doses of epinephrine and steroids, and admitted to the intensive care unit (ICU). Jason has now been in the ICU for the past three days and his latest electroencephalographm (EEG) shows totally flat waves. He remains unable to breathe without the assistance of a ventilator and increasing amounts of pressor agents are needed to maintain his blood pressure. The physicians have consulted with his wife and two adult children and wish to begin to discontinue life care support.

QUESTIONS

What standard of decision-making capacity are the parents using when they allow life-sustaining support to be discontinued and comfort measures to be given Jason? Is there a surrogate decision maker for him, and who is that surrogate decision maker?

Suggested Response

The surrogate decision maker will depend on several factors. If Jason has a valid self-determination document, the person named in that document would have his power of attorney for health care decisions. If there is no such document, then look to statutory law to see if his wife could be considered the statutorily designated decision maker. If the state does not statutorily recognize Jason's wife as his decision maker, then she would most likely be consulted as his clinically designated decision maker.

The standard of decision making is equally vague, given the facts in this scenario. The health care team can determine whether Jason's wife is using the best interest standard or substituted judgment standard by gently querying her about his stated wishes and desires. If Jason had a self-determination document, it would be easier to determine his wishes, because those should be contained in the document. One could also support the futile care standard because the scenario leaves little doubt that medical care at this point in his life is primarily delaying his dying and not contributing to curative care.

SECTION FIVE: Assisted Suicide

Although suicide as a crime has been abolished in all states, most states still prohibit assisted suicide. Some states treat assisted suicide harshly, whereas other states prohibit only causing suicide, not assisting it. Though selected states have tried unsuccessfully through legislation to pass **physician-assisted suicide** (PAS) statutes, Oregon was the first to pass such a statute. A second state has now also voted to adopt such a statute. In November 2008, the citizens of Washington State passed Initiative 1000, which permits physician-assisted suicide in the state, effective March 2009. Proposals to consider assisted suicide were considered in California, Vermont, and Hawaii during the 2007 calendar year, though none of these proposals was formally placed on the 2008 November ballot. Opponents to this type of legislation include the Roman Catholic Church and the American Medical Association as well as the American Nurses Associations.

The Oregon Death with Dignity Act (DWDA) was first narrowly passed by voters in November 1994, with a 51.3% majority. A ballot measure to seek its repeal, Measure 51, was defeated by a 60% vote on November 4, 1997. The first patients to request life-ending medications did so in 1998. In 2002, United States Attorney General John Ashcroft attempted to suspend the license for prescribing drugs of physicians who prescribed life-ending medications under the DWDA. In October 2005, the United States Supreme Court heard arguments in the case of *Gonzales v. Oregon* and on January 17, 2006, that court ruled in favor of Oregon, again upholding the law. There have been no more legal challenges to the law since the Gonzales case.

Since its enactment, 341 patients have died under the terms of the law (Summary of Oregon's Death with Dignity Act, 2007). The most frequently cited reasons for obtaining physician-assisted suicide means were loss of autonomy, decreasing ability to participate in activities that made life enjoyable, and loss of dignity. Additionally, there was a significant increase in the numbers of patients indicating that fear of inadequate pain control prompted their desire for medications to terminate their lives (White, 2007).

The act allows physicians who choose to participate to write lethal drug prescriptions for competent, terminally ill adults who are residents of the state. Box 3–5 outlines the provisions that must be met before a prescription is written.

See Figure 3–2 for the form patients complete under this act.

The question of whether mentally competent, terminally ill patients have a constitutional right to seek a physician's aid in ending their lives had been addressed by the United States Supreme Court in 1997. Early in 1994, Compassion in Dying had initiated a legal challenge of Washington State's prohibition against assisted suicide. The Ninth Circuit Court in March, 1995 had held that the state's attempt to ban physician-assisted suicide violated the constitutional due process rights of terminally ill patients who sought to hasten their deaths by using physician-prescribed medications (*Compassion in Dying v. Washington*, 1995). At the core of the matter was whether states may distinguish between patients who choose to refuse or withdrahw medical treatment (allowing to die) and those who choose to extend this right to include medication-assisted suicide (assisting to die). Additionally, in mid-1994, Compassion in Dying had filed a legal challenge in New York State, also challenging a statute that prohibited physician-assisted suicide. The Second Court of Appeals concurred and struck down the law as it related to physicians and terminally ill persons (*Vacco v. Quill*, 1995). These two cases were then heard concurrently by the United States Supreme Court (*Washington v. Glucksberg*, 1997).

BOX 3–5   Provisions of the Oregon Death with Dignity Act

- Both the attending physician and a consulting physician must certify that the patient is in a terminal state, understands his or her prognosis and feasible alternatives, including, but not limited to, comfort care, hospice care, and pain control.
- The patient must make an oral and written request for the prescription, signed and dated by the patient and witnessed by at least two individuals who, in the presence of the patient, attest that to the best of their knowledge and belief the patient is capable, acting voluntarily, and is not being coerced to sign the request. Note that the witnesses may not be related in any manner to the patient nor may they be recipients under the patient's will. This must be followed by a second oral request 15 days or more after the first request.
- The attending physician must determine that the patient is making an informed and voluntary request, verify that the patient has documentation evidencing Oregon residency, can rescind the request at any time and in any manner, and must offer the patient an opportunity to rescind the request at the end of the 15 day waiting period.
- If in the opinion of either the attending or consulting physician a patient may be suffering from a psychiatric or psychological disorder or depression causing impaired judgment, either physician shall refer the patient for counseling and no medication to end the patient's life shall be prescribed until the counseling determines that the patient is not suffering from a psychiatric or psychological disorder or depression causing impaired judgment.

Source: Oregon State Statues, section 127.800 et seq, 2005

Request for Medication to End My Life in a Humane and Dignified Manner

I, _____, am an adult of sound mind.

I am suffering from _____, which my attending physician has determined is a terminal disease and which has been medically confirmed by a consulting physician.

I have been fully informed of my diagnosis, prognosis, the nature of medication to be prescribed and potential associated risks, the expected result, and the feasible alternatives, including comfort care, hospice care and pain control.

I request that my attending physician prescribe medication that will end my life in a humane and dignified manner.

INITIAL ONE:

_____ I have informed my family of my decision and taken their opinions into consideration.

_____ I have decided not to inform my family of my decision.

_____ I have no family to inform of my decision.

I understand that I have the right to rescind this request at any time.

I understand the full import of this request and I expect to die when I take the medication to be prescribed. I further understand that although most deaths occur within three hours, my death may take longer and my physician has counseled me about this possibility.

I make this request voluntarily and without reservation, and I accept full moral responsibility for my actions.

Signed: _____

Dated: _____

DECLARATION OF WITNESSES

We declare that the person signing this request:

(a) Is personally known to us or has provided proof of identity;
(b) Signed this request in our presence;
(c) Appears to be of sound mind and not under duress, fraud or undue influence;
(d) Is not a patient for whom either of us is attending physician.

_____Witness 1/Date

_____Witness 2/Date

NOTE: One witness shall not be a relative (by blood, marriage or adoption) of the person signing this request, shall not be entitled to any portion of the person's estate upon death and shall not own, operate or be employed at a health care facility where the person is a patient or resident. If the patient is an inpatient at a health care facility, one of the witnesses shall be an individual designated by the facility.

Figure 3–2 ■ Request for Medication to End My Life in a Humane and Dignified Manner. *Oregon Legislative Statutes, 1995 c.3 §6.01; 1999 c.423 §11*

The Supreme Court, in one of the most important decisions of the 1990s, rejected the challenge to the constitutional right of the person to die, and, in essence, said that courts could ban physician-assisted suicides (*Compassion in Dying v. Glucksberg*, 1997, and *Vacco v. Quill*, 1997). Although finding no constitutional right to die, the court explicitly left open the door for states to legalize and regulate physician-assisted suicide, if the state chose to do so. This decision by the Supreme Court came just months before the Oregon voters passed the Death with Dignity Act for the second time. A Model State Act to

Authorize and Regulate Physician-Assisted Suicide was developed to prevent potential managed care abuses with physician-assisted suicide. The model act requires that four conditions be met before one can receive assistance. Box 3–6 displays these requirements, all having the effect of limiting managed care abuses.

Despite the controversy surrounding this legislation, Oregon's experience with assisted suicide has raised awareness of end-of-life care. Oregon has the largest percentage of in-home hospice deaths, and the majority of individuals who die in Oregon have a written directive or other end-of-life planning in place (Skidmore, 2007).

The nurse's role in this area is still developing. The American Nurses Association (ANA) opposes the movement and opposes nurses' participation either in assisted suicide or active euthanasia because they violate the ethical traditions embodied in the *Code of Ethics* (ANA, 2001). If nurses are asked directly by patients to assist with their suicide, the nurse must refuse. But, before closing the door to open communications, look beyond the request to what the patients may be saying. They may be expressing a need for greater pain control or for someone to talk to about the fears of death (Guido, 2006). At this time, nurses must be clear that they cannot assist patients in this aspect, but may be able to assist with procuring medications for more effective pain control or by supplying needed forms to assist patients with advanced directives and POLSTs. Another avenue may be to ensure that patients speak with a chaplain or representative of their faith or with a social worker. Ensure that the patients know that someone cares and assist them in ways that nursing can intervene.

In recognition of the universal need for humane end-of-life care, the American Association of Colleges of Nursing, supported by a Robert Wood Johnson Foundation grant, convened a roundtable of nurse experts and other health care providers to begin communications surrounding this area. This roundtable was in accord with the 1997 International Council of Nurses mandate that nurses have a unique and primary responsibility for ensuring that individuals at the end of life experience a peaceful death. This group of experts in health care ethics and palliative care developed the End-of-Life Competency Statements. While developed as terminal objectives for undergraduate nursing students, they apply to all nursing professionals. These competencies are enumerated in Box 3–7.

BOX 3–7 End-of-Life Competencies

1. Recognize dynamic changes in population demographics, health care economics, and service delivery that necessitate improved professional preparation for end-of-life care.
2. Promote the provision of comfort care to the dying as an active, desirable, and important skill, and an integral component of nursing care.
3. Communicate effectively and compassionately with the patient, family, and health care team members about end-of-life issues.
4. Recognize one's own attitudes, feelings, values, and expectations about death and the individual, cultural, and spiritual diversity existing in these beliefs and customs.
5. Demonstrate respect for the patient's views and wishes during end-of-life care.
6. Collaborate with interdisciplinary team members while implementing the nursing role in end-of-life care.
7. Use scientifically based standardized tools to assess symptoms (such as pain, dyspnea, constipation, anxiety, fatigue, nausea/vomiting, and altered cognition) experienced by patients at the end of life.
8. Use data from symptom assessment to plan and intervene in symptom management using state-of-the-art tradition and complementary approaches.
9. Evaluate the impact of traditional, complementary, and technological therapies on patient-centered outcomes.
10. Assess and treat multiple dimensions, including physical, psychological, social, and spiritual needs, to improve quality at the end of life.
11. Assist the patient, family, colleagues, and oneself to cope with suffering, grief, loss, and bereavement in end-of-life care.
12. Apply legal and ethical principles in the analysis of complex issues in end-of-life care, recognizing the influence of personal values, professional codes, and patient preferences.
13. Identify barriers and facilitators to patients' and caregivers' effective use of resources.
14. Demonstrate skill at implementing a plan for improved end-of-life care within a dynamic and complex health care delivery system.
15. Apply knowledge gained from palliative care research to end-of-life education and care (American Association of Colleges of Nursing, 1999).*

BOX 3–6 Requirements for Limiting Managed Care Abuses

1. The patient must be competent, defined as "based on the patient's ability to understand his or her condition and prognosis, the benefits and burdens of alternative therapy, and the consequences of suicide."
2. The patient must be fully informed.
3. The choice must be voluntary, one that is made independently, free from coercion or undue influences.
4. The choice must be enduring, in that the request must be stated to the responsible physician on at least two occasions that are at least two weeks apart, without self-contradiction during that interval.

Source: Baron et al., 1996, p. 20

*From American Association of Colleges of Nursing, *Peaceful Death: Recommended Competencies and Curricular Guidelines for End-of-Life Nursing Care* (1999). Washington, DC. Used with permission.

SECTION FIVE REVIEW

1. Why is the American Nurses Association against assisted suicide?
   1. Nurses should not be forced to perform actions, such as discontinuing ventilators, that physicians do not wish to perform.
   2. Patients do not have the right to say when their lives will end.
   3. Allowing assisted suicide violates the ethical principles of the ANA *Code of Ethics*.
   4. State law prevents the intentional taking of one's life.
2. In 1999, the American Association of Colleges of Nursing enacted competencies that:
   1. Enhanced peaceful death principles.
   2. Enumerated why assisted suicide was not to be practiced by professional nurses.
   3. Expounded on the need for curative rather than palliative health care measures for patients at the end of life.
   4. Embraced the idea that families must be involved in terminal patients' care.
3. What does Oregon's Death with Dignity Act require?
   1. The attending physician must verify that the patient is within six months of death.
   2. Both an attending and consulting physician must ensure that the patient has been interviewed by a psychologist or psychiatrist before prescribing medications that will end the patient's life.

3. The patient must be fully aware that he or she can rescind the request at any time and in any manner.
4. The patient lived in Oregon at some time in his or her life, but not at the present time.

4. A patient who asks a physician to assist in committing suicide makes the statement, "I am tired of people running my miserable excuse for a life." This situation is an example of which ethical principle? (Select all that apply.)
   1. Autonomy
   2. Nonmaleficence
   3. Paternalism
   4. Fidelity
   5. Veracity
   6. Beneficence
5. Why is there a concern about managed care companies abusing physician-assisted suicide if made legal?
   1. More people will request assisted suicide if it is made legal, thus increasing managed care costs.
   2. Managed care companies will stop paying for hospice and palliative care.
   3. Physicians will refuse to assist patients to commit suicide.
   4. More patients will be asked to consider suicide as a cost-saving measure.

CHAPTER SUMMARY

- Legal issues related to the patient at the end of life concern a person's right to make decisions and determine what the individual will or will not accept regarding health care interventions.
- Court cases beginning in the mid-1970s through the Schiavo cases in the mid-2000s have demonstrated that end-of-life decision making for patients unable to give or deny consent continues to be controversial.
- The Patient Self-Determination Act was passed in 1990 as a means of allowing persons the ability to ensure that their desires and preferences for end-of-life care survive their competency capabilities.
- There are three types of advance directives:
  - Living wills
  - Natural death acts (statutory living wills)
  - Durable power of attorney for health care
- Alternatives to advance directives include:
  - Respecting Choices
  - Physician Orders for Life-Sustaining Treatment

- Communications between health care providers, patients, and family members are essential for advance directives and alternatives to advance directives to be effective.
- Informed consent is the voluntary authorization by a patient or the patient's representative to do something to or for the person.
- Decision-making capacity is generally seen as decision specific and reflects the position that a person may be competent to make some decisions but not other decisions, such as lacking financial decision-making capacity but retaining capacity to determine end-of-life care desires.
- Assisted suicide is now legal in Oregon and Washington State.
- The American Association of Colleges of Nursing, in conjunction with the Robert Wood Johnson Foundation, convened a panel of experts to write standards of competencies for end-of-life care.

CHAPTER REVIEW

Mrs. Duran, a 34-year-old mother of two teen-age sons, was admitted to the hospital for a liver transplant. She is married, lists her occupation as a home-maker, and is a devout Jehovah's Witness. She traveled from her home to a major medical center that performed liver transplants on Jehovah's Witness patients without using blood transfusions. She was placed on the waiting list and she and her husband temporarily relocated to await the transplant.

For the procedure, the patient signed a durable power of attorney for health care, naming as her surrogate a long-time family friend. The reason she signed the durable power of attorney for health care was that she did not want a blood transfusion and was afraid that one might be given over her express objection. Indeed, she several times expressed to the hospital physicians and nurses that she would not accept blood transfusions, regardless of how critical her condition might become.

The surgery was performed and Mrs. Duran rejected the newly trans-planted organ shortly afterward. Her husband, not wanting his wife to die, went to court to override the durable power of attorney for health care and allow blood transfusions to be given. Before the court could rule, Mrs. Duran died, and the court allowed this action to go forward as the question was not moot, but needed as a guide for future patients who might find themselves in such circumstances.

Questions

How do you think the court decided this case? Should Mrs. Duran have had the opportunity to die without the blood transfusions?

Suggested Response

The case example is taken in part from *In re Duran*, 769 A. 2d 497 (Pa. Super., 2001). The court in that case was adamant that there must be a clear-cut expression of the patient's intent; what exactly does the patient want to be done in the event he or she cannot voice that desire for health care providers? In this case, the court held that this patient could not have made her wishes more clear. The durable power of attorney form was not a standard form, but was drafted especially for her. The document stated that she was a Jehovah's Witness, she did not want even her own stored blood auto-transfused and it did not matter to her what her doctors, nurses, family, or friends thought best for her. The court concluded that under no circumstances was blood to be transfused to this patient.

REFERENCES

American Association of Colleges of Nursing. (1999). *Peaceful death: Recommended competencies and curricular guidelines for end-of-life nursing care.* Washington, DC: Author.

American Nurses Association. (2001). *Code of ethics with interpretive statements.* Washington, DC: Author.

Baron, C. H., et al. (1996). A model state act to authorize and regulate physician-assisted suicide. *Harvard Journal on Legislation, 33*, 1–34.

Compassion in Dying v. Glucksberg, 117 S. Ct. 2258 (1997).

Compassion in Dying v. Washington, 49 F. 3d. 586 (1995). 850 F. Supp. 1454 (W. D. Washington, 1994), affirmed 79 F. 3d 790 (9th Cir, 1996), reviewed under the name *Washington v. Glucksberg*, 521 U. S. 702 (1997).

Cruzan v. Director, Missouri Department of Health, 497 U.S. 261, 110 S. Ct. 2841, 111 L.E.D. 2d 224 (1990).

Gonzales v. Oregon, 546 U.S. 243 (2006).

Guido, G. W. (2006). *Legal and ethical issues in nursing* (4th ed.). Upper Saddle River, NJ: Pearson Prentice Hall.

Hammes, B. J., & Rooney, B. L. (1998). Death and end-of-life planning in one midwestern community. *Archives of Internal Medicine, 158*, 383–390.

Harkness, M. & Wanklyn, P. (2006). Cardiopulmonary resuscitation: Capacity, discussion, and documentation. *QJM: An International Journal of Medicine, 99*(10), 683–690.

Hickman, S. E., Hammes, B, J., Moss, A. H., & Tolle, S. W. (2005). Hope for the future: Achieving the original intent of advance directives. *Improving End of Life Care: Why Has It Been So Difficult? Hastings Center Report Special Report 35*(6), S26–S30.

In re Quinlan, 70 N.J. 10, 335 A.2d 647 (1976).

John F. Kennedy Memorial Hospital v. Heston, 58 N.J. 576 (1971).

Lynch, H. F., Mathes, M., & Sawicki, N. N. (2008). Compliance with advance directives: Wrongful living and tort law incentives. *Journal of Legal Medicine, 29*(2), 133–178.

Meisel, A. (2005). The role of litigation in end of life care: A reappraisal. *Improving End of Life Care: Why Has It Been So Difficult? Hastings Report Special Report, 35*(6), S47–S51.

Meisel, A., & Cerminara, K. L. (2004). *The right to die; The law of end-of-life decision-making.* New York: Aspen Press.

Oregon Legislative Statutes, c. 3, sec. 6.01; 1999 c. 423, sec. 11 (1995).

Oregon State Statutes, Death with Dignity Act. Section 127.800 et seq (2005).

Patient Self-Determination Act, Sections 4206 and 4751 of the Omnibus Reconciliation Act of 1990, Public Law 101-508, November 1990.

Physician Orders for Life-Sustaining Treatment State Programs. (2008). Retrieved from http://www.ohsu.edu/ethics/polst/programs/state+programs.htm

Skidmore, S. (2007, October 27). A decade later, Oregon still only assisted suicide state. *The Columbian, 116*(179), A3.

Summary of Oregon's Death with Dignity Act. (2007). Retrieved from http://www.oregon.gov/DHS/ph/pas/docs/year10.pdf

Tulsky, J. A. (2005). Beyond advance directives: The importance of communication skills at the end of life. *Journal of the American Medical Association, 293*(3), 359–365.

Vacco v. Quill, 117 S. Ct. 2293 (1997).

Washington State Legislature, c. 98, sec. 3; 1979 c. 112, sec. 4 (1992).

Washington v. Glucksberg, 521 U.S. 702 (1997).

White, H. (2007). Eighth annual Oregon assisted suicide report shorter with more ambiguous language. Retrieved from http://www.lifesite.net/ldn/printerfriendly.html

Pain at the End of Life

OBJECTIVES   Following completion of this chapter, the learner will be able to:

4.1. Review pain assessment needs for terminally ill individuals.

4.2. Explore how beliefs and practices of diverse populations influence pain management for those patients nearing the end of life.

4.3. Recognize the barriers to pain assessment and interventions that can impair quality end-of-life care.

4.4. Examine the pain scales appropriate for this population.

4.5. Describe holistic pain-management issues for patients at the end of life.

4.6. Identify therapeutic pharmacological and nonpharmacological interventions for pain management in life-limiting conditions.

This chapter explores pain management from the patient's perspective in terminal and life-limiting care states. The importance of a comprehensive pain evaluation is critical to effective pain management for this population of patients. Pain assessment across the age span, including implications for diverse populations, is presented as are unique considerations for aging and cognitively impaired individuals facing death.

The aspects of spiritual, social, and psychological well-being as they influence the management of pain in terminally ill patients are described. Realistic pain-management goals, pharmacological interventions, and complementary and alternative therapies are presented. The chapter concludes with the importance of not undertreating patients who are in pain during their last stages of life.

PRETEST

1. When a patient is dying, pain:
   1. Is easily assessed.
   2. Can be easily treated.
   3. Requires comprehensive assessment and interventions.
   4. Is not synonymous with acute pain.
2. Vital signs in chronic or end-of-life pain:
   1. Match the patient's intensity of pain.
   2. Change and vary in each individual.
   3. Are measurable as the 5th vital sign.
   4. Determine what medications to administer.
3. Pain at the end of life includes aspects of: (Select all that apply.)
   1. Spiritual and psychological care.
   2. Environmental conditions.
   3. Financial needs if they arise.
   4. Family's perception and barriers to pain.

4. Pain at the end of life may be experienced during the last hours, days, weeks, or months of one's life. It usually increases due to:
   1. Cancer or the underlying disease.
   2. Inability to swallow.
   3. Implementing the bowel program.
   4. Family's presence.
5. There are several barriers to pain control, which create further difficulty in management at the end of life. These barriers include:
   1. Location, profession, skill.
   2. Treatment modalities, pain scale usage, adjuvant medications.
   3. Finances, age, culture.
   4. Sibling position within the family.

GLOSSARY

acute pain   Pain that has a sudden onset but usually declines in time (e.g., minutes, hours, days). It occurs following an injury to the body and generally disappears when the injury heals. It is often associated with objective physical signs of autonomic nervous system activity such as tachycardia, hypertension, diaphoresis, and pallor (American Pain Society, 2000).

addiction   (see psychological dependence)

adjuvant analgesic medication   A medication in a different class that has been shown to have analgesic properties but is not a primary analgesic (e.g., antidepressant, anticonvulsant).

anxiolytic   Medication used to reduce anxiety, agitation, or tension.

biofeedback   A process in which a person learns to influence physiologic responses for body systems not ordinarily under voluntary control that may be easily regulated or those whose regulation has broken down because of trauma or disease.

breakthrough pain   Intermittent exacerbations of pain that can occur spontaneously or in relation to activity; pain that increases above the usual level of pain being managed with ongoing analgesics; includes incident pain and end-of-dose failure.

chronic (or persistent) pain   Pain that can range from mild to severe, and persists or progresses over a long period of time.

combination therapy   Method of treating disease through the simultaneous use of a variety of medications to eliminate or control the biochemical cause of the disease.

complementary and alternative medicine (CAM)   A group of diverse medical and health care systems, practices, and products that are not presently considered to be part of conventional medicine or care.

double effect   Providing palliative medications with the intent to relieve pain that might inadvertently hasten death versus providing medication to intentionally cause death.

equianalgesic   Having equal analgesic effect using an appropriate strength of a different medication.

incident pain   A type of breakthrough pain that is related to a specific activity, such as eating, defecating, or walking; also referred to as movement-related pain.

interdisciplinary team   A team of health care professionals and services from relevant clinical disciplines, ideally including the patient and family, whose interactions are guided by specific team functions and processes to achieve team-defined favorable patient outcomes.

life-limiting conditions   Those conditions or illnesses that reduce survival time for patients and shorten chance of recovery.

medication diversion   A transfer of a controlled substance from a lawful to an unlawful channel of distribution or use.

narcotic   An addictive drug, such as opium, that reduces pain, alters mood and behavior, and usually induces sleep or stupor, from the Greek word "narke" for numbness or torpor. Includes prescribed medications as well as drugs such as heroin, phencyclidine (PCP), amphetamines, cocaine, marijuana, Ecstasy, and methamphetamine.

neuropathic pain   Pain that results from a disturbance of function or pathologic change in a nerve; in one nerve, mononeuropathy; in several nerves, mononeuropathy multiplex; if diffuse and bilateral, polyneuropathy.

neuropathy   A disease or abnormality of the nervous system, especially one affecting the cranial or spinal nerves, that produces pain, loss of sensation, and inability to control muscles; examples include phantom pain, diabetic neuropathy, and sympathetic dystrophy.

nociception   The process of pain transmission, usually relating to a receptive neuron for painful sensations.

nonsteroidal anti-inflammatory drug (NSAID)   One of a class of drugs/medication used to reduce inflammation and/or provide pain relief.

nurse-controlled analgesia (NCA)   Analgesics administered by the nurse/clinician via an intravenous, subcutaneous, epidural opioid (e.g., morphine) administration by means of a programmable pump; generally done when the patient is unable to self-administer patient-controlled analgesia (PCA).

opioid   A morphine-like medication that produces pain relief; refers to natural, semisynthetic, and synthetic medications that relieve pain by binding to opioid receptors in the nervous system; *opioid* is preferred to the term *narcotic* or *opiate* because it includes all agonists and antagonists with morphine-like activity, as well as naturally occurring and synthetic opioid peptides.

opioid naïve   Person who has not previously taken an opioid and is using an opioid for the first time.

pain   A symptom of some physical hurt or disorder, emotional distress; a fundamental feeling that people try to avoid or a somatic sensation of acute or chronic discomfort that causes bodily suffering or indisposition.

patient-controlled analgesia (PCA)   Analgesics self-administered by a patient; usually refers to self-dosing with an intravenous, subcutaneous, epidural opioid administered by means of a programmable pump.

persistent (chronic) pain   Constant pain that lasts beyond a three-month time frame.

preemptive analgesia   Preventing pain before it begins or is expected (e.g., lidocaine prior to IV insertion).

psychological dependence (addiction)   A primary, chronic, neurobiological disease characterized by behaviors that include one or more of the following: impaired control over drug use, compulsive use, continued use despite harm, and drug craving (American Pain Society, 2000).

rescue dose   A bolus or extra dose of medication given as needed to relieve pain that occurs despite a regimen of medication given at regularly scheduled intervals.

stoicism   To be free from passion, unmoved by joy or grief, and submissive to natural law, apparently or professedly indifferent to pleasure or pain.

terminal illness Disease or condition that cannot be cured or adequately treated and that is reasonably expected to result in the death of the patient within a six-month time frame or less.

titration The incremental adjustment of a medication in subsequent doses until a desired effect is achieved. Usually intended to reach the patient's level of satisfaction, making the pain as tolerable as possible while minimizing short- and long-term negative effects.

tolerance The state of adaptation in which exposure to a drug induces changes that result in a decrease in one or more of the drug's effects over time.

visceral pain Pain that originates from organs or smooth muscles. thorax, abdomen, or pelvis; characterized by deep, vague, difficult to locate pain that radiates away from the affected organ.

SECTION ONE: Pain Assessment

Importance of Pain Assessment for the Patient Facing the End of Life

Pain at the end of life may be experienced during the last hours, days, weeks, or months or years of one's life. Pain is frequently amplified by anxiety and relationship aspects with the fear of the unknown and the apprehension of losing control. Although physical pain is a priority, it may not be the primary issue for individuals at end of life. Pain is often multifactorial, and can be acute, chronic, or a combination of both. Emotional, spiritual, and psychosocial features of pain are often increased, with the thoughts of facing the loss of life and losing one's loved one becoming a reality. These emotional reactions serve to increase the underlying physical pain. Additional efforts are needed to alleviate the pain and suffering that may accompany end-of-life symptoms. The multidisciplinary team approach becomes more important and enhanced palliative care or comfort care becomes crucial as curative care is no longer effective.

Because pain management and comfort measures become the primary foci of care at the end of life, the American Nurses Association (2003) developed a position statement titled Pain Management and Control of Distressing Symptoms in Dying Patients to emphasize the importance of these two foci:

When the restoration of health is no longer possible, the focus of nursing care is assuring a comfortable, dignified death and the highest possible quality of remaining life. One of the major concerns of dying patients and their families is the fear of intractable pain during the dying process. Overwhelming pain and other distressing symptoms are related to sleeplessness, loss of morale, fatigue, irritability, restlessness, withdrawal and other serious problems for the dying patient. Nurses are essential to the assessment and management of pain and other distressing symptoms as they generally have the most frequent and continuous patient contact. . . . Pain and symptom management must be respected and supported. (paragraph 3)

To implement this nursing mandate, professional nurses must develop the skills necessary to identify and manage pain, understand the myths about pain and pain medications that will help facilitate quality pain management, and appreciate the impact of poor pain control. A thorough understanding of pain and the means of controlling pain in the **terminally ill** person is essential for quality care of this individual.

Defining and Identifying Pain

Pain, which cannot be seen or felt by another person, is a personal subjective experience and there no objective tests to measure its intensity or quality (American Pain Society, 2003). Pain can be measured and described only by the person experiencing it. As Margo McCaffery (1968) so aptly stated, pain is "whatever the experiencing person says it is, and exists whenever he says it does" (p. 3). An earlier definition of pain by the International Association for the Study of Pain (1979) described pain as "an unpleasant sensory and emotional experience associated with actual or potential tissue damage" (p. 249). Pain may or may not include physical changes and may be more intense in one patient with the same physical circumstances than another. Pain tends to be more common as a person ages because of the increase in morbidities, whether acute or chronic (American Geriatric Society, 2002). For instance, a child who has no health issues will more likely experience less pain than an adult who suffers from chronic health conditions. Pain is not a reliable indicator of failing health or advancing disease, and individuals are urged to seek medical attention for any new or worsening pain (Leleszi & Lewandowski, 2005).

Pain is not always associated with a detectable injury or disease in patients at the end of life. Many patients believe that pain must be associated with a specific abnormality and that the pain can be alleviated. **Visceral pain**, however, is characterized by deep, vague, difficult-to-locate pain that radiates away from the affected organ. Unfortunately, chronic pain may occur with no evidence of disease or damage to body tissues and the pain is not easily alleviated.

The effectiveness of pain relief measures relies on effective communication and identification of the pain. Patients and families may be reluctant to discuss the level of pain for a variety of reasons. Some patients may fear that the increasing level and duration of pain indicates that the underlying disease processes are also increasing. Some patients may feel that if they report their pain at a higher level, they will be overmedicated and unable to interact with family members. Other patients may truly be unable to fully perceive the intensity of the pain and fear that if they report a higher pain level early in the disease process, the level of pain will intensify and later pain medications will not be effective. Finally, there are individuals who fear that if they do not report a high level of pain they will not receive adequate pain medications. It may be helpful to begin the pain assessment by reminding patients why it is important that the level of pain be accurately assessed.

To assess pain in the patient capable of verbalizing his or her pain level, pain as the 5th vital sign is recognized using a scale from 0 to 10, with zero being the absence of pain, to 10 being the worst pain possible. Such a scale includes some aspects of quality, but is usually translated into a number or rating for severity and ease of comparing pain levels over time (Pasero & McCaffery, 2005). Other commonly used pain intensity scales are the Wong-Baker scale, which uses faces, words, and numbers, and the Pritchett and Hull scale that has faces for each of the numbers 1–10. The Pritchett and Hull scale is reproduced in Figure 4–1. This latter scale is especially helpful for use with patients who are terminally ill.

Though these scales are most useful in validating a person's pain at various time intervals and newer scales are currently being developed, alternative means of assessing pain in a person can be as simple as a yes or no when asked if pain is present. Equally effective may be asking if the pain is mild, moderate, or severe. Words that form characteristics, such as some, annoying, distracting, or cannot be ignored create further quality to a patient's pain.

Along with this verbal proclamation of pain intensity, observe the person for changes in facial expressions, diminished physical movements, or in nonverbal vocal expressions. Facial expressions include: frowning, grimacing, tearfulness, apprehension, sadness, and/or muscle contractions around the mouth or eyes. Vocalizations include: groaning, moaning, crying, and more labored respirations. Language changes may include: repetitive calling out (such as "help me! help me!"), swearing, excessive laughing, crying, or remaining quieter than is usual for the patient.

Individuals who cannot verbalize their level of pain present a challenge to the assessor of pain. Pain should also be identified in the cognitively impaired by assessing manifestations of physical signs of pain. These include changes in facial expressions such as frowning, grimacing, tearfulness, apprehension, sadness, and/or muscle contractions around the mouth or eyes. It is also helpful to question family members and close personal friends about how the person generally reacts to pain and painful stimuli.

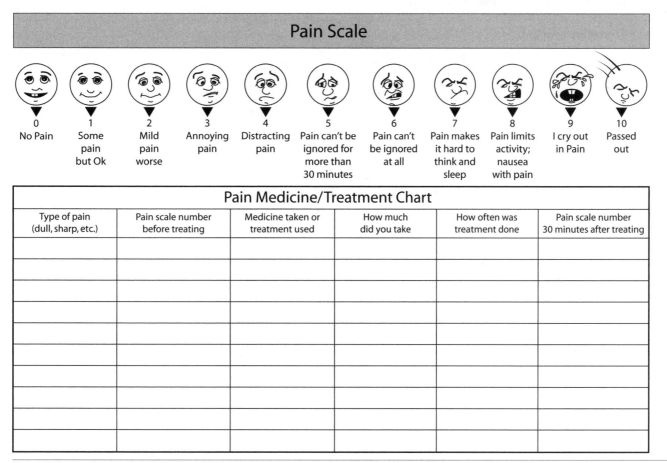

Figure 4–1 ■ Pain Scale. Copyright © 2000, Pritchett & Hull Associates, Inc. Reprinted with permission.

For the nonverbal patient, it is important to use tools and guidelines such as Assume Pain Present (Herr et al., 2006) or other nonverbal pain scales to facilitate objective rating of pain. To overcome difficulties with verbal communication, several observational instruments have been developed to facilitate the detection of pain among cognitively impaired or nonverbal patients. A pain assessment instrument for use in daily practice should be simple and easy to use. A common understanding of the patients' verbal and nonverbal expressions is a prerequisite for proper pain assessment of those patients who are not able to respond verbally (Feldt, 2000; Warden, Hurley, & Volicer, 2003). An example of a nonverbal pain scale is the Checklist of Nonverbal Pain Indicators (CNPI), developed by Feldt (2000) as part of her doctoral dissertation. This tool is reproduced in Box 4–1.

Ongoing studies are in progress to continually develop scales for the cognitively impaired (Herr et al., 2006).

During the patient assessment, consider any comorbidities that the patient may have and his or her past history of illness. Has this type of pain been experienced before? Does it hurt more or less than during previous times? What treatment has been effective and what has not? What was the onset and course of pain at this time? What interventions have been tried? Which ones were useful? One mechanism to assist in the identification of pain for the cognitively able person who has been ill for a period of time is the completion of a pain journal that reflects pain intensity and interventions that have been effective in the past.

Spiritual, Emotional, and Psychological Aspects of Pain

Dame Cicely Saunders (1976), founder of modern hospice care, conceptualized pain associated with the dying process as "total pain," which is the sum of four components: physical pain, spiritual pain (anxiety that may include difficulty facing one's own dying process and death), emotional discomfort (inner pain, suffering), and psychological pain (conflict within one's cognitive self and/or others). Her spiritual, emotional, and psychological aspects of pain are described in the following paragraphs.

Spiritual pain is defined as complex. Spiritual pain can be difficult to assess. Every patient has some degree of spiritual needs, which may be independent of religious orientation or doctrine. The experience of life and suffering's senselessness, personal loss of value, along with situational hopelessness lowers a patient's pain tolerance significantly. Pain is often easier to cope with in the presence of a caring person, which is the role of the nurse as the

---

BOX 4–1   Checklist for Nonverbal Pain Indicators (CNPI)

Checklist of Nonverbal Pain Indicators

Date: _____   Patient Name: _____

(Write a 0 if the behavior was not observed, and a 1 if the behavior occurred even briefly during activity or rest.)

	With Movement	Rest
1. Vocal Complaints: Nonverbal (Expression of pain, not in words, moans, groans, grunts, cries, gasps, sighs)	_____	_____
2. Facial Grimaces/Winces (Furrowed brow, narrowed eyes, tightened lips, dropped jaw, clenched teeth, distorted expressions)	_____	_____
3. Bracing (Clutching or holding onto siderails, bed, tray table, or affected area during movement)	_____	_____
4. Restlessness (Constant or intermittent shifting of position, rocking, intermittent or constant hand motions, inability to keep still)	_____	_____
5. Rubbing: (Massaging affected area) (In addition, record verbal complaints)	_____	_____
6. Vocal Complaints: (Words expressing discomfort of pain—"ouch," "that hurts," cursing during movement, or exclamations of protest— "stop," "that's enough")	_____	_____
Subtotal Scores	_____	_____
Total Scores	_____	_____

Sources: Feldt, K. S., Treatment of pain in cognitively impaired versus cognitively intact post hip fractured elders (Doctoral diss.) Minneapolis: University of Minnesota, 1996. Dissertation Abstracts International 57, 09B: 5574; Feldt, K. S., Checklist of Nonverbal Pain Indicators. Pain Management Nursing 2000;1 (1): 13–21. Used with permission.

primary caregiver. To be able to verbalize the extent of pain and to describe one's own fears, especially in connection with the significance of the actual pain, is very therapeutic. The support of the wider community, including chaplains, pastors, and parish nurses is also helpful. Pain needs to be approached holistically, by observing the patient, asking of his/her burden of suffering, as well as identifying his/her hopes and wishes. It is important not to abandon the patient or have him/her feel left alone or feeling abandoned (Jusić, 2001). Therefore, the importance of spirituality in pain management should not be underestimated.

Newshan (1998) described three spiritual domains: meaning, hope, and love/relatedness. The significance of nurses being closer to their own individual spirituality enhances their ability to care for the patient in pain. Interventions include therapeutic presence, attentive listening, acceptance, and careful self-disclosure (without redirecting the attention from the patient) to promote comfort and diminish pain.

Because all pain has a psychological component, this aspect of pain also affects patients at the end of their lives. And, just as pain affects appetite, sleep, mood, social activities, and sense of well-being, conversely these factors affect pain (Lynn & Harrold, 2006). The presence of physical pain can lead to or intensify clinical depression and anxiety, which in turn can lead to unsatisfactory pain control or relief. Therefore, alleviating all aspects of pain is important in providing quality end-of-life care. Strategies for patients experiencing psychological pain include relaxation techniques, positive imagery, and cognitive behavioral therapy, which may be helpful in reducing physical pain directly or in reducing anxiety that aggravates it (Keefe, Abernethy, & Campbell, 2004). Additionally, interventions that assist to decrease psychological pain include discussing advanced care planning, assessing suffering, and reassuring the person that the needs of the family during the dying process and after the person's death will be addressed (Norlander, 2001).

Dame Cicely Saunders (1970) addressed suffering in her concept of "total pain" as its fourth aspect. Suffering is an extremely personal experience that is directly related to the meaning of pain at the end of life. Suffering is often viewed as the spiritual, emotional, and psychological side of physical pain. A patient's emotional reactions, especially the fear and anxiety produced, increase all aspects of pain.

Nurses should not assume the presence or absence of suffering in patients, especially at the end of their lives. Patients can suffer without physical pain, and physical pain does not necessarily involve aspects of suffering. Common sources of suffering include fear of, or actual, physical pain, the fear of death and dying, changing self-perceptions, relationship concerns, the need to find meaning in any given life experience, and past experiences of witnessing another person's distress (Panke, 2003).

Barriers to Quality Pain Management

Inadequately controlled pain often stems from inability or unwillingness of health care professionals to use knowledge and evidence-based practice in assessing and managing pain. The knowledge and attitudes of health care professionals, as well as patients and families, factor in on the priority placed on pain management. Patients at the end of life should not be allowed to suffer with pain because of barriers to adequate pain management that may be present. Box 4–2 represents a list of these barriers that may be related to patients at the end of life.

BOX 4–2   Barriers to Pain Management

Health Care Professional Barriers to Pain Management

- Lack of training and education in school regarding pain assessment and treatment
- Inadequate knowledge of pain management
- Perceived lack of time to assess and treat pain
- Inability to empathize or establish rapport
- Prejudices and biases about the patient or pain
- Inadequate assessment of pain
- Failure to use validated pain scales
- Rigidity or timidity in interventions
- Concern about side effects of analgesics
- Fear of patient becoming tolerant to analgesic
- Fear that the opioid may hasten death
- Assumption that pain in patients at the end of life may not be relieved

Patient Barriers to Pain Management

- Reluctance to report pain—words, perceptions, subjective, personal nature of the pain experience
- Lack of awareness about the importance of pain assessment and management
- Not wanting to "bother" staff
- Not feeling "believed"
- **Stoicism**—believing that suffering is strength/inevitable, pain is weakness
- Reluctance to take opioids "narcotics"
- Concern that reporting pain may distract physicians from treatment of underlying disease and treating the disease
- Believing "nothing helps"
- Lack of common language/words to describe pain
- Saving medicine in case the pain gets worse
- Fatalism that pain is part of dying

Patient/Family Fears

- Pain means disease is worse
- Addiction or being thought of as an addict
- Costs of medication and treatments
- Unmanageable side effects
- Being labeled a "bad" patient
- Dying in pain

Source: Adapted from Ersek, 1999; McCaffery & Pasero, 1999; Paice & Fine, 2001; Springhouse, 2006.

Comprehensive Pain Assessment

A comprehensive assessment includes the location and type of pain, history, intensity, characteristics, causes, and current treatment interventions. As suggested earlier, the other aspects of pain beyond intensity need to be included to complete a comprehensive pain assessment in patients at the end of life. The McGill-Melzack Pain Questionnaire (MPQ) is a widely used tool that measures subjective pain experience using sensory, affective, and evaluative dimensions of pain. This questionnaire incorporates a series of adjectives to describe the characteristics and intensity of pain. This questionnaire includes other symptoms and other factors besides physical pain (End of Life Nursing Education Consortium [ELNEC], 2008). There are three major measures incorporated into the MPQ: the pain rating index, based on two types of numerical values that can be assigned to each word descriptor; the number of words chosen; and the present pain intensity. It is most useful in the initial assessment and for research, but is generally too burdensome to be used for ongoing pain assessment.

In a comprehensive assessment, it is helpful to be able to evaluate quality of discomfort for those patients with **life-limiting conditions**. OLDCART (ELNEC, 2008) is an acronym that can be used by health care providers to enhance pain management particularly when a patient is nearing death. The key elements of OLDCART (ELNEC, 2008) are depicted in Box 4–3.

While the verbal report is a helpful component of assessment, the physical examination is also essential to complement the data gathering process and paramount in identifying pain for those nearing the end of their lives. Remember that patients may have more than one area of discomfort and these areas

---

BOX 4–3   Key Elements of OLDCART

O = Onset—When did it start? Is it acute or chronic?

L = Location—Where is the pain? Remember, there may be multiple sites.

D = Duration—How long does the pain last? Is it constant? Is it intermittent?

C = Characteristics—Have the patient describe the pain in his or her own words.
  1. Sharp, shooting, burning, electrical—Consider neuropathic or nerve pain.
  2. Sharp, dull, aching—Consider **nociceptive** (also called somatic); bone pain is one example.
  3. Cramping, squeezing—Consider visceral.

A = Aggravating factors (factors that may induce **incident pain**)—breathing, swallowing movement, walking, sitting, turning, defecating, urinating

R = Relieving factors
  1. What makes the pain better or worse?
  2. What medical and nonmedical interventions relieve the pain?

T = Treatment
  1. Medications
  2. Nonpharmacological interventions (e.g., heat, cold, massage, distraction, etc.)

Source: End of Life Nursing Consortium, 2008

TABLE 4–1 Sources of Pain and Possible Drug Interventions

PAIN SOURCE	PAIN CHARACTER	DRUG CLASSIFICATIONS FOR INTERVENTION
Myofacial/Somatic Pain	Constant and well localized.	Muscle relaxants, acetaminophen/nonsteroid pain relievers
Visceral Pain	Injury to sympathetically innervated organs. Pain is vague in quality, deep, dull, and aching.	Opioids
Bone Pain	Axial skeleton with thoracic and lumbar spinal pain the most common.	NSAIDS Corticosteroids Bisphosphonates
Neuropathic Pain Nerve Damage Dysesthesia	Injury to some element of the nervous system (plexus or spinal root). Dysesthesia, burning, tingling, numbing, shooting electrical pain. May not respond well to opioid analgesics.	Tricyclic Antidepressants Anticonvulsants: Corticosteroids Anti-arrhythmics Topical Anesthetic: Opioids

Note: **Nonsteroidal anti-inflammatory drugs** for bone pain and antidepressants or anticonvulsants are but two of many potential co-analgesics. Corticosteroids, neuroleptic agents, bisphosphonates and calcitonin, and some anxiolytic agents may be useful in selected patient populations. Avoid benzodiazepines unless primary anxiety disorder persists after pain relieved.
Source: ELNEC, 2008

require examination as well. A thorough and comprehensive physical assessment is necessary for effective pain management. Table 4–1 illustrates the more common sources of pain to assess expected pain characteristics, and possible medications used to alleviate pain.

SECTION TWO: Pain Management in Special Populations at the End of Life

Pain in Older Adults and Those with Cognitive Impairment

Estimates of elderly patients with significant pain range from 40–80%, depending upon the source (Limaye & Katz, 2006; Zwakhalen, Hamers, Abu-Saad, & Berger, 2006). Some older adults cannot provide an interpretable self-report of pain verbally, in writing, or by other means, even to blink their eyes to answer yes or no questions (Pasero & McCaffery, 2005). This is often seen in patients nearing the end of their lives. Some patients may be able to comprehend and use the numeric pain rating scales, while others may not have cognitive skills to appreciate the scale. Thus, ineffective pain assessment is a major barrier to managing pain in elders. This inability to accurately assess pain requires alternative pain assessment tools and practice (American Geriatric Society, 2002). It is imperative to do comprehensive assessments of the older adult, including those with difficulty understanding the common pain scales. This becomes even more critical as a person nears the end of his or her life.

Even patients who can report pain may appear at times to be confused or agitated or may exhibit changes in behavior, combative behavior, and impaired mobility. At times, health care providers may not even be able to assess pain in the dying patient or those with life-limiting conditions. Pain may present in other ways in the older adult, such as changing their sleep or eating patterns and other behavioral changes. In long-term care, it was found that the higher the behavioral rating of disorientation, withdrawal, or functional impairment, the less analgesics the patient received (Horgas & Tsai, 1998). Patients who are elderly and dying may create further dilemmas for assessment and treatment.

Pain in older patients is often undertreated and misunderstood. One barrier is the assumption that older patients cannot tolerate stronger pain medications or that they do not experience pain as younger patients do. However, many older patients have pain from chronic conditions with daily occurrence that affects their quality of life (Bruckenthal & D'Arcy, 2007). Older adults commonly experience **chronic pain** typically due to chronic, persistent conditions such as osteoarthritis, cancer, diabetic neuropathy, herpes zoster, and osteoporosis. Finally, older adults are less likely than younger people to obtain relief from chronic pain (National Initiative on Pain Control, 2008).

After assessing pain levels, it is important to choose the appropriate medication(s) and therapies based on the older patient's individual characteristics, abilities, and comorbid conditions. Patient aggressiveness and/or resistance in receiving care may be because the patient is guarding against any movement that may cause pain. Achieving appropriate pain relief may be complicated by comorbid diseases and increased risk of adverse drug reaction. Health care providers may lack adequate knowledge in pain management for older adults and those that are dying, leaving these patients underdosed and in pain. The cardinal rule is to begin with lower doses of medications, and titrate slowly but aggressively, remembering that **titration** involves the incremental adjustment of a medication in subsequent doses so that the desired effect is achieved. Many older adults may eventually require doses in the same range as younger adults (American Geriatrics Society, 2002; Davis, Hiemenz, & White, 2002; National Initiative on Pain Control, 2008). Additionally, **complementary and alternative medicine (CAM)** may assist these patients more effectively gain adequate pain control.

Cognitive impairment creates more difficulty in both assessing and treating pain. Patients may have physical reactions such as restlessness (e.g., wandering, looking for family members), fidgeting/rocking, or change or lack of movements, which indicate that they are experiencing pain. Pain may be exhibited by increased or slower movements, rubbing or guarding a body part, rigidity or sleeping in a rigid position, generalized tension, or clenched fist/white knuckles. At times, patients trying to get attention (asking for someone to come, striking out, or even refusing care and pushing away) may be expressing pain issues (Miller, Nelson, & Mezey, 2000).

Many patients with life-limiting diagnoses are in critical care units and may be experiencing pain. Factors compromising the patients' ability to communicate their level of pain verbally include the use of sedating agents, mechanical ventilation, and changes in the level of consciousness. These patients may have underlying pain from their disease etiology as well as from the invasive procedures and equipment that can result in further pain. Patients may be judged to have pain and be managed with infusion of opioids and sedatives (Gélinas, Fillion, Puntillo, Viens, & Fortier, 2006; Shannon & Bucknall, 2003). Conversely, patients not able to express their level of pain may not receive the medications and interventions that they most appropriately need.

Cultural Considerations

Expressions of pain and end-of-life practices and interpretations vary with culture; therefore, assessing pain and implementing pain control modalities can be especially challenging for the health care team. Individuals from some cultures view pain as a weakness and thus do not acknowledge pain when it occurs. Individuals from other cultures allow a few certain members to report pain and other symptoms, while there are cultures that fail to value the administration of medications as an appropriate intervention. With non-English speaking

patients, the degree of assessment, appropriate intervention, and teaching becomes even more complicated (Doka, 2006).

Use of cultural interventions, such as music, prayer, and herbal remedies, must be considered and efforts should be made to integrate these therapies as valid measures to control pain for patients with terminal conditions. Assess pain management in terminology that the patient and family are comfortable using when speaking about pain. Integrate religious and traditional healing practices into pain care as appropriate. Once pain has been assessed, it is important to determine what other interventions can be used in combination with or in place of pain medications (ELNEC, 2008). See Chapter 10 for additional information regarding cultural considerations in terminally ill individuals.

Uninsured, Underinsured, and Underserved

Patients nearing the end of life may be in situations of being uninsured, underinsured, and/or underserved. These individuals may view finances and costs as a major barrier to obtaining effective analgesia at the end of life. Many of the analgesics currently available can be costly and medications may be selected based upon cost rather than appropriateness. Generic and immediate-release medications are generally less expensive than longer-acting and brand name medications (ELNEC, 2008).

In one study (Byock, Sheils-Twohig, Merriman, & Collins, 2006), 22 demonstration projects were employed, representing a wide range of health care settings and patient populations with the goal of developing an innovative model for delivering palliative care that addressed documented deficiencies in the care of patients and families facing the final stage of life. The authors concluded that:

> By individualizing patient and family assessment, effectively employing existing resources and aligning services with specific patient and family needs, it is possible to expand access to palliative services and improve quality of care in ways that are financially feasible and acceptable to patients, families, clinicians, administrators, and payers. (Byock et al., 2006, p. 149)

Patients with a History of Addictive Disease

Addiction, or **psychological dependence**, is a major barrier in treating patients with known pain, even more significant at the end of life and in patients with end-stage diseases. Many of these patients may have had underlying, unresolved chronic, persistent pain. It is critical to use an **interdisciplinary team** approach. In some situations, it may be necessary to include addiction counselors. However, many of these individuals are not experts in pain control and thus a collaborative approach is essential between pain professionals and addiction specialists.

Realistic goals for patients who have addictive disorders at the end of life must be established. Setting limits and maintaining consistency are essential (Ersek, 1999). Comorbid psychiatric disorders are common, particularly depression, personality disorders, and anxiety disorders. Treating these underlying problems may reduce relapse or deviant behaviors, and may make pain control more effective.

Tolerance must also be considered and opioid doses may require more rapid titration and even higher dosing than patients without a history of substance abuse. The use of nonopioids and adjuvant analgesics along with opioids have been shown to be therapeutic. Implementing complementary therapies should be considered. It is important to prevent withdrawal from opioids, benzodiazepines, and alcohol (Berger, Portenoy, & Weissman, 2002; Whitcomb, Kirsh, & Passik, 2002).

A written medication agreement and strong affiliation with dispensing pharmacies are often effective for opioid regulation in patients with addictive disease at the end of life. These practices will help curb **medication diversion** and abuse. Patients and family should be provided education on the differences between addiction, physical dependence, and tolerance at the end of life (Dahl, 2005).

End-of-Life Pain Management in Children and Adolescents

Pain may not be adequately treated in the terminally ill child. There may be fear of hastening a child's death with opioids. It is important for health care professionals to educate themselves and their patients and patients' families in order to correct common misconceptions. Even young infants possess the anatomical and neurological system capabilities to experience pain. Younger children can experience higher levels of pain than older children, as pain tolerance has been shown to increase with age (Initiative for Pediatric Palliative Care, 2008).

Pediatric palliative care studies recognize that a child's physiological, cognitive, and emotional development has an impact on the child's pain perception, available methods of pain management, the roles of the child, parents, and caregivers in pain assessment, and the availability and usefulness of some interventions. Frequently children are not able to provide a self-report of pain. It is important to recognize the role of the parents' observations in pain assessment, and the value of engaging them as part of the team to ensure that a child's pain is managed as early as possible (Wong, Hockenberry-Eaton, Wilson, Winkelstein, & Schwartz, 2001).

Children may be undertreated due to misguided parental fears of addiction or the belief that children do not feel pain due to underdeveloped nervous systems. Opioid fears are common among parents, and if not addressed, can lead to anxiety, distrust, and a breakdown in the collaborative relationships that are needed to provide quality, family-centered care. It is important to recognize the importance of questioning and listening to parents to ascertain the basis of their concerns. This helps to prevent undertreatment that results from a lack of understanding pharmacologic interventions (National Comprehensive Cancer Network, 2005, Solomon et al., 2002, Wolfe et al., 2000).

SECTION TWO REVIEW

1. Older adults may be unable to discuss their level of pain with nurses. Interventions should be based upon:
   1. Assessing for alteration in mental status.
   2. Numerically rating the patient's pain based upon facial expressions and body language.
   3. The understanding that pain is uncommon in the elderly.
   4. Administering pain medications in the same dosage as a younger adult.

2. Pain management and end-of-life practices may differ in cultures unfamiliar to the nurse. As the nurse works with patients of different cultures, he or she recognizes that:
   1. Stoicism may be common in some cultures.
   2. All patients will want to discuss pain if they are experiencing it.
   3. Language is not a barrier when it comes to rating or treating pain.
   4. Medications are valued in all cultures.

3. Finances and costs can be significant barriers to some patients' treatment plan for pain management. Because of this situation:
   1. The uninsured should be treated differently.
   2. Pharmaceutical companies can be contacted for patient assistance programs.
   3. Pain medications should be free to some patients.
   4. Other resources may not be explored to provide adequate pain management.

4. Patients with a history of addictive disease are often treated differently, even at the end of life. Realistic goals for the dying patient include: (Select all that apply.)
   1. Setting limits.
   2. Being consistent.
   3. Treating underlying issues.
   4. Avoiding the use of medications.

5. Children in pain may be difficult to assess and manage. When planning care for a dying child, the nurse understands that:
   1. The parents' fear of opioid addiction is resolved.
   2. Younger children do not have developed sensory systems, so pain is not an issue.
   3. Pain tolerance increases with age.
   4. The health care worker is a better judge of the child's pain than the parents.

SECTION THREE: Goals of Pain Management

Managing pain at the end of life is the culmination of the goals of palliative care. Fishman (1999) summarized this goal with the following words:

> When someone is dying, time as a luxury of wait-and-see is not an option. What matters most in the final days is that patients are free of crippling pain and unbearable suffering so that they can finish their lives in ways that bring comfort, peace, and completion. Concerns about lasting side effects or diminished physical capacity from months of using a drug become secondary to making a patient comfortable. No one has to die in pain. (p. 2)

The World Health Organization (2007) noted that pain relief can most often be provided, without heavy sedation, for 90–95% of people at the end of life. Organizations such as the American Pain Society (APS) and the World Health Organization (WHO), among others, have deemed the goals listed in Box 4–4 as possible and reasonable for the terminally ill patient.

When pain has been chronic and persistent for months to years, and a variety of efforts have failed to provide relief, the clinical challenge becomes even more difficult. Managing chronic pain requires a systematic method, which should include written, structured treatment plans, with clearly stated goals and expectations. Many patients with chronic-pain disorders at the end of life can be treated effectively (Ziegler, 2007). Side effects from pain medication should be anticipated and caregivers should be prepared to treat and manage these to keep the patient comfortable (Hospice and Palliative Nursing Association, 2004).

The ABCDE acronym developed by Jacox and colleagues (1994) for cancer pain assists members of the health care team ensure that the goals of pain are met. The acronym stands for the following:

BOX 4–4   Pain Management Goals

1. Pain should be controlled at all times, 24 hours a day, 7 days a week.
2. Patients should receive frequent pain and symptom assessment by pain management experts, and adjustments made to medications and how medications are delivered, as needed.
3. Pain medications should be provided for continuous pain relief, with other medications immediately available to handle breakthrough pain.
4. Patients and their caregivers should receive complete instructions on managing pain medications, if this responsibility is in their hands; and there should be immediate access to pain professionals if problems or questions arise. They should know who to call and how to reach help, at any hour, 24 hours a day.
5. In general, pain medications should be started with a relatively low dose and increased gradually, to minimize discomfort.
6. Relief of pain should be sufficient in most cases to enable the patient to maintain the quality of life and ability to function as he or she desires at the end of life.

Source: National Comprehensive Cancer Network, 2005

- **A**sk about pain regularly and **A**ssess pain systemically.
- **B**elieve the patient in reports of pains and what relieves the pain.
- **C**hoose pain control options that are appropriate for the patient, family, and setting.
- **D**eliver interventions in a timely, logical, and coordinated fashion.
- **E**mpower patients and family members and **E**nable them to control the course of management to the greatest extent possible.

SECTION THREE REVIEW

1. A goal of pain management should be:
   1. To keep the patient comfortably sedated.
   2. To allow the patient the quality of life and ability to function that the patient desires.
   3. To allow family input on pain management for the patient.
   4. To guard against opioid addiction.
2. The nurse is taking care of a patient with end-of-life pain. The patient is asking about pain control interventions. The nurse recognizes that the patient understands when the patient states which of the following?
   1. "I can only call a health care professional during normal work hours if I have questions on medication."
   2. "I will receive pain medication based upon nursing rounds."
   3. "I will need to ask for pain medication when the pain becomes unbearable."
   4. "I will receive pain medication for continuous pain control with breakthrough medications available as needed."
3. When the patient's current end-of-life pain is exacerbated by chronic pain, which items are important in achieving pain control? (Select all that apply.)
   1. The pain is unlikely to ever be under control.
   2. Frequent assessments
   3. Frequent interventions
   4. Systematic, structured treatment plan

SECTION FOUR: Interventions for Pain at the End of Life

Effective Pharmacotherapy for Pain Management for Patients with End Stage Illnesses

Relieving pain for patients at the end of life with treatments and interventions is as critical as the assessment component. When contemplating the appropriate pain medication, it is important to consider the intensity of the pain, the timing of the pain, the type of pain, and the goals of care.

Immediate-release preparations are used mainly for **acute pain**, determining the correct around-the-clock medication dose, and breakthrough/**rescue dosing**. Immediate release can sometimes be used for long-term management in select patients. The use of as-needed or PRN range orders for opioid analgesics in the management of acute pain or for a breakthrough rescue dose is a common clinical practice. For example, a typical physician order for pain medications could read "morphine immediate release 15–30 mg every 3 to 4 hours as needed for breakthrough pain." This approach provides flexibility in dosing to meet individual patients' unique analgesic requirements. The use of allowing for a range of medications (15–30 mg) to be given enables safe dose adjustments based on an individual's response to medication (Gordon et al., 2005).

Time-released preparations are used for ongoing or chronic pain and to keep a therapeutic level of medication rather than peak and trough levels for patients with ongoing pain. For example, cancer pain and pain at the end of life are chronic in nature and require, with rare exception, both scheduled and rescue dosing. Scheduled dosing will maintain even serum drug levels and provide consistent relief. Rescue dosing should be available on an as-needed basis and can be increased or decreased depending on patient's response. Frequent rescue dosing requires a change in the scheduled long-acting drug dose. In tablet form, these long-acting preparations are usually given every 8 to 12 hours. Transdermal patches are changed every 48 to 72 hours.

The World Health Organization (2007) has devised a ladder of decision making based on the intensity of pain, using a scale that measures pain from mild to severe. This ladder is a guide that can be used to implement the most beneficial drug regimen. For example, if the person reports severe pain, it would not be appropriate to start with acetaminophen and nonsteroidal anti-inflammatory drugs, but to include the appropriate opioid and/or adjuvant.

World Health Organization analgesic ladder is effective in 70–100% of adult patients and consists of three separate steps. Step one concerns medications for mild pain, nonsteroidal anti-inflammatory drugs and acetaminophen. Step two concerns mild to moderate pain medications and indicates that the following medications are appropriate: weak **opioids** (codeine and hydrocondone) and combination analgesics (oxycodone/acetaminophen) plus nonsteroidal anti-inflammatory drugs and adjuvants as needed. The final and third step concerns severe pain and allows for the administration of potent opioids (e.g., morphine, methadone, hydromorphone, fentanyl) plus nonsteroidal anti-inflammatory drugs and adjuvants as needed.

Additionally, the World Health Organization (2007) recommends the following medications for pain relief: adjuvant medications at any level of the ladder; corticosteroids; antidepressants, anticonvulsants, and other agents for neuropathic pain; bisphosphonates and radionuclides for bone pain; antibiotics for pain resulting from ulcerating tumors; nonpharmacologic adjuvant therapy; external-beam radiation; neurosurgical ablative procedures; psychiatric therapy; and anesthesia.

Types of Medications Used for Pain Management

Non-Opioids/Analgesics (Common Over-the-Counter Pain Relievers)

These over-the-counter pain (OTC) medications are used to reduce pain and have fewer side effects than some prescription medications. **Equianalgesic** non-opioids can be used with other types of pain relievers to improve pain control. Most of these medications fall into two categories: acetaminophen and nonsteroidal anti-inflammatory drugs (NSAIDs) (American Pain Society, 2003; Benedetti et al., 2000; McCaffery & Pasero, 1999; Miaskowski et al., 2005; Miyoshi, 2001).

Analgesic drugs such as acetaminophen are mild analgesics that reduce fevers and control mild pain, and may be administered as **preemptive analgesia**. They have no anti-inflammatory action and do not cause stomach irritation. They are often considered first-line treatment in degenerative arthritis or osteoarthritis. When taken long-term at high doses (greater than 4 grams/day), acetaminophen also can cause liver damage and affect hearing.

NSAIDs reduce fever, mild pain, and in high doses are anti-inflammatory, making them useful in conditions such as bone and muscle pain, osteoarthritis, and rheumatoid arthritis. NSAIDs can upset the stomach, cause ulcers, and in rare cases may interfere with coagulation. The most common side effect with NSAIDs is stomach irritation that can be treated. NSAIDs such as aspirin, ibuprofen, and naproxen can cause stomach bleeding as well as kidney or liver problems. The NSAIDs have a ceiling effect, meaning that increasing the dose beyond a certain point will not increase analgesia and will only increase the risk of adverse effects. For example, gastric toxicity through local effects and systemic effects may occur (American Pain Society, 2003; Benedetti et al., 2000; McCaffery & Pasero, 1999; Miaskowski et al., 2005; Miyoshi, 2001).

These medications and other OTC medications can be quite effective and may provide relief from pain in a variety of conditions. However, if patients are taking OTC pain pills on a regular basis, they may be ignoring symptoms of a serious condition. Patients may also be contributing to their pain. For example, taking pain medications every day can lead to rebound headaches. These headaches are actually a symptom of medication withdrawal, caused by taking pain relievers too often over an extended period of time.

Opioids (also known as Narcotics)

The term **narcotic** is slowly being replaced with the word *opioid* in an attempt to enhance the pharmacological value in intervention and to eliminate the stigma of street drug terminology. Opioid analgesics are generally used for moderate to severe pain. These medications may be used in combination with acetaminophen, NSAIDs, or COX II inhibitors to provide better pain control. Opioids work by keeping sensory messages from traveling through the body to the brain, where they are interpreted as pain. Different drugs block different nerves at different levels of the nervous system. This process affects pain relief and the type of side effects a person develops. Common opioids include morphine, hydrocondone, hydromorphone, fentanyl, methadone, oxycodone, codeine, and combinations of these with other analgesics. (See Table 4–2 for a more complete list of pain medications.)

Methadone has unique properties in pain management. Methadone has very specific analgesic properties that make it useful in both complex, chronic cancer pain and **neuropathic pain** issues. Methadone has a long half-life, which may be beneficial, but requires expert dosing. Methadone can usually be given every eight hours, which provides long-lasting relief and allows most patients the ability to sleep through the night. However, this long half-life can make titration difficult. Increasing dosage should be done gradually. Methadone is available in oral tablets and liquids. Another attribute of Methadone is that it is very inexpensive (Bruera et al., 2004; Bruera & Sweeney, 2002; Ripamonti & Bianchi, 2002; Stephenson, 2004).

Adverse Effects. Allergic reactions to opioids are extremely rare and are not usually due to the opioid itself, but to preservatives, dyes, and other additives. Patients may state they are allergic; further questioning may reveal that they may have developed nausea and vomiting, itching, or sedation when given a particular opioid at a certain dose. Learning these facts provides an opportunity to educate patients regarding allergic responses versus adverse effects that can be controlled by changing the dose, the medication, or controlling the symptoms. The only absolute contraindication to the use of an opioid is a history of a hypersensitivity reaction (e.g., wheezing, edema). Allergic reactions are limited almost exclusively to the morphine derivatives. In the rare event that a patient describes a true allergic reaction, the recommendation is to begin therapy with a low dose of a short-acting synthetic opioid (e.g., intravenous fentanyl) (Doka, 2006; Dickerson et al., 2001; ELNEC, 2008; Kaye, 1990; Watson, Lucas, Hoy, & Black, 2005).

Nausea and vomiting can occur. Treatment includes antiemetics or changing to a different opioid. Tolerance of the opioid can occur and these adverse effects diminish, but pain control will continue.

Pruritus (itching) can occur, more commonly with spinal delivery of opioids. Tolerance occurs within a few days. Antihistamines can be helpful; however, sedation may result from the use of these drugs.

Respiratory depression is greatly feared by patients, families, and health care providers, yet rare. Respiratory depression is almost always preceded by sedation, thus in most cases, the health care professional has a warning. In terminal conditions, it is important for the family to understand that the medication is given for comfort, not to hasten death. The time of greatest prevalence of respiratory depression is after the first dose of the opioid in an **opioid-naïve** patient. Respiratory depression can also occur after a change in dose of the opioid. Patients with respiratory rates as low as 6 or 8/minute can be considered normal if the oxygenation seems normal, the oxygenation saturation is within normal range, the patient is arousable, and the patient is comfortable. This is particularly true if the patient is sleeping. Opioid reversal may be considered if the patient is unarousable, has a low respiratory rate, and has poor oxygenation (one can use pulse oximeters or evaluate perfusion in the fingernails) (ELNEC, 2008; Institute for Clinical Systems Improvement, 2007).

If the patient has true opioid-induced respiratory depression, the opioid can be reversed using an antagonist (naloxone or Narcan®). Strict care must be taken to avoid opioid withdrawal and reverse all the analgesic effect of the drug. Signs and symptoms of opioid withdrawal syndrome include sweating, anxiety, restlessness, dilated pupils, chills, tachycardia, hypertension, nausea/vomiting, crampy abdominal pains, diarrhea, and muscle aches and pains. To prevent withdrawal while reversing the respiratory depressant effect, mix 1 ampule of naloxone (0.4 mg) in 10 ml of sterile water or saline. Administer 1 ml increments slowly to reverse the sedative/respiratory depressant effect without reversing the analgesic effect. Remember that the duration of action of naloxone is approximately 30–60 minutes, while the duration of effect of most opioids is much longer. Thus, naloxone may need to be readminstered once its antagonist effect wears off. In some patients, the dose may need to be administered every 10 to 15 minutes. Thus, careful monitoring of the patient's sedation, respiratory status, and analgesic state is indicated (Doka, 2006; Dickerson et al., 2001; ELNEC, 2008; Kaye, 1990; Watson et al., 2005).

Constipation is a major adverse effect of opioid therapy, often leading to reducing or stopping opioids if not well managed. Opioids reduce gut motility and peristalsis as well as increase the re-absorption of water from the stool back into the lining of the intestines. The result is slow moving, dry fecal material. A laxative with stool softener combination is needed to offset this effect. Much like opioid dosing, the dose of laxative/softener is titrated based upon the frequency and consistency of bowel movements. Bowel regimen should be administered regularly to prevent constipation, not only when the patient has not had a bowel movement for a period of time. It is much easier

TABLE 4–2 Pharmacological Agents Used in Treatment of Persistent Pain Indications and Common Uses

CLASS/AGENT/(BRAND NAME)	INDICATIONS/COMMON USE
Analgesic, P-Aminophenol, Paracetamol, APAP **Acetaminophen** (Tylenol®)	Mild to moderate pain
Analgesic, topical **Lidocaine Patch 5%** (Lidoderm®)	Postherpetic neuralgia, diabetic neuropathy, osteoarthritis, low back pain
Anticonvulsants **Carbamazepine** (Tegretol®) **Gabapentin** (Neurontin®) **Lamotrigine** (Lamictal®) **Phenytoin** (Dilantin®) **Pregabalin** (Lyrica®)	Trigeminal neuralgia, postherpetic neuralgic, diabetic neuropathy, fibromyalgia
Antidepresants, Serotonin-Norepinephrine Reuptake inhibitors (SNRIs) **Duloxetine** (Cymbalta®) **Venlafaxine** (Effexor®)	Peripheral neuropathic pain, chronic pain
Antidepressants, Tricyclic **Amitriptyline** (Elavil) **Amoxapine** (Asendin®, Asendis®, Defanyl, Demolox®, Moxadil®) **Desipramine** (Norpramin, Pertofrane) **Doxepin** (Aponal, Adapine, Deptran, Sinquan®, Sinequan®) **Nortriptyline** (Sensoval®, Aventyl®, Pamelor®, Allegron®, Nortrilen®) **Protriptyline** (Vivactil®)	Postherpetic neuralgia, phantom limb pain, diabetic neuropathy, trigeminal neuralgia, osteoarthritis, rheumatoid arthritis
Counterirritants, topicals **Capsaicin** (Icy Hot®, Capsin®, Pain Enz®, Sportsmed®)	Temporary relief—osteoarthritis, rheumatoid arthritis, postherpetic neuralgia, diabetic neuropathy, intractable pruritis, postmastectomy, and phantom limb pain
COX-2 inhibitors **Celecoxib** (Celebrex®)	Rheumatoid arthritis, osteoarthritis, primary dysmenorrhea
Muscle relaxants, centrally acting **Baclofen** (Kemstro®, Lioresal®)	Intrathecally administered—intractable spasticity
N-methyl-d-aspartate (NMDA) **Ketamine** (Ketanest S®)	Some use for breakthrough pain in chronic pain
Nonsteroidal antiinflammatory (NSAIDS) **Diclofenac, Ibuprofen** (Advil®, Motrin IB®) **Naproxen** (Aleve®) **Salsalate** (Disalcid®)	Rheumatoid arthritis, osteoarthritis, inflammatory processes, acute headaches, ankylosing spondylitis
Opioids, Opioid-like agent **Tramadol** (Ultram®)	Moderate to moderately severe pain
Opioids, oral **Hydrocodone/APAP** (Norco®, Vicodin®/Lortab®) **Hydromorphone** (Dilaudid®); **Levorphanol** **Morphine** (MS Contin®, Oramorph®, Kadian®, Avinza®, Roxanol®) **Oxycodone** (OxyContin®, Roxicodone®, Roxifast®) **Methadone** (Dolophine®) **Oxymorphone** (Opana®, Numorphan®, Numorphone®)	Moderate to severe chronic pain in opioid-tolerant patients
Opioids, transdermal **Fentanyl** (Duragesic®);	Management of chronic pain in patients requiring continuous opioid analgesic

Source: Institute for Clinical Symptoms Improvement, 2007; National Initiative on Pain Control, 2008; Paice & Fine, 2006; Springhouse, 2006

to prevent the onset of constipation than to treat it once it occurs. When constipation develops, various medications can be used for treatment, including stimulants, laxatives, enemas, and other therapies. Tolerance does not develop to the constipating effect of opioids; it will always be a symptom to be addressed (Doka, 2006; Dickerson et al., 2001; ELNEC, 2008; Kaye, 1990; Watson et al., 2005).

In 2008, the Federal Drug Administration approved methylnaltrexone bromide subcutaneous injection (Relistor®) for the treatment of opioid-induced constipation in patients with advanced illness who are receiving palliative care. Use of the peripherally acting μ-opioid antagonist is reserved for patients who have had insufficient response to laxative therapy. Methylnaltrexone should be administered once every other day, as needed, but no more frequently than once every 24 hours. The recommended doses are 8 mg for patients weighing 38 to less than 62 kg (84 to < 136 lbs) and 12 mg for patients weighing 62 to 114 kg (136 to 251 lbs) (Thomas et al., 2008).

Opioid sedation can occur, but usually wanes within hours or days. Many times patients are exhausted from unrelieved pain and require restful sleep. Once their pain is relieved, they are finally able to rest. If they continue to be sleepy just from the opioid, treatment may require changing to a different opioid. Methylphenidate (Ritalin®) can be given at doses of 5–10 mg orally in the morning and at lunch to provide less sedation and allow more awareness/wake time (Dickerson et al., 2001; ELNEC, 2008; Kaye, 1990; Watson et al., 2005).

Urinary retention is more common in opioid-naïve patients and is most common with spinal delivery of medications (e.g., epidural or intrathecal). Tolerance occurs to this effect, usually within a few days (ELNEC, 2008).

Adjuvants

There are some drugs that are not usually ordered for pain, but are effective in enhancing the effects of other pain medications. Several major categories of **adjuvant analgesic medications** are used in pain control. They include antidepressants, anticonvulsants, and anti-anxiety drugs (Dickerson et al., 2001; Institute for Clinical Systems Improvement, 2007; ELNEC, 2008; Watson et al., 2005).

Antidepressants.   Patients with depression, including patients at the end of life, frequently have concomitant pain complaints. Antidepressant medications increase the activity of the brain chemicals serotonin and norepinephrine, to help relieve both depression and chronic pain. Common antidepressants include sertraline (Zoloft®), bupropion (Wellbutrin®), venlafaxine (Effexor®), desipramine (Norpramin®), amitriptyline (Elavil®), paroxetine (Paxil®), fluoxetine (Prozac®), mirtazapine (Remeron®), and nefazodone (Serzone®). Atypical antidepressants block serotonin and weakly block norepinephrine reuptake. Agents such as venlafaxine (Effexor®) and duloxetine (Cymbalta®) are being used for chronic neuropathic pain.

Anticonvulsants.   These drugs were originally developed to prevent seizures in patients, but have been shown to be effective for chronic pain. Pain may cause the nervous system to react by becoming overly sensitive. These medications quiet the overly activated neurons within the brain. Common anticonvulsants include Nefazodone (Dilantin®), Carbamazepine (Tegretol®), divalproex (Depakote®), gabapentin (Neurontin®), Clonazepam (Klonopin®), topiramate (Topamax®), and duloxetine (Cymbalta®).

Anti-anxiety (anxiolytics).   Just as there is a strong connection between depression and pain, there is also a strong connection between anxiety and pain. Stress and anxiety, often symptoms at the end of life, can directly increase pain. Anti-anxiety medications can reduce muscle tension that may increase pain in patients. A reduction in stress level can enhance the effectiveness of the pain medications. These drugs are better used for only short periods of time. Common anti-anxiety medications include diazepam (Valium®), alprazolam (Xanax®), lorazepam (Ativan®), and buspirone (Buspar®).

Corticosteroids.   Corticosteroids inhibit prostaglandin synthesis and reduce edema surrounding many types of tissues. These drugs are useful when treating neuropathic pain, bone pain, and visceral pain. Dexamethasone (Decadron®) produces the least amount of mineralcorticoid effect (changes in sodium and potassium excretion due to effect of the drug on the adrenal glands), and is often preferred at the end of life. Standard doses may range widely, with doses as high as 16–24 mg/day or higher.

Side effects may include psychosis and proximal muscle wasting. Benefits include improved energy and appetite. Due to its long half-life, dexamethasone should be ordered every morning. This prevents sleeplessness, which is encountered when this medication is administered in the evening hours.

Antispasmodic.   Baclofen is useful in the relief of spasm-associated pain. Doses begin at 10 mg/day and are titrated gradually based upon patient response and adverse effects. Table 4–3 illustrates sample orders for pain management at the end of life.

Inappropriate Choices for Persistent, End-of-Life Pain

There are two very common medications prescribed for pain control that are inappropriate for long-term, chronic pain. The drugs are meperidine (Demerol®) and propoxyphene (Darvocet® and Darvon®). These two medications are poorly absorbed, produce metabolites, and therefore are considered unsuitable for long-term pain management. They should be discontinued after any extended use.

Meperidine is not indicated in end-of-life care. Meperidine is metabolized to normeperidine in the liver, which is then

TABLE 4–3 Sample Orders for Pain Management at the End of Life

Mild Pain: Acetaminophen (Tylenol®) 650 to 1000 mg three to four times daily.

Moderate Pain—The above plus:

Oxycodone 5 to 10 mg every three to four hours as needed for pain.

OR (with maximum daily dose of acetaminophen 4 grams)

Oxycodone/acetaminophen (Percocet®) 1 to 2 tablets every three to four hours as needed for pain.

Hydrocodone/acetaminophen (Norco®, Vicodin®, Lorcet®) 1 to 2 tablets every four to six hours as needed for pain.

Severe Pain:

Morphine 10 to 20 mg orally every three to four hours as needed for pain.

Hydromorphone (Dilaudid®) 2 to 4 mg orally every three to four hours as needed for pain.

Oxycodone 10 to 20 mg orally every three to four hours as needed for pain.

OR

Morphine 0.5 to 2 mg IV every two hours as needed for pain.

Hydromorphone (Dilaudid®) 1 to 0.3 mg every two hours as needed for pain.

Fentanyl 20 to 30 mcg IV every two hours as needed for pain.

Bowel Program: (if opioids prescribed): If long-acting opioids are prescribed, the bowel medications should be scheduled.

Senna or Senna Plus 1–4 tablets BID.

Bisacodyl (Dulcolax®) 5 to 10 mg by mouth daily or 10 mg pr daily.

Magnesium hydroxide (Milk of Magnesia®) 30 ml by mouth daily

70% Sorbitol 15 to 30 ml daily.

Lactulose 15 to 30 ml daily.

Neuropathic Pain:

Amitriptyline 10 to 25 mg daily at bedtime. Titrate up as tolerated (most sedating; avoid in elderly).

Nortriptyline 10 to 25 mg daily at bedtime. Titrate up as tolerated.

Desipramine 10 to 25 mg daily at bedtime. Titrate up as tolerated.

Gabapentin (Neurontin®)—**elderly:** 100 mg at bedtime, then increase to 100 mg twice daily, 100 mg three times daily; increase dose every several days as tolerated (adjust dosage for renal dysfunction).

Gabapentin (Neurontin®)—**non-elderly:** 100 to 300 mg at bedtime, then increase to 300 mg twice daily, then 300 mg three times daily; increase dose every few days as tolerated (adjust dosage for renal dysfunction).

Pregabalin (Lyrica®) 75 mg twice daily. Adjust dose upward as tolerated (adjust dosage for renal dysfunction).

Bone Pain:

Ibuprofen 400 to 800 mg every four hours as needed or scheduled (max dose 3200 mg/day)

Naproxen 200 to 500 mg twice daily as needed or scheduled (max dose = 1500 mg/day)

Source: Adapted from the Institute for Clinical Systems Improvement, 2007

excreted through the kidneys. In the face of renal dysfunction, normeperidine is not excreted, and therefore accumulates in the bloodstream and may become toxic. Because normeperidine is toxic to the central nervous system, these patients are at risk for seizures, and seizures have been reported in healthy individuals receiving just a few doses of meperidine. Meperidine's oral bioavailability is poor, such that 50 mg of oral meperidine is approximately equal to 650 mg of aspirin. Finally, meperidine is painful when given by injection (Dickerson et al., 2001; ELNEC, 2008; Kaye, 1990; Watson et al., 2005).

Propoxyphene is considered a very mild analgesic that also produces toxic metabolites and therefore is not recommended for end-of-life care. Similar to meperidine, propoxyphene is converted to norpropoxyphene, which is renally cleared.

Accumulation of this byproduct in the presence of renal disease can cause tremors and seizures. Furthermore, propoxyphene is a very weak analgesic. Finally, propoxyphene admixtures often contain large amounts of acetaminophen, which, in turn, can cause liver damage (Dickerson et al., 2001; ELNEC, 2008; Kaye, 1990; Watson et al., 2005).

Routes of Administration

The preferred route of administration for pain medications is typically oral. It is the most noninvasive and a majority of patients prefer this route. However, absorption and the patient's ability to swallow at the end of life may affect the efficacy of the medication delivery. Medications can be given around the clock for **persistent (chronic) pain** and as needed for management of breakthrough short-lived pain. Rescue doses for **breakthrough pain** are given along with long-acting, around-the-clock medications. Symptoms of nausea and vomiting may not only affect the absorption of oral medication taken, but the patient's ability and willingness to take the medication. As patients weaken during their final days and weeks, often swallowing becomes an issue (Dickerson et al., 2001; ELNEC, 2008; Kaye, 1990; Watson et al., 2005).

The oral transmucosal or sublingual delivery of medication is effective for those with difficulty swallowing or who have gut dysfunction (Gordon, 2006). It is frequently used for breakthrough pain in patients at the end of life. Enteral feeding tubes can be used to administer oral medications when patients can no longer swallow; however, there are many ethical issues surrounding the use of feeding tubes in end-of-life care, and it is advised not to place one just for medication administration.

Other choices for home use at the end of life include transdermal and topical routes and these routes may be preferred. Fatty layers of the skin and sweaty secretions can change the level and rate of absorption for medications delivered in patches, thus some patients may require an increase in dose and/or more frequent applications of patches. Placement of a patch over a bony region may decrease absorption. Currently, the only formulation for transdermal delivery is fentanyl, and the patch should be placed every 72 hours over nonhairy skin that has good capillary flow and no edema. The upper chest, shoulders, or upper arms are the optimal sites. Because an initial patch dose may take 18–24 hours to reach peak onset, this medication is not recommended for acute or escalating pain (Dickerson et al., 2001, ELNEC, 2008; Kaye, 1990; Watson et al., 2005).

Topical capsaicin can be used for neuropathic pain. Gloves should be worn and one's hands washed after application to prevent accidental contact with eyes or any open tissues that may result in burning. Topical lidocaine and other local anesthetics can be used for isolated, brief pain conditions. A new formulation consists of a patch with 5% lidocaine (Lidoderm®). This is approved for the relief of pain associated with post-herpetic **neuropathy** and has been used for other pain sites, such as cancer, bone, and arthritis pain (Ferrini & Paice, 2004).

The use of compounded topical opioids (not to be confused with transdermal delivery) is controversial. Most opioids (except for fentanyl and related opioids) are water soluble, which prevents their absorption through the fat tissues of the skin. One exception is morphine cream, used for painful decubiti. The open skin of the ulcer allows morphine to be absorbed locally (ELNEC, 2008). Local anesthetics can be useful in relieving neuropathic pain. Local anesthetics may be administered intravenously (e.g., lidocaine) or via the spinal column (e.g., epidurally or intrathecally, usually bupivacaine—Marcaine®).

The rectal route (also stomal/vaginal) is usually considered for limited use only. This route can be an appropriate route for short-term use of long-acting opioids when the patient is no longer able to swallow or is having gastrointestinal difficulties, such as nausea and vomiting. Because the rectum is a part of the digestive tract, medications given via this route have been shown to have similar efficacy in absorption, especially long-acting opioid tablets (Dickerson et al., 2001).

The parenteral routes, subcutaneous or IV, are preferred for acute pain, such as surgical or trauma, as well as being feasible for long-term therapy. It is the most invasive route and requires access either short term to a few weeks with peripheral lines, midlines or peripherally inserted central catheter lines, to long term access, via port-a-caths or central lines. IV administration may be accomplished using **patient-controlled analgesia (PCA)** or **nurse-controlled analgesia (NCA)**. Risks using this route of administration include phlebitis, infection, and thrombosis. Once at home, this route may require interventions of home health or hospice team members, infusion specialists, and extensive management training for the caregivers. Parenteral infusions are useful when patients cannot swallow or when absorption through the gastrointestinal tract is altered.

Subcutaneous boluses have a slower onset and lower peak effect when compared with intravenous boluses. Subcutaneous infusions may be administered in amounts not to exceed 5–10 ml/hour, although 1–3 ml is ideal (Institute for Clinical Systems Improvement, 2007). Intramuscular mediations are not recommended due to wide variability in absorption, potential delays in vascular uptake of the drug, and pain (Paice & Fine, 2001). Similarly, nasal administration is not recommended for chronic pain management. Currently, the only nasal preparation is the mixed agonist-antagonist butorphanol (Stadol®) (Dickerson et al., 2001; ELNEC, 2008; Kaye, 1990; Watson et al., 2005).

Epidural or intrathecal routes allow delivery of drugs in combinations, including opioids, local anesthetics, and/or alpha-adrenergic agonists. The technology is complex, requiring specialized knowledge for health care professionals. Risk of infection and cost are additional concerns. There is little advantage to using intraspinal opioids alone if the patient can tolerate these agents when given systemically. Thus, the time to select intraspinal delivery is when patients cannot tolerate adverse systemic opioid effects (Smith, Kemp, Hamphill, & Vojir, 2002).

Approaches to pain requiring anesthesia are very invasive, including blocks and pain pumps, with single or multiple medications. This route by injection or surgically placed by a specialist. Ongoing management is done as an outpatient, which may require filling the pump placed under the skin and adjusting medications as needed. The timeliness of a life-limiting condition may influence the choice to include this intervention and treatment plan for a patient at the end of life. Table 4–4 illustrates some of the more frequently administered pain medications and the frequency of administration.

Evaluation of Pharmaceutical Interventions

Effective pain management requires careful individual titration of analgesics based on a valid and reliable assessment of pain and pain relief. The nurse who is competent in pain assessment

TABLE 4–4 Pain Medications, Available Strengths, and Frequency of Administration

MEDICATION	AVAILABLE STRENGTHS	FREQUENCY OF DOSING
Morphine	**Immediate Release Tablets**	
	MSIR – 15, 30 mg	q 3–6 hrs
	Sustained Release Tablets	
	MS Contin® – 15, 30, 60, 100, 200 mg	q 12 hrs
	Kadian® – 20, 30, 50, 60, 100 mg	q 24 hrs
	Oramorph SR® – 15, 30, 60, 100 mg	q 12 hrs
	Oral Liquid	
	MSIR Oral Solution – 2 mg/ml, 4 mg/ml	q 3 hrs
	MSIR Oral Concentrate – 20 mg/ml	q 3 hrs
	Roxanol® Concentrate – 20 mg/ml	q 1 hr
	Suppository	
	Rectal Morphine Sulfate (RMS) – 5, 10, 20, 30 mg	q 4 hrs
Hydromorphone	**Tablets**	
	Dilaudid® – 2, 4, 8 mg	q 3 hrs
	Liquid	
	Dilaudid® – 2 mg/ml	q 3 hrs
	Dilaudid® – 10 mg/ml	q 3 hrs
	Suppository	
	Dilaudid® – 3 mg	q 6 hrs
Oxycodone	**Immediate Release Tablets**	
	Oxy IR® – 5 mg	q 3 hrs
	Roxicodone – 5 mg	q 3 hrs
	Oxycodone/Acetiminophen	
	Percocet® –5/325, 7.5/500, 10/500 mg	q 3 hrs
	Roxicet® –5/325, 5/500 mg	q 3 hrs
	Sustained Release Tablets	
	Oxycontin® – 10, 20, 40, 80 mg	q 8–12 hrs
	Liquid	
	Roxicodone – 1 mg/ml, 20 mg/ml	q 1 hr
	OxyFAST ® – 20 mg/ml	q 1 hr
Fentanyl Transdermal	**Skin Patch**	
	Duragesic® – 25, 50, 75, 100 mcg/hr	q 48–72 hrs
Fentanyl Transmucosal	**Oral Lozenge**	
	Actiq® – 200, 400, 600, 800, 1200, 1600 mcg	
Methadone	**Tablet**	
	Dolophine® – 5,10 mg	q 4–12 hrs
	Liquid	
	Generic Methadone – 1, 2 mg/m	q 4–12 hrs

(continued)

TABLE 4–4 Pain Medications, Available Strengths, and Frequency of Administration *(continued)*

Hydrocodone	**Hydrocodone/Acetaminophen Tablets**	
	Vicodin® –5/500 mg	**q 4–6 hrs**
	Vicodin ES® – 7.5/750 mg	**q 4–6 hrs**
	Lorcet® or Vicodin HP® – 10 mg/650 mg	**q 4–6 hrs**
	Lortab® – 2.5/500 mg, 5/500 mg, 7.5/500 mg, 10/500 mg	**q 4–6 hrs**
	Norco® – 5/325 mg, 7.5/325 mg, 10/325 mg	**q 4–6 hrs**
	Hydrocodone/Ibuprofen	
	Vicoprophen® – 7.5/200 mg	**q 4–6 hrs**

Source: Delaware Pain Initiative, 2007; Institute for Clinical Symptoms Improvement, 2007

and analgesic administration can safely interpret and implement analgesic medications as ordered. The American Society for Pain Management Nursing (2002) and the American Pain Society (2000) support safe medication practices and the appropriate use of opioid analgesic orders in pain management, especially when there is a range order. Nurses should base their decisions about a specific dose on their knowledge of the drug, thorough pain assessment, including level of sedation produced and resulting respiratory effort, along with the knowledge of the drug to be administered.

Pain assessment should also include pain intensity, type of pain, location, and the patient's previous response to this or other analgesics (e.g., pain relief, side effects, and impact of function). The nurse should be familiar with the anticipated time of onset of the medication, time of peak effect, duration of action, and side effects of the analgesic to be administered, based on dose and route of administration. Evaluate and document the patient's response to the analgesic dose and dosing interval. Reevaluation includes patient's continued response and this may be dependent on route and frequency of delivery of opioids, other adjuvant medications, and nonpharmacological interventions.

SECTION FOUR REVIEW

1. The WHO Cancer pain relief ladder:
   1. Is effective only for acute pain.
   2. Does not rely on the intensity of pain, just location.
   3. Combines non-opioids, opioids, and adjuvants for pharmacotherapy.
   4. Includes opioids as the first intervention for mild pain.
2. Timing is an important aspect of pharmacotherapy intervention. To enhance pain management in patients at the end of life, nurses should:
   1. Give appropriate doses in a timely manner.
   2. Use time-released medications only in chronic pain.
   3. Treat constipation only when it occurs.
   4. Start Fentanyl patches on patients with acute pain.
3. The type of pain, as well as the intensity of pain, will influence the choice of medications. Non-opioids:
   1. Are only used for minor pain.
   2. Can be used in combination with opioids.
   3. Are not effective later in treatment.
   4. Do not cause rebound pain.
4. When preparing for patient teaching for the patient receiving opioids, the nurse needs to know that:
   1. Opioids are different than narcotics.
   2. Morphine is the only addictive drug.

3. Many people are truly allergic to opioids.
4. Methadone is known for addiction withdrawal, but is also useful in chronic cancer and neuropathic pain.
5. There are numerous medications that potentiate, or enhance, other pain medications. These adjuvants:
   1. May not be needed if the patient has underlying depression as well.
   2. Should only be used if the patient has the disease or problem for which it is primarily used.
   3. May effectively be given in combination with primary pain medications.
   4. Should be used cautiously, when combined with pain medication, in patients with the underlying disease or condition for which it is primarily used.
6. Propoxyphene and meperidine are considered poor choices for persistent and end of life pain. They have poor efficacy and:
   1. Are hard to administer.
   2. Have toxic metabolites.
   3. No side effects.
   4. Have no equianalgesic conversion.

SECTION FIVE: Complementary and Alternative Therapies

Non-Pharmacological Interventions

Frequently, when patients at the end of life are taking medications and may still be experience on-going moderate to severe pain, other methods for the treatment of pain are pursued. These include complementary modalities as alternatives for pain management therapies and interventions in conjunctions with their current regime of medications. This **combination therapy** allows nurses and patients to utilize choice as well as trial of medications along with **complementary and alternative medicine** (CAM) techniques in diagnosing, treating and/or preventing pain and other symptoms (Khatta, 2007). Because there may be interactions with some forms of CAM and the patient's pain medications, all complementary and alternative therapies should be discussed with the health care team prior to their use.

Rehabilitative therapy that includes physical and/or occupational therapy, exercise, and other treatment interventions is one form of CAM that may be useful in pain management. Usually this therapy assists a patient to recover from trauma or surgery while relieving pain. However, for the terminally ill individual, this therapy may help the person to maintain strength, relaxation, and relief of pain. In a study of the effectiveness of massage therapy in hospice patients, relaxation was achieved as measured by blood pressure, heart rate, and skin temperature. A 10-minute back massage was found to relieve pain in male cancer patients (Ernst, 2004; Smith et al., 2002; Stephenson, Weinrich, & Tavakoli, 2000; Syrjala, Donaldson, Davis, Kippes, & Carr, 1995; Wilkie et al., 2000).

Psychological approaches target the mental and emotional aspects of pain. For example, psychologists and psychiatrists may include behavioral interventions and use cognitive-behavioral therapies in addition to analgesic therapies. The use of cognitive and behavioral interventions is considered beneficial after administering a breakthrough dose of immediate-release opioid. Even though there may be a delay in response to the opioid, the nonpharmacological techniques can begin to help reducing pain during this delay period (Grealish, Lomasney, & Whiteman, 2000). Examples of cognitive and behavioral techniques include: relaxation, guided imagery, distraction, cognitive reframing, support groups, and pastoral counseling/prayer.

There are numerous CAM interventions that can be helpful for patients across the lifespan. These interventions vary from gentle touch to skilled professional or specialist interventions. Some easy, brief nursing interventions (back rub, hand massage, repositioning a patient, diversion, and conversation) can be implemented without a physician's order and should be individualized and tailored to each patient. Other treatments may

BOX 4–5	Common Examples of Complementary and Alternative Therapies

Aerobics/exercise
Acupressure
Acupuncture
Ancient Indian healing arts
Animal-assisted therapy (pet therapy)
Aromatherapy
Biofeedback
Chinese medicine (traditional Chinese medicine, TCM)
Chiropractic care
Cognitive reframing
Color light therapy
Cutaneous stimulation
Deep breathing exercises
Diet-based/nutrition therapies
Distraction
Energy healing therapy
Folk medicine
Guided imagery
Healing touch
Herbal medicine
Homeopathy
Hypnosis
Imagery
Magnetic therapy
Massage
Meditation
Megavitamin therapy
Music therapy
Naturopathic treatment
Native American healing system–Native American medicine
Osteopathic care
Prayer/pastoral counseling
Progressive muscle relaxation
Reflexology
Relaxation
Ta'i chi
Transcutaneous electrical nerve stimulation (TENS)
Trigger points
Ultrasound
Yoga

include the multidisciplinary team. Box 4–5 outlines some of the more common modalities that may assist patients with reducing pain.

Complementary therapies are frequently culturally based. Discussions and requests for information should be handled in a nonjudgmental manner and patients should be encouraged to discuss the use of any CAM in conjunction with the health care team.

SECTION FIVE REVIEW

1. Adjuvant therapies may include: (Select all that apply.)
   1. Pharmacology
   2. Relaxation techniques.
   3. Rehabilitative approach.
   4. Prayer.
2. The nurse is evaluating the effectiveness of the adjuvant therapy massage. It is important that the nurse review which of the following prior to deciding if the therapy has been effective?
   1. Documentation of the patient's response to treatment

2. Documentation of the patient's intake and output
3. The family's cultural background
4. The patient's medical history
3. Nonpharmacological interventions that might be employed in an effort to relieve pain include: (Select all that apply.)
   1. Surgical intervention.
   2. Medications.
   3. Diversion.
   4. Deep breathing.

Case Study 1

Mrs. Sanchez is concerned that the health care providers are not providing adequate pain control to her 3-year-old, Jaime, who has a Wilm's tumor. However, she has been very reluctant to let the nurses give any opioids because of her past experiences with her brother's drug addiction. She doesn't want "drugs" in the home. Jaime's pain experience is preventing him from getting sleep and he cries frequently. He misses his dog, Chewie, and wants to see him. Mrs. Sanchez is asking if there is anything else that can be used to halt the pain.

Suggested Responses

Distraction, relaxation, pet therapy, sleep routines/comfort, nutritional considerations, aromatherapy, skin care–massage, oxygen if breathless, parent's involvement in care, support groups, and more! And remember, Jaime's pain affects the family's level of comfort.

Question

What complementary or alternative therapies may be effective for a 3-year-old in pain at the end of life?

SECTION SIX: Undertreatment of Pain at the End of Life

Impact of Inadequate Pain Control

Inadequate pain control can be a major issue facing patients at the end of life. Despite dramatic advances in research treatment for conditions such as cancer, arthritis, and neuropathy, diseases continue to cause devastating pain and suffering to the hundreds of thousands at the end of life each year in the United States (Agency for Health Care Research and Quality, 2002). The fear of pain is common among cancer patients and the impact of pain is immense. Pain can impact on all areas of a person's life, reducing the quality of his or her physical, mental, social, and spiritual life. Pain may cause reduced mobility, fatigue, sleeplessness, loss of appetite, and decreased physical functioning. Pain can cause distancing in relationships, as friends and family may be uncomfortable when they do not know how to

interact with a patient in pain. Suicidal wishes in patients with advanced disease are closely linked to unrelieved pain and to mood alterations such as depression and anxiety, which like pain, frequently respond to clinician treatment if the clinician identifies and addresses them (Foley, 1995).

At present, physicians and nurses are often reluctant to give large doses of analgesics to dying patients, perhaps fearing that they will be subject to lawsuits if the medications contribute to respiratory arrest. Laws and regulations provide protection for health professionals to aggressively treat pain with analgesic drugs, and when needed, with terminal sedation, even if these treatments may potentially hasten death. Regulations specify that the intent to relieve pain is supported by documentation of the patient's report of pain or behaviors that suggest pain justifies higher doses of analgesics or sedatives, even if these treatments could also depress respiratory effort or hasten death in any way. Such treatment is based on ethical principles that are widely accepted by health professionals and ethicists and should not be considered an act of assisted suicide or euthanasia. Review Chapters 2 and 3 for additional information.

When deciding the need for increasing pain medications in terminally ill patients, remember the following:

Patients at the end of life need not have unrelieved pain. Thorough assessment and multidisciplinary treatment can provide comfort with a minimum of adverse effects. Patients and their families can be freed to accomplish their final goals, and the bereaved families can be spared the pain of memories of loved ones who suffered in their final days. (Abraham, 2001, p. 100)

Pain and symptom relief may be the only achievable goal when curative therapy has failed. Relief of pain can help to restore decision-making capacity and enhance the patient's right to self-determination. Constant pain may cause a spiritual crisis as the patient tries to find meaning in suffering. Patients may begin to question their lives in an attempt to explain their pain. Patients in pain are not as able or willing to enjoy normal activities. They may have difficulty concentrating and have feelings of anxiety and fear. Often patients express concerns about feeling out of control or of feeling helpless. Depression commonly results from long periods of untreated pain and can cause thoughts of and attempts at suicide.

Some of the more harmful effects of pain include decreased quality of life and cognitive disruption and pulmonary, cardiovascular, gastrointestinal, genitourinary, muscular, endocrine, and and metabolic complications (Whitecar, Jonas & Clasen, 2000).

Double Effect

The principal of **double effect** distinguishes between providing palliative medications with the intent to relieve pain that might unintentionally hasten death versus the provision of medication to deliberately cause death. However, opioid administration at end of life has not been shown to be associated with shorter survival rates (Sykes & Thorns, 2003; Thorns & Sykes, 2000). Health care professionals have the responsibility to be aware of the potential risks of treating pain with opioids and other analgesics. In clinical practice, the risk is quite small that opioid doses might hasten death. Both the American Nurses Association (2003) and the Hospice and Palliative Nurses Association (2004) have acknowledged that this is an acceptable risk in the delivery of quality nursing care to terminally ill individuals.

SECTION SIX REVIEW

1. The impact of inadequate pain control is very significant at the end of life. Fear of pain alone can intensify pain. Other factors that are a result of poor pain control include:
   1. Reducing the quality of life physically as well as socially.
   2. Reduction of suicidal thoughts.
   3. More energy.
   4. Low heart rate.
2. Pain can have harmful effects on humans. These include:
   1. Decreased anxiety.
   2. Increased pulmonary function.
3. Decreased gastric motility.
4. Increased output.
3. Physicians and nurses are aware of the potential harm of giving opioids. At the end of life this becomes even more of an issue, with the intent to relieve pain that might unintentionally hasten death versus providing medication to deliberately cause death. This dilemma is called:
   1. Double blind.
   2. Double effect.
   3. Equianalgesia.
   4. Justice over competency.

CHAPTER SUMMARY

- Pain is multifactorial and can be acute, chronic, or a combination of both; pain at the end of life is often a combination of acute and chronic pain.
- Pain is wholly subjective and there are no objective tests to measure its intensity or quality.
- Effectiveness of pain relief measures begin with effective communication and identification of the pain.
- There are multiple pain scales to assess pain in individuals who are cognitively alert and those who are cognitively impaired.
- A comprehensive assessment of pain includes the location and type of pain, history, intensity, characteristics, causes and current treatment interventions.
- Pain in older patients is often under treated and misunderstood; similarly pain in terminally ill children may not be adequately treated.

- Managing pain at the end of life is the culmination of the goals of palliative care.
- When contemplating pain medication in the terminally ill person, it is important to consider the intensity of the pain, the timing of the pain, the type of pain and the goals of care.
- Multiple medications and routes of administration are available for pain relief in the terminally ill person.
- Complementary and alternative therapies may be used in conjunction with pain medications to relieve pain in patients at the end of life.
- The impact of inadequate pain control concerns all aspects of a person's life, reducing the quality of one's physical, mental, social, and spiritual life.

CHAPTER REVIEW

Helen Anderson is a 73-year-old woman with advanced metastatic breast cancer and her prognosis is poor. She has been on 300 mcg Fentanyl patches for several months, using hydromorphone 8 mg every 4 hours for break-through pain. She states her chest pain and upper abdomen pain are intolerable, she is rating it at 10+, and denies any relief with any interventions. Helen has been admitted to the hospital for intractable pain control.

Understanding the benefits of pain control infusions, the nurse asked the physician about discontinuing the patches and starting Fentanyl IV 50 mcg/hr. However, the physician felt the patches should be left on, unless they were due to be changed. He started Helen on Fentanyl 25 mcg/hr without any demand dose.

Several hours later, the nurse phoned the doctor to report that Helen's pain was still so out of control she felt she needed to "jump out of the window." Nurses who had known Helen from previous admissions are quite sure her pain can be controlled. Helen had not had issues of psychological tolerance, just escalating cancer issues. The nurses know that Helen is not suicidal. However, the on-call physician was hesitant to change her medications, concerned that Helen may stop breathing and need Narcan.

Questions

Which of the realistic pain management goals for a terminally ill patient were not being met? What would you recommend for adequate pain control for Helen?

Suggested Response

Four factors are relevant: Helen's pain is not controlled; assessment and interventions are not being made frequently enough to adequately assess her pain; she has not been provided demand or **patient-controlled analgesia** (PCA) doses as needed to control her pain; and, because of the continuing level of pain, Helen does not have quality of life.

The palliative care resource nurse and/or pain management team should be consulted if present or available. The fentanyl patches were continued for her baseline pain and her infusion was changed to an equianalgesic hydromorphone infusing with patient-controlled analgesia (PCA) demand every 10 minutes and titrated every few hours until Helen was able to achieve satisfactory pain control. In time, her pain was controlled and titrated to the appropriate fentanyl patch dosing, with hydromorphone for breakthrough pain.

REFERENCES

Abraham, J. (2001). Pain management for dying patients: How to assess needs and provide pharmacologic relief. *Postgraduate Medicine, 110*(2), 99–100, 108–109, 113–114.

Agency for Health Care Research and Quality. (2002). Management of cancer symptoms: Pain, depression and fatigue. Retrieved from http://www.ahrq.gov/downloads/pub/evidence/pdf/cansymp/cansymp.pdf

American Geriatric Society. (2002). The management of persistent pain in older persons. *Journal of the American Geriatrics Society, 50*(s6), 205–224.

American Nurses Association. (2003). *Position statement: Pain management and control of distressing symptoms in dying patients.* Washington, DC: Author.

American Pain Society. (2000). *Treatment of pain at the end of life: A position statement from the American Pain Society.* Retrieved from http://www.ampainsoc.org/advocacy/treatment.htm

American Pain Society. (2003). *Principles of analgesic use in the treatment of acute pain and cancer pain* (5th ed). Glenview, IL: Author.

American Society of Pain Management Nurses. (2002). *Position statement on end of life care.* Retrieved from http://aspmn.org/Organization/documents/EndofLifeCare.pdf

Benedetti, C., Brock, C., Cleeland, C., Coyle, N., Dube, J. E., Ferrell, B. R., et al. (2000). NCCN practice guidelines for cancer pain. *Oncology (Huntington), 14*(11A), 135–150.

Berger, A., Portenoy, R. K., & Weissman, D. E. (2002). *Principles and practice of palliative care supportive oncology* (2nd ed.). New York: Lippincott Williams & Wilkins.

Bruckenthal, P., & D'Arcy, Y. (2007). Assessment and management of pain in older adults: A review of the basics. *Topics in Advanced Practice Nursing eJournal, 7*(1). Retrieved from http://www.medscape.com/viewarticle/556382

Bruera, E., Palmer, J. L., Bosnjak, S., Rico, M. A., Moyano, J., Sweeney, C., et al. (2004). Methadone versus morphine as a first-line strong opioid for cancer pain: A randomized, double-blind study. *Journal of Clinical Oncology, 22*(1), 185–192.

Bruera, E., & Sweeney, C. (2002). Methadone use in cancer patients with pain: A review. *Journal of Palliative Medicine, 5*(1), 127–138.

Byock, I., Sheils-Twohig, J., Merriman, M., & Collins, K. (2006). Promoting excellence in end-of-life care: A report on innovative models of palliative care. *Journal of Palliative Medicine, 9*(1), 137–151.

Dahl, J. (2005). How to reduce the fears of legal/regulatory scrutiny in managing pain in cancer patients. Available online from http://www.supportiveoncology.net/journal/articles/0305384.pdf

Davis, G., Hiemenz, M., & White T. (2002). Barriers to managing chronic pain of older adults with arthritis. *Journal of Nursing Scholarship, 34*(2), 121–126.

Delaware Pain Initiative. (2007). Equianalgesic chart. Retrieved from http://www.endpain.org/dosage.html

Dickerson, E., Benedetti, C., Davis, M., Grauer, P., Santa-Emma, P., Zafirides, P., et al. (2001). *Palliative care pocket consultant.* Dubuque, IA: Kendall/Hunt.

Doka, K., ed. (2006). *Pain management at the end of life.* Washington, DC: Hospice Foundation of America.

End-of-life Nursing Education Consortium (ELNEC). (2008). *Advanced end of life nursing care: ELNEC supercore training program 2008. Washington, DC: American Association of Colleges of Nursing.*

Ernst, E. (2004). Manual therapies for pain control: Chiropractic and massage. *Clinical Journal of Pain, 20*(1), 8–12.

Ersek, M. (1999). Enhancing effective pain management by addressing patient barriers to analgesic use. *Journal of Hospice and Palliative Nursing, 1*(3), 87–96.

Feldt, K. (2000). The checklist of nonverbal pain indicators. *Pain Management Nursing 1*(1), 13–21.

Ferrini, D., & Paice, J. (2004). How to initiate and monitor infusional lidocaine for severe and/or neuropathic pain. *Journal of Supportive Oncology, 2*(1), 90–4.

Fishman, S. (1999). *War on pain.* New York: Harper Collins.

Foley, K. (1995). A review of ethical and legal aspects of terminating medical care. *American Journal of Medicine (84),* 291–301.

Gélinas, C., Fillion, L., Puntillo, K., Viens, C., & Fortier, M. (2006). Validation of the critical-care pain observation tool in adult patients. *American Journal of Critical Care, 1*(4), 420–427.

Gordon, D. (2006). Fast facts and concepts #53, sublingual morphine (2nd ed.). EPERC-End-of-Life/Palliative Education Resource Center. Retrieved from www.eperc.mcw.edu

Gordon, D. B., Dahl, J., Phillips, P., Frandsen, J., Cowley, C., Foster, R. L., et al. (2005). The use of "as-needed" range orders for opioid analgesics in the management of acute pain: A consensus statement of the American Society of Pain Management Nursing and the American Pain Society. *Pain Management Nursing, 5*(2), 53–58.

Grealish, L., Lomasney, A., & Whiteman, B. (2000). Foot massage: A nursing intervention to modify the distressing symptoms of pain and nausea in patients hospitalized with cancer. *Cancer Nursing, 23*(3), 237–243.

Herr, K., Coyne, P., Key, T. R., Manworren, R., McCaffery, M., Merkel, S., et al. (2006). Pain assessment in the nonverbal patient: Position statement with clinical practice recommendations. *Pain Management Nursing, 7*(2), 44–52.

Horgas, A., & Tsai, P. (1998). Analgesic drug prescription and use in cognitively impaired nursing home residents. *Nursing Research, 47*(4), 235–242.

Hospice and Palliative Nursing Association (HPNA). (2004). HPNA position paper: Pain. *Journal of Hospice and Palliative Nursing 6*(1), 62–64.

Initiative for Pediatric Palliative Care. (2008). Module 2: Relieving pain and other symptoms. Retrieved from http://www.ippcweb.org/module2.asp

Institute for Clinical Systems Improvement. (2007). Palliative care health order set. Retrieved from http://www.icsi.org//guidelines_and_more/guidelines__order_sets___protocols/

International Association for the Study of Pain (IASP) Task Force on Taxonomy. (1979). Pain terms: A current list with definitions and notes on usage. *Pain 6*(3), 249–252.

Jacox, A., Carr, D. B., Payne, R., Berde, C. B., Breitbart, W., Cain, J. M., et al. (1994). *Management of cancer pain: Clinical practice guideline, No 9. AHCPR Publication No. 94-0592*. Rockville, MD: Agency for Healthcare Research and Quality, U.S. Department of Health and Human Services, Public Health Service.

Jusić, A. (2001). Psychological, emotional, spiritual and social aspects of pain. *Lijec Vjesn, 123*(1–2), 46–50.

Kaye, P. (1990). *Symptom control in hospice and palliative care*. Essex, CT: Hospice Education Institute.

Keefe, F., Abernethy, A., & Campbell, L. (2004). Psychological approaches to understanding and treating disease-related pain. *Annual Review Psychology, 56*, 601–630.

Khatta, M. (2007). A complementary approach to pain management. *Topics in Advance Practice Nursing eJournal, 7*(1). Retrieved from http://www.medscape.com/viewarticle/556408

Leleszi, J., & Lewandowski, J. (2005). Pain management in end-of-life care. *Journal of the American Osteopathic Association. 105*(3), 6–11.

Limaye, S. S., & Katz, P. (2006). Challenges of pain assessment and management in the minority elder population. *Annals of Long-Term Care, 14*(11). Retrieved from http://www.annalsoflongtermcare.com/article/6408

Lynn, J., & Harrold, J. (2006). *Handbook for mortals: Guidance for people facing serious illness*. Retrieved from http://www.mywhatever.com/cifwriter/library/mortals/mort2495.html

McCaffery, M. (1968). *Nursing practice theories related to cognition, bodily pain, and man-environment interactions*. Los Angeles: University of California at Los Angeles Students' Store.

McCaffery, M., & Pasero, C. (1999). Assessment: Underlying complexities, misconceptions, and practical tools. In M. McCaffery & C. Pasero (Eds.) *Pain: clinical manual* (2nd ed.). St. Louis: Mosby.

Miaskowski, C., Cleary, J., Burney, R., Coyne, P., Finley, R., Foster, R., et al. (2005). *American Pain Society Clinical Practice Guideline Series, No. 3: Guide for the management of cancer pain in adults and children*. Glenview, IL: American Pain Society.

Miller, C. C., Nelson, C. C., & Mezey, M. (2000). Comfort and pain relief in dementia: Awakening a new beneficence. *Journal of Gerontological Nursing, 26*(9), 32–40.

Miyoshi, H. R. (2001). Systemic nonopioid analgesics. In D. Loeser, S. H. Butler, R. Chapman, & D. C. Turk (Eds.). *Bonica's management of pain* (3rd ed.). Philadelphia: Lippincott Williams & Wilkins.

National Comprehensive Cancer Network (NCCN) Practice Guidelines. (2005). Oncology: Adult cancer pain: Version 1. Retrieved from http://www.nccn.org/professionals/physician_gls/PDF/pain.pdf

National Initiative on Pain Control. (2008). *Optimizing pain management in the older patient syllabus*. Secaucus, NJ: Professional Postgraduate Services.

Newshan, G. (1998). Transcending the physical: Spiritual aspects of pain in patients with HIV and/or cancer. *Journal of Advanced Nursing 28*(6), 1236–1241.

Norlander, L. (2001). *To comfort always: A nurse's guide to end of life care*. Washington, DC: American Nurses Association.

Paice, J. A., & Fine, P. G. (2001). Pain at the end of life. In B. F. Ferrell & N. Coyle (Eds.) *Textbook of palliative nursing* (2nd Edition, pp. 76–90). New York: Oxford University Press.

Panke, J. (2003). Difficulties in managing pain at the end of life. *Journal of Hospice and Palliative Nursing 5*(2), 83–90.

Pasero, C., & McCaffery, M. (2005). No self-report means no pain-intensity rating. *American Journal of Nursing, 105*(10), 50–55.

Prichett and Hull Associates, Inc. (2000). Pain scale. [Handout]. Atlanta: Authors.

Ripamonti, C., & Bianchi, M. (2002). The use of methadone for cancer pain. *Hematology-Oncology Clinics of North America, (16)*3, 543–555.

Saunders, C. (1970). Nature and management of terminal pain. In E. Shotter (Ed.) *Matters of life and death* (pp. 15–26). London: Darton Longman & Todd.

Saunders, C. (1976). The challenge of terminal care. In T. Symington & R. L. Carter (Eds.) *Scientific foundations of oncology* (pp. 673–679). London, England: Heinemann.

Shannon, K., & Bucknall, T. (2003). Pain assessment in critical care: What have we learned from research? *Intensive and Critical Care Nursing, 19*(3), 154–162.

Smith, M. C., Kemp, J., Hamphill, L., & Vojir, C. P. (2002). Outcomes of therapeutic massage for hospitalized cancer patients. *Journal of Nursing Scholarships, 34*(3), 257–262.

Solomon, M., Dokken, D., Fleishman, A., Heller, K., Levetown, M., Rushton, C., et al. (2002). The initiative for pediatric palliative care: Background and goals. Newton, MA: Education Developmental Center.

Springhouse. (2006). *End of life: A nurse's guide to compassionate care*. Philadelphia: Author.

Stephenson, N. L., Weinrich, S. P., & Tavakoli, A. S. (2000). The effects of foot reflexology on anxiety and pain in patients with breast and lung cancer. *Oncology Nursing Forum, 27*(1), 67–72.

Stephenson, R. (2004). Opioids in end of life care: Promises and problems. *North Carolina Medical Journal, 65*(4), 229–234.

Sykes, N., & Thorns, A. (2003). The use of opioids and sedatives at the end of life. *The Lancet Oncology, 4*(5), 312–318.

Syrjala, K. L., Donaldson, G. W., Davis, M. W., Kippes, M. E., & Carr, J. E. (1995). Relaxation and imagery and cognitive-behavioral training reduce pain during cancer treatment: A controlled clinical trial. *Pain, 63*(2), 189–198.

Thomas, J., et al. (2008). Methylnaltrexone for opioid-induced constipation in advanced illness. *New England Journal of Medicine, 358*(22), 2332–2343, 2400–2402.

Thorns, A., & Sykes, N. (2000). Opioid use in last week of life and implications for end-of-life decision-making. *Lancet, 356*(9227), 398–399.

Warden, V., Hurley, A. C., & Volicer, L. (2003). Development and psychometric evaluation of the pain assessment in advanced dementia scale. *Journal of the American Medical Association, 4*, 9–15.

Watson, M., Lucas, C., Hoy, A., & Back, I. (2005). *Oxford handbook of palliative care*. New York: Oxford University Press.

Whitcomb, L. A., Kirsh, K. L., & Passik, S. D. (2002). Substance abuse issues in cancer pain. *Cancer Pain and Headache Reports, 6*(3), 183–190.

Whitecar, P., Jonas, A., & Clasen, M. (2000). Managing pain in the dying patient. *American Family Physician, 61*(3), 755–770.

Wilkie, D. J., Kampell, J., Cutshall, S., Halabisky, H., Harmon, H., Johnson, L.P., et al. (2000). Effects of massage on pain intensity, analgesics and quality of life in patients with cancer pain: A pilot study of a randomized clinical trial conducted within hospice care. *The Hospice Journal, 15*(3), 31–53.

Wolfe, J., Grier, H. E., Klar, N., Levin, S. B., Ellenbogen, J. M., Salem-Schatz, S., et al. (2000). Symptoms and suffering at the end of life in children with cancer. *New England Journal of Medicine, 342*(26), 326–333.

Wong, D. L., Hockenberry-Eaton, M., Wilson, D., Winkelstein, M. L., & Schwartz, P. (2001). *Wong's essentials of pediatric nursing* (6th ed.). St. Louis: Mosby.

World Health Organization (WHO). (2007) WHO's Pain Ladder. *Cancer pain relief and palliative care*. Retrieved from http://www.who.int/cancer/palliative/painladder/en/

Ziegler, P. (2007). Chronic pain conundrums in primary-care practice *Pain Treatment Topics*. Retrieved from http://www.pain-topics.org/clinical_concepts/comments.php#Ziegler

Zwakhalen, S., Hamers, J., Abu-Saad, H. H., & Berger, M. (2006). Pain in elderly people with severe dementia: A systematic review of behavioral pain assessment tools. *BMC Geriatrics, 6*(3), 1471–1486.

USEFUL WEBSITES

American Academy of Hospice and Palliative Medicine
http://www.aahpm.org/

American Academy of Pain Medicine: Contains valuable fast fact sheets, which are peer-reviewed, up-to-date, one-page outlines of key information on important end-of-life clinical topics for end-of-life educators and clinicians.
http://www.painmed.org

American Alliance of Cancer Pain Initiatives
http://aspi.wisc.edu

American Geriatrics Society
http://www.americangeriatrics.org/

American Society of Pain Management Nursing
http://www.aspmn.org/

Cochrane Pain, Palliative and Supportive Care Collaborative Review Group
http://www.jr2.ox.ac.uk/cochrane/topics.html

End-of-Life Nursing Education Consortium Project (ELNEC)
http://www.aacn.nche.edu/elnec/

End of Life/Palliative Education Resource Center (EPERC)*
http://www.eperc.mcw.edu
http://www.eperc.mcw.edu/ff_pa.htm

Hospice and Palliative Nurses Association
http://www.hpna.org/

The Initiative for Pediatric Palliative Care (IPPC)
www.ippcweb.org.

National Comprehensive Cancer Network
www.nccn.org/professionals/physician_gls/PDF/pain.pdf

National Consensus Project for Quality Palliative Care Releases Clinical Practice Guidelines
http://www.nationalconsensusproject.org/

Palliative Care & JCAHO Standards
http://www.capc.org/content/279/J.pdf

Palliative Care Nursing
http://www.palliativecarenursing.net/index.html

World Health Organization (WHO) Pain and Palliative Care Communications Program
http://www.WHOcancerpain.wisc.edu

Non-Pain Symptom Management at the End of Life

OBJECTIVES   Following completion of this chapter, the learner will be able to:

5.1. Identify and describe non-pain symptoms commonly seen in patients at the end of life.

5.2. Describe specific assessment and treatment options based on these individual symptoms.

5.3. Compare and contrast disease processes with anticipated symptom needs.

The focus of this chapter is on the multiple non-pain physiological and other symptoms that may affect a patient at the end of life. Each of these symptoms is discussed separately and in depth, including the specific nursing interventions and treatment options that are appropriate for patients experiencing these symptoms at the end of life. The chapter concludes by comparing and contrasting these symptoms with disease processes that may occur in terminally ill patients.

PRETEST

1. Which is the most common symptom seen at the end of life?
   1. Pain
   2. Anorexia
   3. Fatigue
   4. Constipation
2. Which three symptoms are often confused?
   1. Depression, anxiety, asthenia
   2. Depression, delirium, and anxiety
   3. Anxiety, agitation, and anorexia
   4. Nausea, vomiting, and diarrhea
3. Manifestations of delirium include poor concentration, misinterpretations, and: (Select all that apply.)
   1. Rambling incoherent speech.
   2. Impaired level of consciousness.
   3. Clear speech.
   4. Impaired short-term memory.

4. Nonpharmacological interventions for dyspnea include:
   1. Fan, cool environment, and diversion.
   2. Heat, massage, and uncontrolled breathing.
   3. Wheelchair when the patient is not in bed, lying flat while in bed, and reading.
   4. Lying laterally, breathing into brown bag, and increased activity.
5. Symptoms become more severe as renal disease progresses. Which of these may be a symptom of renal failure? (Select all that apply.)
   1. Hiccups
   2. Muscle cramps
   3. Infections
   4. Metallic taste

GLOSSARY

agitation   The term refers to an unpleasant state of extreme arousal, increased tension, and irritability and is usually outwardly seen as restless behavior.

angina   Chest pain due to an inadequate supply of oxygen to the heart muscle, described as heaving, squeezing, severe and crushing, a feeling just behind the sternum of pressure and suffocation.

anhedonia   Absence of pleasure from the performance of acts that would ordinarily be pleasurable.

anorexia   An eating disorder characterized by markedly reduced appetite or total aversion to food.

anxiety   Feeling fear, stress, tension, apprehension, shortness of breath with or without underlying respiratory distress.

aphasia   Defect or loss of the power to express by speech, writing, or signs, or a defect or loss of the power of comprehension of spoken or written language.

ascites   Abnormal accumulation of fluid in the abdomen, serous fluid in the peritoneal cavity.

asthenia   Weakness, lack or loss of energy and strength.

cachexia   Physical wasting with loss of weight and muscle mass caused by disease.

debility   Weakness, loss of strength, an infirmity producing the state of being weak in health or body.

delirium   A sudden state of severe confusion with a rapid change in brain function, sometimes associated with hallucinations, hyperactivity, or reduced level of consciousness, in which the patient is inaccessible to normal contact.

depression   Medical illness characterized by persistent sadness, discouragement, and loss of self-worth. These feelings are accompanied by reduced energy and concentration, insomnia, decreased appetite and weight loss, bodily aches and pains.

dry eyes (xerophthalmia)   Lack of tears, necessary for the normal lubrication of eyes, to wash away particles and foreign bodies, with a feeling of burning, scratching, or stinging.

dysphagia   Difficulty when swallowing or the sensation that food is retained in the throat or upper chest.

dyspnea   Difficulty breathing, breathlessness, observed shortness of breath.

extrapyramidal symptoms   Physical symptoms, including tremor, slurred speech, akathesia (inner restlessness and the inability to sit or stand still), dystonia (involuntary muscle contractions, which force certain parts of the body into abnormal, sometimes painful, movements or postures, anxiety, distress, paranoia, and bradyphrenia (a slowing of thought processes), that are primarily associated with improper dosing of or unusual reactions to certain medication.

fatigue   Lessened capacity for work and reduced efficiency of accomplishment, usually accompanied by a feeling of weariness and tiredness, in response to physical exertion, emotional stress, boredom, or lack of sleep, or a nonspecific sign of a more serious psychological or physical cause.

insomnia   Patient's perception of inability to sleep, get rest, sleeplessness.

laser therapy   Any treatment using intense beams of light to precisely cut, burn, or destroy tissue.

orthopnea   The inability to breathe easily when lying down and is relieved when sitting up straight or standing erect.

paracentesis   The removal of fluid from a body cavity using a needle, trocar, cannula, or other hollow instrument, such as from inside the abdominal cavity—abdominal tap.

pleurodesis   A procedure that causes the membranes around the lung to stick together and prevents the buildup of fluid in the space between the membranes.

radiation therapy   The treatment of a disease by means of radiation. *External beam radiation* is the most common form, which aims high-powered X-rays directly at the tumor from outside of the body. *Internal beam radiation* uses radioactive seeds that are placed directly into or near the tumor; also called interstitial radiation or brachytherapy.

sleep disturbance   A disturbance of the normal sleep pattern, including difficulty falling or staying asleep, falling asleep at inappropriate times, disturbances in the amount, quality, or timing of sleep, disruption in sleep pattern or inability to sleep.

stomatitis   Literally means inflammation of the mouth or of the mucous lining of any of the structures in the mouth.

supportive therapy   Treatment given to prevent, control, or relieve complications and side effects and to improve the patient's comfort and quality of life.

thoracentesis   Removal of fluid in the pleura/chest cavity through a needle; pleural tap.

xerostomia   Dry mouth, the condition of not having enough saliva to keep the mouth wet, resulting from thickened or reduced saliva flow.

SECTION ONE: Common Non-Pain Symptoms in End-of-Life Care

In palliative nursing, common symptom management as well as **supportive therapy** at the end of life can have a positive impact on a patient's physical, emotional, psychosocial and spiritual well-being (International Association of Hospice and Palliative Care, 2006). For example, a patient with severe dyspnea could be expected to have difficulty maintaining a satisfactory conversation with family members. Conversely, successful symptom management would ideally have a positive impact on both the physical and social aspects of the same patient. Treatment of distressing symptoms and associated side effects incorporates pharmacological, nonpharmacological, and complementary/supportive therapies and mandates a holistic approach (DeLima, 2006; Grocott & Dealey, 2004; International Association of Hospice and Palliative Care, 2006).

The goals of care and anticipated outcomes are based on the patient's quality of life and individualized, personal goals. Members of the health care team consider and monitor all aspects of care ensuring that the terminally ill person's comfort needs are met and that the individual and family members receive appropriate supportive care. A multisymptom approach is extremely important to consider as a patient is nearing the end of life. Assessment, plan, intervention, and evaluation are key components to offset the multiple symptoms that have an impact on the quality of life for patients facing terminal illness and their families (Institute for Clinical Symptoms Improvement, 2007).

This section is divided into an overview of the more commonly seen symptoms in these patients. The reader is cautioned to remember that signs and symptoms are not distinguished, but the more generic term *symptoms* is used to incorporate both signs and symptoms. Secondly, the symptoms are arranged alphabetically, not in order of priority or incidence. A preview of the presented symptoms may be found in Box 5–1.

Agitation

Agitation refers to an unpleasant state of extreme arousal, increased tension, and irritability and is usually outwardly seen as restless behavior. Extreme agitation can lead to confusion, hyperactivity, and outright hostility, which affects the quality of life for patients, families, and care providers. Agitation can come on suddenly or gradually and can last for minutes, weeks, or months. Pain, stress, and fever can all increase agitation. Agitation by itself may not have great clinical significance, but in combination with other symptoms can be an indicator of a disease state. Agitation is often closely associated with infections, anxiety, depression, bipolar disorder, and schizophrenia (Quijada & Billings, 2002).

As with other symptoms, it is important to identify any specific underlying cause or contributing factors. Multiple factors may lead to agitation, including but not limited to pain, hypoxia, metabolic/electrolyte abnormalities, infection, urinary retention,

---

BOX 5–1   Common Non-Pain Symptoms Encountered by Patients at the End of Life

- Agitation
- Anorexia/Cachexia
- Anxiety
- Constipation
- Cough
- Delirium
- Depression
- Diarrhea
- Dry eyes/dry nose
- Dyspnea
- Fatigue
- Fever
- Hiccups
- Nausea/Vomiting
- Secretions
- Sleep disturbances
- Skin and wound care
- Stomatitis
- Xerostomia

---

and constipation. Additional causes of agitation may include trauma, sleep and sensory deprivation, and medications, both prescribed and recreational drugs. Disruption of one's usual routine or familiar surroundings along with psychological, emotional, and spiritual distress may also contribute to agitation (Inouye, 2006; Watson, Lucas, Hoy, & Black, 2005; Weissman, 2005a).

The health care provider can initiate simple strategies to manage agitation. For example, if appropriate, ensure the patient uses prescribed glasses or hearing aids as needed. Sensory stimulation in the environment can be controlled by keeping doors closed to noisy halls or decreasing the volume to low on electronic equipment. Maintaining the patient's usual routine as closely as possible promotes comfort and lessens agitation. Avoid the use of any type of physical restraint, as these increase a person's agitation.

Medications may also be employed to lessen agitation. Some of the more frequently used medications for agitation include haloperidol (Haldol®) 0.5 to 5 mg every 30 minutes as needed and lorazepam (Ativan®) 0.5 to 2 mg every 2 hours. These two medications are recommended for patients withdrawing from alcohol or benzodiazepines and who can clearly articulate symptoms of anxiety. The medications should be used with caution in older patients, as they may cause paradoxical agitation (Elsayem, Driver, & Bruera, 2003; Institute for Clinical Symptoms Improvement, 2007; Quijada & Billings, 2002; Watson et al., 2005; Wiseman, 2005a).

Anorexia and Cachexia

Anorexia refers to the loss of desire to eat, while **cachexia** refers to the weight loss. Each may significantly impair the patient's ability to continue with further therapy. Both of these symptoms are found in many severe medical conditions, including cancer, AIDS, chronic obstructive pulmonary disease, congestive heart failure, chronic liver and kidney disease, and infections. Anorexia is a common symptom at the end of life and decreased intake is almost always seen in the last few weeks of life (Cline, 2006).

Treatable causes of anorexia and cachexia should be identified and addressed. Causes may include pain, depression, gastrointestinal tract dysfunction, and cognitive impairment. Stimulation of appetite through the use of progesterones and corticosteroids may help. However, these agents are associated with an increased risk of thromboembolic events, peripheral edema, hyperglycemia, hypertension, and Cushing's syndrome and each should be used with careful observation (International Association of Hospice and Palliative Care, 2007). Corticosteroids may provide a temporary improvement in appetite and food intake. However, because of significant side effects, this category of drugs should probably be used in those patients who may simultaneously benefit from the antiemetic and analgesic properties of the steroids (End of Life Nursing Consortium [ELNEC], 2008).

In some cases the patient is less disturbed than the family by poor nutritional intake and lack of appetite (Cline, 2006). To prevent family conflict, staff should explore the meaning of food within the context of the family's cultural and religious background, and help identify alternate steps to take to promote congenial participation in the patient's care. Additionally, help the patient and family to understand that dehydration and malnutrition/starvation do not cause suffering, but that abstinence from food and fluids can be a normal process (International Association of Hospice and Palliative Care, 2007). A more in-depth discussion on this topic may be found in Chapter 6.

Strategies to control or diminish anorexia include offering cold, appealing, and smaller portions of foods and drinks, minimizing dietary restrictions, and utilizing a dietician/nutritionist. Large portions served in a large plate are often overwhelming, causing further reluctance to eat. Decreasing odors is beneficial, as some aromas that might be stimulating for healthy individuals can become unpleasant to ill individuals, particularly in the late stages of disease. Offering alcoholic drinks can be appealing and increase appetite; wine, sherry, and beer have significant calories and are well-known appetite stimulants, especially in small quantities. Caution should be used with alcohol ingestion if the patient is taking multiple medications, because the intake of alcohol with prescribed medications could trigger adverse effects.

Artificial hydration and/or nutrition should be implemented, if the treatment is not medically futile, for a time-limited trial with an endpoint and goals. It is important to attempt to honor patient/family wishes if risks, benefits, outcomes, and goals of care are understood (Center to Advance Palliative Care [CAPC], 2005b). See Chapter 6 on hydration and nutrition for a more in-depth discussion on this topic area.

Medications that may assist the individual who is experiencing anorexia and cachexia include Dexamethasone 2–6 mg daily, megestrol acetate (Megase®)160 mg, with a maximum dose of 800 mg/day, medroxyprogesterone acetate (Depo-Provera®) 100 mg 3 times a day, metoclopramide (Reglan®)10–20 mg 4 times a day, or dronabinol (Marinol®) 2.5–5 mg 2 to 3 times a day. For the patient experiencing multisymptoms such as depression or respiratory complications in conjunction with anorexia and cachexia, the medication of choice is mirtazapine (Remeron®) 15–45 mg at bedtime. If the patient has chronic obstructive pulmonary disease or AIDS, anabolic steroids should also be administered (CAPC, 2007; Elsayem et al., 2003; Finnish Medical Society, 2005; Watson et al., 2005).

Anxiety

Affective disorders such as **anxiety** and depression are common in seriously ill patients and can adversely affect their quality of life. Not only can both conditions cause physical symptoms such as nausea, dyspnea, and **insomnia,** but the presence of these physical symptoms can exacerbate anxiety and depression as well. Even undertreated pain can exacerbate psychological distress, including shortness of breath and dyspnea (Watson et al., 2005).

Benzodiazepines are often helpful in the treatment of anxiety. Lorazepam is preferred since it does not have active metabolites. Some individuals may manifest a paradoxical reaction to benzodiazepines, becoming more agitated. Patients with chronic anxiety frequently respond more favorably to the use of antidepressants, such as serotonin-specific or serotonin-norepinephrine reuptake inhibitors. However, these antidepressants require treatment for weeks before the patient reaches a therapeutic level.

Additional medications to consider for treatment of anxiety include: lorazepam (Ativan®) 0.25–2 mg every 4 hours; alprazolam (Xanax®) 0.25–0.5 mg 3 times a day; clonazepam (Klonopin®) 0.25–0.5 mg 2 times a day; sertraline (Zoloft®) 25–50 mg 1 time a day; and citalopram (Celexa®) 20–30 mg 1 time a day (Center to Advance Palliative Care [CAPC], 2005a, 2007; Elsayem et al., 2003; Finnish Medical Society, 2005; Watson et al., 2005).

Health care providers should remember that the more effective means of treating anxiety is to use a team approach and involve social services, psychology, and chaplaincy services as appropriate. Educate patients and families about use of non-pharmacologic interventions such as guided imagery, effective breathing techniques, and relaxation techniques.

Constipation

Constipation is a common and troublesome symptom for seriously ill patients. Immobility, decreased oral intake, and medications, as well as underlying medical conditions, can contribute to decreased gastrointestinal motility. Abdominal distention or bloating, less frequent movement, fullness, pressure, and pain are common complaints. As many as 95% of patients treated with opioids will experience constipation; all opioids are associated to some degree with constipation. Therefore a prophylactic bowel regime with stool softeners and/or laxatives is needed (Economou, 2006).

Constipation can exacerbate other symptoms common at the end of life, including nausea and anorexia. Constipation can also cause hemorrhoids or anal fissures that are painful and potential sites for infection. Strategies to prevent or alleviate constipation include adding prunes or other fibrous fruits to the patient's diet and ensuring adequate hydration. Some patients have reported that coffee and licorice serve as stimulants. Stool softeners and stimulant laxatives, such as bisacodyl and senna, can be effective in preventing continuing constipation. Patients on scheduled opioids should prophylactically and routinely receive stool softeners and stimulant laxatives on a daily basis, unless contraindicated. Some patients, particularly those with neurogenic bowels, benefit from scheduled suppositories or enemas (Hallenbeck, 2005a). Because of inadequate fluid intake, fiber supplements are generally not used in seriously ill patients.

Medications that can assist with preventing or treating constipation include: docusate (Colace®) 100–400 mg 2 times a day; glycerin or bisacodyl (Dulcolax®) suppository daily; senna 1–4 tablets 2 times a day; combination senna/docusate (Senokot S®) 1–4 tabs 2 times a day; bisacodyl 5–10 mg 1 time a day; magnesium hydroxide (Milk of Magnesia®) 30 ml at bedtime; 70% sorbitol 15–30 ml 1 time a day; and lactulose 15–30 ml 1 time a day (CAPC, 2005a; Elsayem et al., 2003; Finnish Medical Society, 2005; Hallenbeck, 2005a; Watson et al., 2005). For patients whose constipation is opioid induced, methylnaltrexone bromide (Relistor®) 8 or 12 mg (weight based) every other day and continue with other bowel regimen (Thomas et al., 2008).

Cough

Thirty-nine to eighty percent of palliative care patients will experience cough-related problems (Dudgeon, 2006; Estfan & LeGrand, 2004). Cough, similar to dyspnea, can be very frustrating and debilitating for the patient, leading to pain, fatigue, vomiting, and insomnia. An ongoing cough can be a frequent reminder of the progression of the disease process. Cough is frequently present in advanced diseases such as bronchitis, congestive heart failure, HIV/AIDS, and various cancers; however, the greatest incidence is in patients diagnosed with lung cancer. Coughs vary in intensity and there are three types of cough: acute; chronic or persistent; or nocturnal.

The primary goal of care is to treat the underlying cause, if possible. Pain may prevent the patient from coughing effectively and thus exaggerate the cough. Gastroesophageal reflux disease can produce an irritating cough. Reducing the pH of refluxed gastric fluid may minimize irritation of the airways. Postnasal drainage from chronic sinusitis is a common cause of cough. Dysphagia can result in aspiration of liquids. Thickening the consistency of fluids for patients having difficulty swallowing may reduce aspiration and cough (Estfan & LeGrand, 2004).

Medications that can assist the patient with cough control include: guaiafenesin with dextromethorphan (100 mg/10 mg per 5 ml), 5 to 10 ml every 2 hours; guaiafenesin with codeine (100 mg/10 mg per 5 ml), 5 to 10 ml every 2 hours; benzonatate

(Tessalon Perles®), 200 mg 3 times a day; and lidocaine 20 mg in 2 ml (premixed), nebulized, every 4 hours as needed for cough. When administering this latter medication, avoid administration within two hours of eating to decrease the risk of aspiration (CAPC, 2005a, 2007; Dudgeon, 2006; Elsayem et al., 2003; Finnish Medical Society, 2005; Watson et al., 2005).

Delirium

Delirium is an acute state of confusion and the incidence of delirium rises with age. While delirium can occur in any clinical setting, delirium is more frequently seen in hospitalized patients, with a prevalence of up to 24% upon admission and an overall incidence of up to 50% during the hospitalization (Inouye, 2006). Some settings present an even greater risk. It is estimated that 50% of older patients may develop delirium after surgery with another 75% of elders developing delirium in the intensive care unit setting (Inouye, 2006).

Delirium is a clinical syndrome, not a disease in itself. Its etiology is usually multifactorial, and includes central nervous system injury, fluid and electrolyte abnormalities, hypoxia, and other metabolic abnormalities. Additional causes of delirium include infection and pain (International Association of Hospice and Palliative Care, 2007). Functional dependence, polypharmacy, sensory impairments, and the existence of chronic health problems are factors that increase the risk for delirium (Quijada & Billings, 2002). Acute changes in mental status, with disorientation, fluctuations of attentiveness, and rambling incoherent speech are hallmarks of delirium. Paranoid ideas, restlessness, disorientation, and hallucinations may also be observed. Patients often present with hyperactivity, agitation, and combativeness, though hypoactive delirium marked by lethargy is equally serious (Kuebler, English, & Heidrich, 2006). Delirium is particularly prevalent in patients with preexisting dementia (Grocott & Dealey, 2004).

Patients with a diagnosis of delirium tend to have a poorer prognosis. For example, in-hospital mortality rates for patients with delirium range from 22% to 76%, and the one-year mortality rates approach 40% (Inouye, 2006). There are no specific diagnostic tests, but assessment should include review of all medications, especially psychoactive drugs, general physical evaluation, including vital signs, hydration status, and oxygenation, presence of pain, and recent alcohol or substance use. A focused search for infection, metabolic abnormalities, and other acute illness is critical. In elders, delirium may be the only harbinger of serious illness or complications (Dahlin & Coyne, 2006).

Treatment of delirium requires correction of underlying abnormalities, decreasing insomnia, fear, noise, and unfamiliar surroundings. Reorientation or familiarity with family and objects, along with a restful environment, may be helpful. Some patients may find touch helpful; others withdraw or become further agitated. When behavioral symptoms threaten the safety of the patient or the ability to receive therapy, psychotropic medications may be used with caution, because many of the medications administered to patients with delirium may cause **extrapyramidal symptoms.**

Haloperidol remains the first drug of choice, with the best evidence base supporting its effectiveness. Lower doses are recommended in the elderly. Benzodiazepines are not recommended for single therapy because the risk of paradoxical stimulation, over-sedation, and possibly prolonging delirium, but can be useful adjuncts if haloperidol alone is not effective (Morrison & Liao, 2007). No solid evidence exists for the use of other psychotropic drugs for delirium (Weissman, 2005a).

Medications that are indicated in patients with delirium may be found in Box 5–2.

Depression

Most patients who are terminally ill develop sadness at some point during their illness. These feelings can be very intense and may be associated with a sense of hopelessness and helplessness. An estimated 22 to 75% of patients at the end of life experience clinical **depression** (Periyakoil & Hallenbeck, 2002). However, depression is not inevitable and should not be considered a normal part of the dying process. Diagnosing depression can be challenging because many of the typical somatic symptoms, including fatigue, insomnia, anorexia, weight loss, and irritability,

can be caused by the underlying medical illness or medications (Pasacreta, Minarik, & Nield-Anderson, 2006). Psychological symptoms such as apathy, **anhedonia,** as well as feelings of worthlessness and hopelessness may suggest the diagnosis.

Sadness and grief are often confused with depression and it is important to differentiate grief from depression. Grieving can be an appropriate response to loss, but if it persists in conjunction with apathy and feelings of hopelessness and affects the patient's quality of life, it mandates consideration of depression. Simply asking a patient, "Are you depressed?" can be a useful screening tool. Evaluation of depression requires a careful interdisciplinary team assessment and approach (Arnold, 2005). Consider involving a medical counselor or therapist as well as a spiritual counselor.

Nonpharmacologic measures for affective disorders such as depression are often beneficial. Some of the interventions that assist persons who are depressed include counseling, support groups, and/or talking about the feelings of depression with members of the interdisciplinary team. Additional measures to assist with depression are activities such as walking, listening to music, reading a favorite book, or watching a favorite movie or television show. Some patients find keeping a journal allows them an acceptable avenue for expressing their feelings.

There are also pharmacological measures that assist with depression. Serotonin-specific reuptake inhibitors are drugs of first choice, including older and frail patients. However, it may take weeks to reach a therapeutic response. Psychostimulants such as methylphenidate (Conserta® or Ritalin®) can produce a more rapid response, and are well tolerated in most patients. In patients with a life expectancy of more than a few weeks, a successful therapeutic trial of psychostimulants should be followed by an antidepressant medication such as a serotonin-specific reuptake inhibitor (Warm & Weissman, 2005).

Additional medications to be considered with patients who are depressed include: serotonin-specific reuptake inhibitors (SSRI), usually given no more than 1 time a week; escitalopram (Lexapro®), 5–10 mg 1 time a day; citalopram (Celexa®), 10 mg 1 time a day; sertraline (Zoloft®), 25–50 mg 1 time a day; and a psychostimulant such as methylphenidate (Concerta®, Ritalin®), 5 mg 30 to 60 minutes before breakfast and lunch. Other medications that may be effective include mirtazapine (Remeron®), 7.5 to 15 mg 1 time a day (Arnold, 2005; Elsayem et al., 2003; Pasacreta et al., 2006; Watson et al., 2005; Warm & Weissman, 2005).

BOX 5–2   **Medications for Patients Experiencing Delirium**

- Haloperidol (Haldol®) 0.5–1.0 mg; titrate at 2.0–5.0 mg every hour, then administer two or three times per day with a maximum dose of 30 mg per day; IV haloperidol may cause less extrapyramidal symptoms than oral haloperidol
- Chlorpromazine (Thorazine®) 10–25 mg every 4–6 hours, maximum dose 600 mg/day
- Midazolam (Versed®) 0.5 mg every 1–2 hours
- Oisperidone (Risperdol®) 0.5–1 mg at bedtime or twice daily (age related); *avoid in patient with cerebrovascular disease*
- Methotrimeprazine (Levomeprom®) 12.5–50 mg at bedtime or twice daily
- Olanzapine (Zyprexa®) 2.5–5 mg at bedtime; *avoid in patient with cerebrovascular disease*
- Quetiapine (Seroquel®) 25–50 mg twice a day
- Promazine (Sparine®) 25 mg at bedtime

For patients who are acutely disturbed, violent, aggressive:

- Haloperidol (Haldol®) 2.5–5 mg with lorazepam 0.5–2 mg; may repeat every 20 to 30 minutes (but risk of paradoxical agitation), then every 1 to 2 hours, to a maximum dose of 10 mg per day

Source: Elsayem et al., 2003; Inouye, 2006; Kuebler et al., 2006; Weissman, 2005a; Quijada & Billings, 2002; Watson et al., 2005

Diarrhea

Diarrhea, less common than constipation at the end of life, can have a significant impact on quality of life. Diarrhea increases the risk for dehydration, electrolyte imbalance, skin breakdown, and fatigue. Causes of diarrhea may include: medications such as laxatives, antibiotics, chemotherapy, antacids, magnesium supplements, malignancy, fistula, ileal resection, gastrectomy or colectomy, and other diseases, including inflammatory bowel disease and AIDS. The presence of diarrhea does not exclude the possibility of bowel impaction as the effect of gut flora on fecal material can cause liquefaction and subsequent passage of loose stool. Diarrhea due to *Clostridium difficile* infection must be excluded. When present, this can be difficult to treat, and an individual may require more than one round of treatment if symptoms persist.

Assessment of the underlying causal factor is the first step to treatment. Ensure adequate hydration; encourage sips of clear liquids if tolerated; IV hydration should be considered for severe dehydration. Simple carbohydrates such as toast or crackers replenish small amounts of electrolytes and glucose. Milk, dairy products, and other lactose containing products should be avoided (Alderman, 2003). Additional foods to avoid include carbonated beverages or sorbitol, foods high in fat, spicy, high-fiber foods, and those high in sugar and caffeine content (Economou, 2006).

Medications that assist in preventing diarrhea include: kaolin and pectin (Kaopectate®); loperamide (Imodium®), 4 mg to 4 to 8 mg 1 time per day, though up to 54 mg per day of loperamide have been used in palliative care settings with few adverse effects; diphenoxylate hydrochloride/atropine sulfate (Lomotil®), 2 tab or 10 mL of solution 4 times a day; octreotide (Sandostatin®) 10–80 g per hour; and psyllium (Metamucil®, Fibersure®) stool bulking agents (Alderman, 2003; Economou, 2006; Elsayem et al., 2003; Watson et al., 2005).

Dry Eyes/Dry Nose

Drying of eyes and nose are common symptoms in terminally ill persons. Contributing factors for both symptoms include dry air, medications, dehydration, environmental conditions, and oxygen use. Treatment for **dry eyes (xerophthalmia)** includes the addition of humidity in the room, and medications that assist with this condition include artificial tears. Treatment for dry nose includes the addition of humidity in the room or to the oxygen source, and medications include saline nasal spray or gel as needed (Elasyem et al., 2003; Institute for Clinical Systems Improvement, 2007; Watson et al., 2005).

Dyspnea

Dyspnea is often experienced at the end of life and is defined as the subjective sensation of difficult breathing. Neither the patient's respiratory rate nor the level of oxygenation by oximetry can predict the severity of dyspnea. Some of the common causes include obstructing tumors, radiation therapy, chemotherapy, pulmonary embolism, pleural effusions, **thoracentesis,** diuresis, infections, heart failure, fluid overload, abdominal **ascites,** and superior vena cava syndrome. Dyspnea is also caused by severe lung or heart disease, anemia, anxiety, and electrolyte imbalance (Weissman, 2005b).

The endpoint for managing dyspnea should be the patient's self-report of diminished breathlessness. Oximetry, pulmonary function tests, chest imaging, and other diagnostic evaluations should be performed only if they are required for treatment interventions. The impact on function and the patient's level of satisfaction toward quality of life drives the goals of care. It is important to evaluate the patient's ability to sleep, perform activities of daily living, and engage socially with family and friends. Patients may report breathlessness in spite of adequate oxygenation levels or less severe disease states (Dudgeon, 2006).

Treatment of dyspnea should be focused on eliminating the underlying cause, when possible, and managing symptoms. Pharmacologic methods include oxygen, opioids, and anxiolytics. Oxygen is generally better tolerated via a nasal cannula than by mask, as patients have reported a feeling a suffocation when oxygen is delivered via a mask (Weissman, 2005b). Benzodiazepines, such as lorazepam, are useful when anxiety is a significant contributing factor. However, patients need to be monitored for sedation when combining benzodiazepines and opioids (Weissman, 2005). Low-dose opioids are often used for relieving dyspnea. Morphine sulfate is the best studied and most used medication for dyspnea and may be administered by the oral, buccal, subligual, or intravenous route. Morphine decreases dyspnea by dilating capacitance vessels, decreasing preload and oxygen consumption, and lowering sympathetic tone (Jantarakupt & Porock, 2005; Weissman, 2005b). Other opioids likely have a similar mechanism of action and can be used if morphine is contraindicated. Respiratory suppression, which may be reversed by administering naloxone (Narcan®), is a potential side effect, especially in opioid naive patients. Careful titration of the opioid dose to treat the patient's symptoms usually avoids this problem. Additional medications to be considered may be found in Box 5–3.

Basic nursing care for the patient with dyspnea may be as simple as elevating the head of the bed or having the patient

---

BOX 5–3   Medications for Patients Experiencing Dyspnea

- Oxygen per nasal cannula, 2 liters/minute and titrate as needed
- Morphine sulfate, 2.5–10 mg PO/SL or 1–2 mg IV every 1 hour prn
- Oxycodone, 2.5–10 mg every hour
- Lorazepam (Ativan®), 0.25–1 mg every 2 hours

For patients with rales:

- Furosemide (Lasix®), 20–40 mg 1 time

For patients who experience wheezing:

- Nebulized albuterol, every 4 hours
- Nebulized ipatropium (Atrovent®), every 4 hours
- Albuterol and ipatropium can be combined (e.g., Duoneb®)

Source: Del Fabbro, Dalal, & Bruerea, 2006; Elsayem et al., 2003; International Association of Hospice and Palliative Care, 2007; Watson et al., 2005; Weissman, 2005b

sit forward in an upright position. This reduces the sensation of choking and promotes expansion of the lungs. Teaching the patient pursed lip breathing slows respiratory rate and decreases small airway collapse. Having the patient inhale completely and exhale slowly decreases the rate of respirations and aids in distraction. Nonpharmacologic treatment may include repositioning, improving air circulation, maintaining cool room temperatures, and using relaxation techniques. Finally, for some patients, prayer promotes comfort and relaxation (International Association of Hospice and Palliative Care, 2007).

Performing continuous oximetry, pulmonary function tests, chest imaging, and other diagnostic evaluations should only be implemented if the results would support a change in therapeutic interventions. Other means of aggressive and invasive treatments include thoracentesis, **pleurodesis**, stent tube placement, and radiation or **laser therapy. Paracentesis** may be employed if dyspnea is secondary to ascites.

Fatigue

Fatigue is defined with decreased vitality in physical functioning and may affect mental functioning. Fatigue is reported by more than 90% of patients at the end of life and is frequently the most distressing symptom for these patients (Bailey, 2004). Activity is decreased and there is increased dependency and a diminished sense of control and self-determination. Physical symptoms include generalized weakness, feeling of heavy limbs, insomnia, and unrestful sleep. Cognitively, patients may have short-term memory loss, diminished concentration and attention (Bailey, 2004). Assessment tools that assist in determining the degree of patient fatigue include the Memorial Symptom Assessment Scale, the Edmonton Functional Assessment Tool, the Multidimensional Fatigue Symptom Inventory, and the Profile of Mood States (ELNEC, 2008).

Causes of fatigue may include infection, hypoxemia, anemia, electrolyte abnormalities, sedating medications, and chemotherapy. Fatigue may be a symptom of nutritional imbalance/impairment, cachexia and anorexia, deconditioning, and weakness. Sleep disturbance, depression, and emotional or psychological distress contribute to fatigue. Uncontrolled pain as well as progression of the underlying disease processes may be directly linked to fatigue (Reisfield & Wilson, 2007).

Managing fatigue includes treating the underlying causes, if possible, as well as using nonpharmacologic and pharmacologic therapies directed toward the symptom itself. Nonpharmacologic treatment includes patient education, modifying the activities of daily living, and scheduling frequent rest periods during the day. Keeping a daily log or journal of sleep/rest/fatigue patterns may be helpful. Clinicians should counsel patients to prioritize activities and pace themselves accordingly. Mild exercise for brief periods may be beneficial in reducing the perception of fatigue for some patients (Agency for Health Care Research and Quality, 2002).

Pharmacologic treatment of fatigue includes erythropoietin, psychostimulants, and corticosteroids. Psychostimulants such as methylphenidate, dextroamphetamine, and modafanil may also be beneficial in managing fatigue. Due to significant side effects, corticosteroids should be reserved for terminally ill patients who may complain of nausea and vomiting. Medications that may make the patient more tired should be administered at bedtime rather than in the morning (Anderson & Dean, 2006). For example, sedatives and opioids taken to manage other symptoms may increase lethargy and fatigue.

Specific medications may be used to treat fatigue that has a specific etiology. Data to support the use of mediations to treat nonspecific fatigue are limited (Institute for Clinical Systems Improvement, 2007). The following medications are recommended: methylphenidate (Concerta®, Ritalin®), 5 mg every 2 hours; dextroamphetamine (Dexadrine®), 5–60 mg in 2 to 3 divided doses daily; prednisone, 7.5–10 mg daily; dexamethasone, 1–2 mg 1 time a day; methylprednisolone, 32 mg 1 time a day; and megestrol acetate (Megase®), 160 mg 3 times a day (Bailey, 2004; Elsayem et al., 2003; Institute for Clinical Systems Improvement, 2007; Reisfield & Wilson, 2007; Watson et al., 2005).

Fever

Fevers are common at the end of life. Because patients near the end of life often have concomitant medical conditions, it can be difficult to establish the cause of a fever and the treatment options. If the fever is a new onset, the cause may be an infection. Patients near the end of life may choose not to treat the cause of the fever, but only to receive comfort measures, such as cool baths, a cool washcloth placed on the person's forehead, and adequate fluid intake.

Fevers often respond to analgesics. Acetaminophen is a relatively nontoxic method to decrease fever, and enhance comfort. Daily doses in excess of 4 grams per day have been associated with liver toxicity. For fever that is unresponsive to acetaminophen, a nonsteroidal anti-inflammatory drug (NSAID) may be alternated with the acetaminophen so that the patient either receives a NSAID or acetaminophen every 2 hours. NSAIDs should be used cautiously in patients with renal impairment and history of gastrointestinal bleeding. To decrease the risk of NSAID-induced gastrointestinal bleeding, a proton-pump inhibitor may be prescribed (Elsayem et al., 2003; International Association of Hospice and Palliative Care, 2007; Watson et al., 2005).

Hiccups

Hiccups, also called singultus, can be common at the end of life. They are distressing to patients and families and have a significant impact on quality of life, disrupting sleep, causing fatigue, anxiety, depression, and inability to eat (Dahlin & Goldsmith, 2006). An involuntary reflex involving the respiratory muscles of the chest and diaphragm, a single episode can last for a few seconds to as long as several days. If they last longer than 48 hours hiccups are termed persistent; longer than one month, intractable (Farmer, 2007). Causes of hiccups include stress/excitement, cancer, myocardial infarction, esophageal or gastric distension, liver disease, uremia, IV steroids, and central nervous system lesions (Smith & Busracamwongs, 2003).

If the cause of hiccups can be identified, it is preferable to direct the treatment at the specific cause. However, many times a cause cannot be identified and general symptom measures are implemented. Nonpharmacologic treatments include holding one's breath, breathing into a paper bag, biting a lemon, swallowing sugar, taking long and slow drinks of water, compression of the nose while swallowing, acupuncture, and valsalva maneuver.

Pharmacologic approaches are often the most rational therapies for these patients, although treatment options can include nonpharmacologic agents well as. Unfortunately, the same agents that are used to treat hiccups may also cause them. Chlorpromazine (Thorazine®) 25–50 mg every 6 hours is the only FDA approved drug for hiccups. Baclofen 5 mg every 8 hours seems to be a promising drug for use with both palliative care and perioperative patients, and using garabentin as an addition to baclofen may also be a reasonable option to consider. While baclofen does not eliminate hiccups, it does provide symptomatic relief for some patients. Other agents that have been used include: haloperidol, promethazine, prochlorperazine, metoclopramide, gabapentin, nifedipine and sertraline, amitriptyline, amantidine, quinidine, ranitidine, and clonazepam (Elsayem et al., 2003; Farmer, 2007; Smith & Busracamwongs, 2003; Watson et al., 2005).

Nausea and Vomiting

Nausea and vomiting can have a profound effect on physical and mental functioning and thus have a profound impact on one's quality of life. Nausea and vomiting are generally more debilitating in patients with cancer, AIDS, and hepatic and renal failure. Causes of nausea and vomiting include medications, gastrointestinal obstruction, uremia, psychological distress (particularly those related to odors and secondhand smoke) and vestibular stimuli. All triggers that cause nausea and vomiting should be controlled or eliminated if possible.

Treatment consists of nonpharmacologic and pharmacologic treatment, while evaluating and treating the underlying cause. Nonpharmacologic treatment consists of relaxation, acupuncture, and transcutaneous electrical wave stimulation. Dietary interventions with ginger, ginger ale, tea, sips of clear liquids, sports drinks, and crackers are often effective. Because of their effectiveness, bananas, rice, applesauce, and toast are referred to as the BRAT diet, an effective combination of dietary foods in alleviating nausea and vomiting (Hallenbeck, 2005a).

Pharmacologic therapy centers on the central neurotransmitters of nausea and vomiting (dopamine, serotonin, histamine and substance P), though peripheral mechanoreceptors and chemoreceptors located in the gut, liver, and viscera also play an important role in preventing nausea and vomiting. Generally, the following medications are used: prochlorperazine (Compazine®) 5–10 mg 4 times a day; prochlorperazine (Compazine®) 25 mg suppositories every 12 hours; promethazine (Phenergan®) 6.25–25 mg every 6 hours; droperidol (Inapsine®) 0.625–1.25 mg every 6 hours; haloperidol (Haldol®) 1 mg 2 times a day; metoclopramide (Reglan®)10–20 mg 4 times a day; and lorazepam (Ativan®) 0.25–2 mg every 4 hours (Elsayem et al., 2005; Institute for Safe Medication Practices, 2006; Watson et al., 2003).

Secretions

Increased oral secretions are very prevalent as patients near the end of life. Numerous underlying conditions can cause excessive secretions at the end of life, including infections, pulmonary edema, and aspiration or by pooling of normal oropharyngeal secretions in a patient who is weak, in pain, unable to swallow or cough effectively, or has a reduced state of consciousness. As patients lose their ability to swallow and clear oral secretions, each respiration produces a gurgling or rattling noise, sometimes referred to as a death rattle. This can be very distressing for family and friends.

Educating the family about the physiological inability for their loved one to swallow saliva normally and about approaches to managing secretions can be comforting. Patients who can cough effectively may benefit from measures to thin or mobilize secretions. Techniques include: hydration/humidification, expectorants, positioning, chest physiotherapy, pain management, and oral suctioning. A Yaunker's suction can easily be used by the patient or family as well. Suctioning of the oropharynx is sometimes recommended, but its effectiveness has not been well studied, and it may cause patient distress. Repositioning the patient from side to side in a semi-upright position is recommended as a nursing strategy for patients in the last stages of life, though evidence to support this intervention is scant (Bickel & Arnold, 2008).

Anticholinergic agents are the most commonly used pharmacological agents, but side effects often include: dry mouth, urinary retention, confusion/sedation, and mucus plugging. Postnasal drainage from chronic sinusitis may respond to inhaled steroids or anticholinergic agents. Additional medications to consider are listed in Box 5–4.

Sleep Disturbance/Insomnia

Sleep disturbance is a generalized term to indicate changes from restful sleep, causing sleep deprivation, and is a common symptom seen in patients nearing the end of life. Insomnia is the difficulty in falling or staying asleep, the absence of restful sleep, or poor quality of sleep. Multiple factors may disturb sleep and

---

BOX 5–4   Medications to Decrease Patient Secretions

For thick secretions:

- Guaifenesin (100 mg/5 ml, or 600 mg extended release tablet) 200–400 mg every 4 hours or 600–1,200 mg extended release tablet every 1–2 hours, as needed for thick secretions

For excessive secretions:

- Atropine 1% ophthalmic drops, 1–4 drops SL every 2 hours
- Hyoscyamine (Levsin®) 0.125–0.25 mg SL every 6 hours
- Scopolamine (Transderm-scop®) 1.5 mg transdermal patch every 72 hours; apply behind ears
- Glycopyrrolate (Robinul®) 1–2 mg every 8 hours

Source: Bickel & Arnold, 2008; Elsayem et al., 2003; Hsin & Hallenbeck, 2006; International Association of Hospice and Palliative Care, 2007; Watson et al., 2005; Wiseman, 2006

BOX 5–5   Common Causes of Impaired Skin Integrity

- Pressure over bony prominences
- Immobility
- Dryness (xerosis) of the skin
- Poor skin hygiene
- Poor nutrition
- Underlying skin disease or lesions
- Medications
- Cholestasis (failure of bile flow)
- Uremia
- Malignancy
- Hematologic conditions

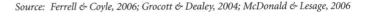

Source: Ferrell & Coyle, 2006; Grocott & Dealey, 2004; McDonald & Lesage, 2006

---

prevent adequate rest; two primary causes are pain and restless legs syndrome. Other causes include medications, worsening of chronic medical conditions (e.g., congestive heart failure and chronic obstructive pulmonary disease), respiratory distress, bladder or bowel disturbance, nausea and/or vomiting, cognitive impairment disorders, an unfamiliar environment, and altered bedtime routine. Emotional/psychological distress such as depression, anxiety or fear (e.g., fear of not waking up) greatly affect a patient's rest (Glass, Lanctot, & Hermann, 2006; Miller & Arnold, 2003).

The underlying cause for sleeplessness and insomnia should be the first course of action as appropriate. Non-pharmacologic therapy includes provision of a quiet, comfortable environment, including natural sounds or white noise according to patient preference. The use of relaxation therapies as well as stimulus control therapy may assist the patient to achieve restful sleep. Caffeine and alcoholic beverages, especially in the evening hours, should be avoided, as both are stimulants.

Medications that are recommended include: diphenhydramine (Benadryl®) 25–50 mg at bedtime, except in the elderly patient; lorazepam (Ativan®) 0.5–2 mg at bedtime and every 2 hours; zolpidem (Ambien®) 5–10 mg at bedtime; temazepam (Restoril®) 15 mg at bedtime; and quetiapine (Seroquel®) 50–100 mg at bedtime. For the most elderly patients, the medications include trazadone (Desyrel®) 25–100 mg at bedtime and mirtazapine (Remeron®) 7.5–15 mg at bedtime (CAPC, 2005a, 2007: Elsayem et al., 2003; Miller & Arnold, 2003, 2004; Watson et al., 2005).

Skin and Wound Care

Major symptom issues of the skin are common for terminally ill patients. There are many causes of skin impairment near the end of life; Box 5–5 lists these causes.

The overall goals of care are based on the patient's condition, stage of illness, and preference (Schim & Cullen, 2005). Meticulous skin care contributes to well-being; education of the patient and family centers on the importance of sufficient hydration and nutrition, including adequate amounts of protein and vitamin C. Ensure comfortable room temperature and humidity. Keep fingernails trimmed, suggest oatmeal baths, particularly for pruritis, and topical over-the-counter moisturizing lotions.

The following topical medications for pruritis are recommended: Camphor/menthol lotion (e.g., Sarna®); hydrocortisone 1% cream or lotion; and triamcinolone 0.1% cream. Systemic medications that are specific for pruritis include: diphenhydramine (Benadryl®) 25 mg every 4 hours; hydroxyzine (Atarax®)10–25 mg every 4 hours; doxepin (Sinequan®) 10–25 mg at bedtime; dexamethasone 1–4 mg 1 time a day; and cholestyramine (Questran®) 4 g 1 time a day or 2 times a day. Care should be taken with prescribed antihistamines and anticholinergics in the more elderly patients, as they are more susceptible to side effects of these drugs including sedation and confusion (CAPC, 2005a; Institute for Safe Medication Practices, 2006).

Wound care presents more of a challenge and wounds are most often caused by neuropathic, venous, and/or arterial dysfunction. Malignant wounds are common in patients with cancer. Wound care includes meticulous assessment and care of the skin, remembering that patients should be premedicated with opioid analgesics prior to performing dressing changes. Some patients also benefit from the implementation of complementary therapies such as music, acupuncture, visualization, and guided imagery during painful wound dressing changes.

When performing dressing changes, cleanse the wound with gentle irrigation using a preservative-free normal saline or a noncytotoxic wound cleaner. If needed, morphine hydrogel may be applied to the wound surface to control pain. Exudate from wounds may be controlled with the use of hydrocolloid or foam dressings or the application of an ostomy appliance.

Medications that assist with wound care include metronidazole (Flagyl®) 500 mg 3 times a day and silver sulfadiazine (Silvadene®) cream used 1 time a day (Institute for Safe Medication Practices, 2006; Seaman, 2006).

Preventive measures are important to avoid bleeding and further wound decline. Moisten dressings with normal saline before removal and exclusively use nonadherent absorbing dressings. If active wound bleeding is observed, the recommended intervention is to apply gauze saturated with a 1:1000 solution of epinephrine. Consult wound care specialists or enterostomal nurse specialists for patients who have complicated or poorly responding wounds (McDonald & Lesage, 2006; von Gunten & Ferris, 2005).

Stomatitis

Stomatitis is a distressing inflammation of the oral tissues and frequently presents in patients at the end of life. The condition may be caused by **radiation therapy,** chemotherapy, infection, dryness, and administration of antibiotics. Stomatitis causes pain, difficulty swallowing, and decreased oral intake (Henson & Arnold, 2004), and can result in candida infections. Nursing interventions include educating the patient and family about food preparation, noting that foods should be served at lukewarm temperature and that soft, bland foods are usually more comforting than very cold, very hot, or textured foods (Henson & Arnold, 2004; Rosielle, 2005).

Four medications assist with stomatitis, including: 2% topical viscous lidocaine; salt-sodium bicarbonate mouthwash; clotrimazole (Lotrimin®) 10 mg; and 2% viscous lidocaine, diphenhydramine elixir, Maalox® mouth wash.

If the patient has candida or an oral herpes infection, topical treatments include nystatin suspension 500,000 u mouthwash and miconazole (Monistat®) gel 2%.

Fluconazole (Diflucan®) 200 mg 1 time a day is used for systemic treatment of stomatitis (Elsayem et al, 2003; Henson & Arnold, 2004, 2005; National Guideline Clearinghouse, 2008; Rosielle, 2005; Watson et al., 2005).

Xerostomia (Dry Mouth)

There are many causes of **xerostomia** (dry and sore mouth); most are easily treatable. This is a common symptom seen in patients in life-limiting conditions. Causes may include head and neck surgery, radiation to head and neck, medication side effects, infections, autoimmune processes, cancer and chemotherapy as well as decreased intake (Henson, 2004). Dehydration from other causes such as anorexia, vomiting, oxygen therapy, diabetes, and fever can also result in (Dahlin & Goldsmith, 2006). Prevention includes measures that keep the teeth and the oral cavity clean, and prompt treatment of any tooth decay or painful mouth lesions (Quinn, 2007).

Interventions that assist in providing relief from xerostomia include the use of lip balm, mouth moisturizer gel, sore throat sprays, throat lozenges, and sugarless gum and candy. Avoid using lemon/glycerin swabs, which further dry the oral mucosa, and strong mouth rinses or toothpastes, which can irritate a dry mouth (Reisfield, Rosielle, & Wilson, 2007).

SECTION ONE REVIEW

1. Raising the head of the bed or having the patient sit forward in an upright position are basic nursing care treatments for:
   1. Pain.
   2. Fatigue.
   3. Dyspnea.
   4. Nausea and vomiting.
2. A patient with metastatic lung cancer comes to the hospital. He has had the disease for about one year and has managed his symptoms effectively at home until now. He presents with the following symptoms: increased shortness of air, anorexia with weight loss, fatigue, insomnia, and constipation. Which concept for a nursing diagnosis might be appropriate?
   1. Alteration in body elimination
   2. Comfort alteration
   3. Knowledge deficit of disease process
   4. Airway clearance impairment
3. Potential interventions for a patient with stomatitis are:
   1. Offering the patient cold foods, such as gelatin and ice cream.
   2. Offering the patient water only.
   3. Offering the patient his or her typical foods, such as hamburger and roast beef.
   4. Offering the patient lukewarm, bland foods such as nonspicy mashed potatoes and gravy.
4. The terminally ill patient who presents with a significant wound requires clarification of the goal for wound care. Which goals might be appropriate for this patient? (Select all that apply.)
   1. Relief of distressing symptoms
   2. Wound healing
   3. Prevention of further skin breakdown
   4. Elimination of the disease process

SECTION TWO: Comparison and Contrast of Diseases and Symptoms

Knowledge of the more common symptoms seen in terminally ill patients according to the disease etiology assists nurses in better assessment and treatment options. This section compares and contrasts the more common symptoms reported by patients with selected disease diagnoses. The specific treatment and nursing interventions for these symptoms have been addressed in the preceding section of this chapter.

Cancer

Cancer, often thought of as the most common end-stage disease, is the second leading cause of death in the United States (Centers for Disease Control, 2007). There are in excess of 300 different types of cancers, affecting almost every body system. Often cancer patients have 16 or more symptoms at any given time, thus aggressive symptom management is imperative for these patients. Fatigue is the leading symptom reported by 80–90% of cancer patients, with 70–90% of cancer patients experiencing pain, 60–90% experiencing oral symptoms, and 70% reporting respiratory symptoms (Tadman & Roberts, 2007).

Other symptoms typically seen in patients with cancer include skin integrity impairment, insomnia, weakness, anorexia, malnutrition, nausea, vomiting, and constipation or diarrhea. Sleep disturbances, depression, and anxiety account for other significant symptoms experienced by patients with cancer (Meier, 2002; Solano, Gomes, & Higginson, 2006; Tadman & Roberts, 2007). Box 5–6 lists the more common causes of respiratory symptoms seen in patients diagnosed with cancer.

Cardiac

The major cause of death in the United States today involves cardiac diseases (Centers for Disease Control, 2007). In patients with cardiomyopathies, the most common symptoms reported are shortness of breath, **orthopnea,** dyspnea with exertion and fatigue. In coronary artery disease, symptoms include **angina** with radiating pain, palpitations, and dyspnea on exertion (Goodlin, Hauptman, & Arnold, 2004; Solano et al., 2006). Patients with end-stage congestive heart failure report multiple symptoms, including edema, anxiety, severe shortness of breath, dyspnea, nausea, vomiting, and constipation (Brooks, 2003; Pantilat & Steimle, 2004).

Pulmonary

Chronic obstructive pulmonary disease (COPD), also known as chronic obstructive lung disease (COLD), is the predominant

---

BOX 5–6	**Causes of Respiratory Symptoms in Cancer Patients**

- Chronic lung diseases
- Airway obstruction
- Pneumonia
- Pain
- Edema or obesity
- Stress or anxiety
- Surgery
- Anemia
- Side effects of chemotherapy or radiation therapy
- The cancer itself
- Fluid in the lungs

Source: Elsayem et al., 2003; Ferrell & Coyle, 2006; Grocott & Dealey, 2004

BOX 5–7	**Symptoms of End-Stage Respiratory Disease**

- Tachypnea
- Breathlessness, short of breath (subjective) on a scale 0–10
- Dyspnea (difficult, rapid, or labored breathing—objective)
- Tachycardia
- Hypoxemic
- Confusion
- Diaphoretic
- Cyanosis
- Hypercapnia (cause headaches and sleepiness)
- Apnea
- Cough

Source: Elsayem et al., 2003; Ferrell & Coyle, 2006; Grocott & Dealey, 2004

---

end-stage disease affecting the pulmonary system (Campbell & Coyne, 2006). Major symptoms associated with either emphysema or chronic bronchitis, the two major divisions of COPD, include shortness of breath, rapid respirations, dyspnea, chronic cough, confusion, purulent sputum, wheezing, fatigue, weight loss, sleep disturbances, and cyanosis. Patients who are close to death may also experience apnea and Cheyne-Stokes respirations. Box 5–7 depicts some of the more common symptoms of end-stage respiratory disease.

Renal

Renal failure can be an end-stage disease diagnosis for patients nearing the end of their lives. Renal failure, similar to respiratory and cardiac failure, impacts the majority of body systems. For example, renal failure has been known to precipitate hypertension, anemia, osteoporosis, and cardiac arrhythmias (Gorman & Coyne, 2005; Solano et al., 2005).

Major symptoms reported by patients with end stage renal disease include weakness, fatigue, confusion, depression, behavioral changes, muscle cramps, pain, shortness of breath, dyspnea, nausea, vomiting, stomatitis, and pruritis (Gorman & Coyne, 2005, Solano et al., 2005).

Neurological

One of the most life-threatening neurological diseases is amyotrophic lateral sclerosis (ALS), most often referred to as Lou Gehrig's disease. ALS is also the leading cause of end-stage diseases from a neurological perspective (Centers for Disease Control, 2007). This disease is a progressive neurodegenerative disease that affects nerve cells in the brain and the spinal cord. With voluntary muscle action progressively affected, patients in the later stages of the disease may become totally paralyzed. Symptoms are based on the stage of the disease and include cramping, or stiffness of muscles, muscle weakness affecting a specific limb, slurred and nasal speech, muscle atrophy, spasticity, dysphagia, depression, anxiety, and paralysis stages (Elsayem et al., 2003, Watson et al., 2005; Wicks, Abrahams, Masi, Hejda-Forde, Leigh, & Goldstein, 2005).

Cerebrovascular

Cerebrovascular vascular accident (CVA) is the third leading cause of death in the United States and the leading cause of adult disability (Centers for Disease Control, 2007). CVA can be the primary diagnosis for terminally ill individuals, but more often complicates other end-stage disease diagnoses. Symptoms depend upon the areas of the brain affected and may include muscular spasticity, weakness, tremors, and atrophy. Other symptoms include **aphasia,** fatigue, depression, anxiety, sleep disturbances, anorexia, malnutrition, and behavioral changes. In severe cases, dyspnea, apnea, seizures, and loss of consciousness may occur (Davies & Higginson, 2007; Rogers & Addington-Hall, 2005; Payne, Hall, Burton, Hendra, & Jones, 2007; Traue & Ross, 2005).

Dementia

Dementia, though not an end-stage disease in itself, frequently complicates other end-stage disease diagnoses. Since the patient is unable to care for himself or herself in severe dementia, it could become an end-stage disease state. Symptoms of dementia depend upon the severity of the disease state and generally include increasing impairment of mental abilities, mood swings, behavioral changes, depression, constipation, problems with skin integrity, **dysphasia,** forgetfulness, malnutrition, sleep disturbances, anorexia, and increased susceptibility to infections

(Bailey, 2004; Dahlin & Coyne, 2006). This topic is covered in more depth in Chapter 11.

HIV/AIDS

Human immunodeficiency virus (HIV) is a viral infection that gradually destroys the immune system, resulting in infections that are hard for the body to fight. This disease often leads to severe immunosuppression and constitutional disease, neurological complications, and opportunistic infections and neoplasms (Corless, Keller, Strand, & Coyne, 2007).

Symptoms that can be seen months to years after the initial infection include lack of energy, weight loss, frequent fevers, night sweats, persistent or frequent yeast infections (oral or vaginal), persistent skin rashes, or flaky skin. Also, frequent episodes of severe herpes infections and shingles can be expected and short-term memory loss may occur (Harding, Easterbrook, & Higginson, 2005).

Acquired immunodeficiency syndrome (AIDS) is the final and most serious stage of HIV disease, causing severe damage to the immune system. Symptoms commonly seen in patients with AIDS may be found in Box 5–8.

Some Final Notes

General **debility** is a common thread for all the diseases that have been discussed in this section. Often patients report some general, vague, or subtle comment of symptoms such as "not doing well," or "I'm just feeling under the weather." Such comments are particularly common in the more elderly individual who has

---

BOX 5–8   **Symptoms Associated with Aids**

- Extreme fatigue
- Dyspnea and shortness of breath
- Cough
- Weight loss
- Nausea, abdominal cramps, and vomiting
- Seizures and lack of coordination
- Difficult or painful swallowing
- Mental symptoms such as confusion and forgetfulness
- Severe and persistent diarrhea
- Fever
- Vision loss
- Severe headaches
- Coma
- Prone to developing various cancers
- Pain
- Depression
- Shingles

Source: Ferrell & Coyle, 2006; Grocott & Dealey, 2004; Harding et al., 2005

been diagnosed with a terminal illness for some period of time. These comments are reflective of chronic concurrent diseases and functional impairments. Debility denotes functional decline, progressive apathy, and a loss of willingness to eat and drink that culminates in death. Symptoms that the patient is nearing the end of life include increasing pain, a new onset of pain, anorexia, cachexia, **asthenia,** increasing levels of depression, and severe anxiety. Box 5–9 lists the more commonly seen symptoms in patients experiencing general debility.

BOX 5–9   Symptoms of General Debility

- Pain
- Asthenia-impaired physical function—immobility and inactivity
- Anorexia—decreased appetite
- Decreased intake—malnutrition
- Cachexia—weight loss > 5% of baseline
- Decreased swallowing ability
- Depression
- Anxiety
- Decreased cognitive ability
- Increase in decubitus ulcers

Source: Ferrell & Coyle, 2006; Grocott & Dealey, 2004

Palliative care is often the most beneficial care in treating symptoms accompanying debility. Evaluating these symptoms includes managing underlying physical symptoms that may be poorly controlled, identifying needs for additional supportive services, and providing education for family members. To manage symptoms, a plan of care is developed that will aid in palliating symptoms, though disease-modifying therapies may also be included. The disease progression itself is generally an accumulation of the individual's underlying health issues, although not one specific disease may be the terminal one (CAPC, 2007; Institute for Clinical Systems Improvement, 2007).

Treatment for symptoms in terminally ill individuals associated with a diagnosis of specific disease states begins with the recognition that curative measures may induce additional symptoms and further diminish quality of life. Conversely, some more curative measures could enhance quality of life, at least temporarily. Thus, goals of care and realistic expectations must be discussed before embarking on either curative or palliative measures. Patients and their families have the decision to initially accept, continue, or reject treatment and interventions at any time (ELNEC, 2008). Sometimes the severity of symptoms helps to assist patients in the decision-making process to forgo further interventions. For example, side effects associated with chemotherapy or increasing severity of pain may cause patients to forego further curative treatment and allow the natural course of disease to evolve. Review Chapters 2 and 3 for more information.

SECTION TWO REVIEW

1. Interventions for end stage renal disease (ESRD) may include: (Select all that apply.)
   1. Treating the itching
   2. Haldol (haloperidol)
   3. Morphine
   4. Fan
2. For most terminal diseases, treatment of _____ yields the greatest benefit for the patient, creating a better quality of life.
   1. distressing symptoms
   2. pain
   3. clinical depression
   4. the underlying disease
3. Besides the management of symptoms, what other nursing roles are vital for the nurse to perform on behalf of the patient to ensure optimum patient care? (Select all that apply.)
   1. Patient advocacy
   2. Assist with activity of daily living tasks
   3. Frequent patient assessments
   4. Communication with other health care providers

Case Study

Tina Clark is a 36-year-old single female who was admitted to the hospital on an emergency basis. She is in the end stages of AIDS. She had been exhibiting profound dyspnea, an oxygen saturation of 78%, and she is currently on a re-breather face mask at 100% oxygen at a 15 liter flow. She is unable to walk and was admitted via ambulance. She is confused and is delirious. She is coughing profusely, but nonproductively at this time. Her temperature is 39°C., heart rate 120, respiratory rate 36, and blood pressure 165/102.

Saturation on the re-breather mask now is currently 84%. She is holding her abdomen and has vomited once in the emergency center.

Her mother accompanied Tina and reports that Tina has had frequent fevers, chills, and sweats. Tina has had a persistent oral thrush infection for over a month and has been unable to eat anything substantial, only consume bites of food and take small sips of fluids. She has complained of difficulty and pain with swallowing and has lost 40 pounds in the past 2 months. She has had severe and persistent diarrhea. Tina also has had a persistent skin rash on her arms. Her vision has diminished to the point where she can no longer read. Tina has severe headaches and her mother reports that she has become much more depressed over the past week, refusing to associate with any of her friends or colleagues.

Questions

1. Should Tina be transferred to the intensive care unit?
2. What are the health care provider's priorities in her care?
3. What are the symptoms that will need to be managed?
4. What other team members should be called?
5. What information will the health care providers share with her mother regarding symptom management?

Suggested Responses

1. A review of her code status is a priority; then discuss with her mother the options of care. Does Tina have an advance directive? Is her mother listed as next of kin on the release of information list? Because Tina is in end-stage failure and aggressive treatments may be futile and ineffective, an intensive care unit transfer is inappropriate. Symptom management would be the appropriate direction for the health care providers to take.

2. Dyspnea should be an immediate concern, and a morphine infusion with patient controlled analgesia demand dosing could be initiated. Review her medications to see if she has used any opioids and convert the oral dose of morphine to infusion. Add lorazepam if needed for breathlessness and anxiety. Hypoxia may be causing the altered mental status. Respiratory therapy can also assist in converting her re-breather mask to a more appropriate source of oxygen.

3. Breathlessness, pain if any, fever, oral integrity, hydration needs, anorexia and cachexia, cough, delirium, altered mental status, diarrhea, impaired skin integrity, asthenia/weakness, fatigue, headaches, depression, social isolation, helplessness.

4. Physician, chaplain, social worker/case manager, next of kin (if not her mother). The nurse may need to arrange a family conference regarding goals of care and prognosis discussion, with support for family and others. Care associates may assist with details of positioning in bed and other bedside needs (e.g., diarrhea).

5. Based on the patient record and the Health Insurance Portability and Accountability Act of 1990 (HIPAA) standards, it would be important to establish the mother's relationship and role in Tina's care. If Tina's mother is not directly involved, start with a description of the basic interventions being implemented to make Tina comfortable and manage her symptoms. Further discussion will be based on a need-to-know basis.

CHAPTER SUMMARY

- Multiple physiological and nonphysiological symptoms accompany end-of-life disease states; each presents unique challenges for multidisciplinary team members.
- Goals of care and anticipated outcomes are based on the patient's quality of life and individualized, personal goals.
- Symptoms commonly seen in patients at the end of life include agitation, anorexia and cachexia, anxiety, constipation, cough, delirium, depression, diarrhea, dry eyes/dry nose, fatigue, fever, hiccups, nausea and vomiting, secretions, sleep disturbance/insomnia, skin and wound care, stomatitis, and xerostomia.
- Treatment for these symptoms include both pharmacological and nonpharmacological interventions; initial interventions include identifying and treating the underlying cause or contributing factors, if possible.

- The most commonly seen end-stage diseases include diagnoses of cancer, cardiac, pulmonary, renal, neurological, cerebrovascular, dementia, and HIV/AIDS.
- General debility, though not a disease state in itself, is a common thread that pervades end-stage diseases.
- Treatment for symptoms in terminally ill patients associated with a diagnosis of a specific disease state begins with the recognition that curative measures may induce additional symptoms and further diminish the individual's quality of life.

CHAPTER REVIEW

Ben Johnson is a 55-year-old gentleman with known metastatic lung cancer, including metastasis to the bone. He presents to the clinic with increased shortness of breath, weakness, and fatigue. His pain has been adequately managed with morphine sulfate extended release 60 mg q12 hr, with morphine immediate release 15 mg q 4 hr as needed, which he uses 1 time or 2 times a day. His appetite has diminished and he has lost 12 pounds in the past 6 weeks. He complains of not sleeping well for several days and has noted an increase in shortness of breath.

Ben has become increasingly anxious and unable to do his usual outdoor yard work, which he attributes to his breathlessness. He has not had a bowel movement for 5 days, but thought it could be related to his decreased intake and sore mouth. He has developed a productive cough with yellow phlegm in the past 2 weeks, but denies hiccups. He reports no fever, chills or sweats; no nausea or vomiting. He does not have any skin breakdown, rashes, or bruises. His last chemotherapy was 5 days ago.

Ben also reports his mood has changed; he has been very sad, discouraged, and does not have any motivation. His wife and children are worried that he is becoming more depressed as evidenced by the fact that he is staying home and not going to work daily.

Questions

1. What other measurements or tests should be considered?
2. What are Ben's symptoms that can be managed?
3. What might you expect to see or write as physician's orders?

Suggested Responses

1. Assess vital signs, including oxygen saturation, skin, weight, assess lung sounds, oral cavity for thrush, cough secretions, depression assessment

2. Breathlessness, anorexia, insomnia, fatigue, constipation, question the presence of stomatitis, cough, diet, possible hydration

3. Assessment of his overall condition should include a metabolic panel due to his weight loss and either a complete blood count or arterial blood gases based on the severity of his symptoms. Additionally a chest X-ray should also have been ordered. Treatments such as nebulizer treatments for wheezing, furosemide for rales if present on physical examination, possibly home oxygen, increased morphine dosages, and a prescription for lorazepam would be expected. Additionally, medications such as Senokot S 1-4 tabs bid, lactulose, docusate suppository, Fleet's enema, guaiafenesin or benzonatate could be ordered by the primary health care provider.

REFERENCES

Agency for Health Care Research and Quality. (2002). Management of cancer symptoms: Pain, depression and fatigue. Retrieved from http://www.ahrq.gov/downloads/pub/evidence/pdf/cansymp/cansymp.pdf

Alderman, J. (2003). Fast facts and concepts #96: Diarrhea in palliative care. Retrieved from www.eperc.mcw.edu

Anderson, P., & Dean, G. (2006). Fatigue. In B. R. Ferrell & N. Coyle (Eds.) *Textbook of palliative nursing*. (pp. 155–168). New York: Oxford University Press.

Arnold, R. (2005). Fast fact and concept #146: Screening for depression in palliative care. Retrieved from www.eperc.mcw.edu

Bailey, A. (2004). *The palliative response.* [Ebook] Retrieved from http://www.hospice.va.gov/Amosbaileybook/index.htm

Bickel, K., & Arnold, R. (2008). Fast facts and concepts #109: Death rattle and oral secretions. Retrieved from www.eperc.mcw.edu

Brooks, L. (2003). More end-of-life services needed for heart failure patients. Retrieved from http://www.medscape.com/viewarticle/462462

Campbell, M., & Coyne, P. (2006). *Compendium of treatment of end stage non-cancer diagnoses: Pulmonary.* Dubuque, IA: Kendall/Hunt Publishers.

Centers for Disease Control. (2007). *United States health, 2007.* Atlanta, GA: Author.

Center to Advance Palliative Care (CAPC). (2005a). Medication guidelines for symptom relief. Retrieved from http://www.capc.org/tools-for-palliative-care-programs/clinical-tools/policies-procedures/medication-guidelines.doc

Center to Advance Palliative Care (CAPC). (2005b). Palliative care treatment algorithms for symptom management. Retrieved from http://www.capc.org/tools-for-palliative-care-programs/clinical-tools/policies-procedures/palliative-algorithms.ppt

Center to Advance Palliative Care (CAPC). (2007). Moving palliative care into the emergency room: Ensuring the right care for seriously ill patients right from the beginning. Retrieved from http://www.michigancancer.org/PowerPoints/CtrToAdvancePallCare/AudioConfSlides-011107.ppt

Cline, D. (2006). Nutrition issues and tools for palliative care. *Home Healthcare Nurse, 4*(1), 54–57.

Corless, I., Keller, L., Strand, C., & Coyne, P. (2007). *Compendium of treatment of end stage renal disease: HIV/AIDS.* Dubuque, IA: Kendall/Hunt Publishers.

Dahlin, C., & Coyne, P. (2006). *Compendium of treatment of end stage non-cancer diagnoses: Dementia.* Dubuque, IA: Kendall/Hunt Publishers.

Dahlin, C., & Goldsmith, T. (2006). "Dysphagia, Xerostomia and Hiccups." In B. R. Ferrell, & N. Coyle (Eds.) *Textbook of palliative nursing.* (pp. 195–218) New York: Oxford University Press.

Davies, E., & Higginson, I. (Eds.) (2007). *The solid facts: Palliative care.* Retrieved from http://www.euro.who.int/document/E82931.pdf

Del Fabbro, E., Dalal, S., & Bruerea, E. (2006). Symptom control in palliative care: Part III: Dyspnea and delirium. *Journal of Palliative Medicine, 9*:422–436.

DeLima, L. (2006). International Association for Hospice and Palliative Care List of essential medicines for palliative care. *Annals of Oncology, 18*(2), 395–399.

Dudgeon, D. (2006). Dyspnea, death rattle and cough. In B. R. Ferrell & N. Coyle (Eds.) *Textbook of palliative nursing* (pp. 249–264). New York: Oxford University Press.

Economou, D. (2006). Bowel management: Constipation, diarrhea, obstruction, and ascites. In B. R. Ferrell & N. Coyle (Eds.) *Textbook of palliative nursing* (pp. 219–238). New York: Oxford University Press.

Elsayem, A., Driver, L., & Bruera, E. (Eds.). (2003). *The M. D. Anderson symptom control and palliative care handbook.* Houston, TX: University of Texas MD Anderson Cancer Center.

End of Life Nursing Consortium. (2008). *Advanced end of life nursing care: ELNEC supercore training program 2008. Washington, DC: American Association of Colleges of Nursing.*

Estfan, B., & LeGrand, S. (2004). Management of cough in advanced cancer. *The Journal of Supportive Oncology, 2*(6), 523–527.

Farmer, C. (2007). Fast facts and concepts #81: Management of hiccups (2nd ed.). Retrieved from http://www.eperc.mcw.edu/fastFact/ff_81.htm

Ferrell, B. R., & Coyle, N. (Eds.). (2006). *Textbook of palliative nursing.* New York: Oxford University Press.

Finnish Medical Society Duodecim. (2005). Palliative treatment of cancer. In EBM guidelines: Evidence-based medicine. [CD-ROM]. Retrieved from http://www.guideline.gov/summary/summary.aspx?ss=15&doc_id=8240&nbr=004598&string=symptom+AND+management+AND+palliative+AND+care

Glass, J., Lanctot, K., & Hermann, N. (2006). Sedative hypnotics in older people with insomnia: Meta-analysis of risks and benefits. *British Medical Journal, 331*, 1169.

Goodlin S., Hauptman, P., & Arnold, R. (2004). Consensus statement: Palliative and supportive care in advanced heart failure. *Journal of Cardiac Failure, 10*(3), 200–209.

Gorman, L., & Coyne, P. (2005). *Compendium of treatment of end stage non-cancer diagnoses: Renal.* Dubuque, IA: Kendall/Hunt Publishers.

Grocott, P., & Dealey, C. (2004). Symptom management: Nursing aspects. In D. Doyle, G. Hanks, N. Cherney, & K. Calman (Eds.) *Oxford textbook of palliative medicine* (3rd ed., pp. 628–640). Oxford, UK: Oxford University Press.

Hallenbeck, J. (2005a). Fast facts and concepts #5: Causes of nausea and vomiting (2nd ed.). Retrieved from www.eperc.mcw.edu

Hallenbeck, J. (2005b). Fast facts and concepts #15: Constipation: What makes us go (2nd ed.). Retrieved from www.eperc.mcw.edu

Harding, R., Easterbrook, P., Higginson, I. J. (2005). Access and equity in HIV/AIDS palliative care: A review of the evidence and responses. *Palliative Medicine, 19*(3), 251–258.

Henson, D., & Arnold, R. (2004). Fast facts and concepts #121: Oral mucositis: Diagnosis and assessment. Retrieved from www.eperc.mcw.edu

Henson, D., & Arnold, R. (2005). Fast facts and concepts #130: Oral mucositis: Prevention and treatment. Retrieved from www.eperc.mcw.edu

Hsin, G., & Hallenbeck, J. (2006). Fast facts and concepts #158: Respiratory secretion management. Retrieved from www.eperc.mcw.edu

Inouye, S. (2006). Delirium in older persons. *New England Journal of Medicine, 354,* 1157–1165.

International Association of Hospice and Palliative Care. (2006). IAHPC List of essential medicines for palliative care. Retrieved from http://www.supportiveoncology.net/journal/articles/0408409table.pdf

Institute for Clinical Systems Improvement. (2007). Palliative care health order set. Retrieved from http://www.icsi.org//guidelines_and_more/guidelines_order_sets_protocols/

Institute for Safe Medication Practices. (2006). Promethazine conundrum: IV can hurt more than IM injection! Retrieved from http://www.ismp.org/newsletters/acutecare/articles/20061102.asp?ptr=y

Jantarakupt, P., & Porock, D. (2005). Dyspnea management in lung cancer: Applying the evidence from chronic obstructive pulmonary disease. *Oncology Nursing Forum, 32*(4), 785.

Kuebler, K. K., English, N., & Heidrich, D. E. (2006). Delirium, confusion, agitation, and restlessness. In B. R. Ferrell & N. Coyle (Eds.) *Textbook of palliative nursing.* (pp. 401–428). New York: Oxford University Press.

McDonald, A., & Lesage, P. (2006). Palliative management of pressure ulcers and malignant wounds in patients with advanced illness. *Journal of Palliative Medicine, 9*(2), 285–295.

Meier, D. (2002). Overview of cancer pain and palliative care. *Journal of Pain and Symptom Management, 24*(2), 265–269.

Miller, M., & Arnold, R. (2003). Fast facts and concepts #101: Insomnia: Patient assessment. Retrieved from www.eperc.mcw.edu

Miller, M., & Arnold, R. (2004). Fast facts and concepts #104: Insomnia: Non Pharmacological treatments and #105: Insomnia: Pharmacological therapies. Retrieved from www.eperc.mcw.edu

Morrison, L., & Liao, S. (2007). Fast facts and concepts #174: Dementia medications in palliative care. Retrieved from www.eperc.mcw.edu

National Guideline Clearinghouse. (2008). Palliative Treatment of Cancer. Available online from http://www.guideline.gov/summary/summary.aspx?ss=15&doc_id=11041&nbr=5820

Pantilat, S., & Steimle, A. (2004). Palliative care for patients with heart failure. *Journal of the American Medical Association, 291,* 2476 –2482.

Pasacreta, J., Minarik, P., & Nield-Anderson, L. (2006). Anxiety and depression. In B. R. Ferrell & N. Coyle (Eds.) *Textbook of palliative nursing* (pp. 375–399). New York: Oxford University Press.

Periyakoil, V., & Hallenbeck, J. (2002). Identifying and managing preparatory grief and depression at the end of life. *American Academy of Family Physicians, 65*(5), 884–890.

Payne, S., Hall, A., Burton, C., Hendra, T., & Jones, A. (2007). Palliative care after stroke. Retrieved from, http://www.stroke.org.uk/research/funded_research/research_projects_programme_grants/research_region/north_east_england/palliative_care.html

Quijada, E., & Billings, J. A. (2002). Fast facts and concepts #60: Pharmacologic management of delirium: Update on newer agents. Retrieved from www.eperc.mcw.edu

Quinn, T. (2007). Xerostomia: Dry mouth. Retrieved from http://yalecancercenter.org/education/download/YaleCares%20June%202007.pdf

Reisfield, G., & Wilson, G. (2007). Fast facts and Concepts #173: Cancer-related fatigue. Retrieved from www.eperc.mcw.edu

Reisfield, G., Rosielle, D., & Wilson, G. (2007). Fast facts and concepts #182: Xerostomia. Retrieved from www.eperc.mcw.edu

Rogers, A., & Addington-Hall, J. (2005). Care of the dying stroke patient in the acute setting. *Journal of Research in Nursing, 10*(2), 153–167.

Rosielle, D. (2005). Fast facts and concepts #147: Oropharyngeal candidiasis. Retrieved from www.eperc.mcw.edu

Schim, S., & Cullen, B. (2005). Wound care at the end of life. *Nursing Clinics of North America, 40,* 281–294.

Seaman, S. (2006). Management of malignant fungating wounds in advanced cancer. *Oncology Nursing, 22,* 185–193.

Smith, H., & Busracamwongs, A. (2003). Management of hiccups in the palliative care population. *American Journal of Hospital and Palliative Care, 20,* 149–152.

Solano, J. P., Gomes, B., & Higginson, I. J. (2006). A comparison of symptom prevalence in far advanced cancer, AIDS, heart disease, chronic obstructive pulmonary disease and renal disease. *Journal of Pain and Symptom Management, 31*(1), 58–69.

Tadman, M., & Roberts, D. (Eds.) (2007). *Oxford handbook of cancer nursing.* New York: Oxford University Press.

Thomas, J., et al. (2008). Methylnaltrexone for opioid-induced constipation in advanced illness. *New England Journal of Medicine, 358*(22), 2332–2343, 2400–2402.

Traue, D., & Ross, J. (2005). Palliative care in non-malignant diseases. *Journal of Research in Social Medicine, 98*(11), 503–506.

von Gunten, C., & Ferris, F. (2005). Fast facts and concepts #40: Pressure ulcers: Prevention and management and #41: Pressure ulcers: Debridement and dressings (2nd ed.). Retrieved from www.eperc.mcw.edu

Warm, E., & Weissman, D. (2005). Fast facts and concepts #7: Depression in advanced cancer (2nd ed.). Retrieved from www.eperc.mcw.edu

Watson, M., Lucas, C., Hoy, A., & Black, I. (Eds.) (2005). *Oxford handbook of palliative care.* New York: Oxford University Press.

Wicks, P., Abrahams, S., Masi, D., Hedja-Forde, S., Leigh, P. N., & Goldstein, L. H. (2005). The prevalence of depression and anxiety in motor neuron disorders. *Amyotrophic Lateral Sclerosis and other Motor Neuron Disorders, 6* (Supp. 1), 147.

Weissman, D. (2005a). Fast facts and concepts #1: Diagnosis and management of terminal delirium (2nd ed.). Retrieved from www.eperc.mcw.edu

Weissman, D. (2005b). Fast facts and Concept #27: Dyspnea at End-of-Life. (2nd Edition). Retrieved from www.eperc.mcw.edu

Wiseman, M. (2006). The treatment of oral problems in the palliative patient. *Journal of the Canadian Dental Association, 76,* 453–458.

CHAPTER 6

Hydration and Nutrition in Terminal Care

OBJECTIVES
Following completion of this chapter, the learner will be able to:

6.1. Describe artificial nutrition and hydration.

6.2. Compare and contrast the risks and benefits of hydration and nutrition for patients who are at the end of life.

6.3. Describe alternate treatment options for hydration and nutrition in terminal care.

6.4. Enumerate and analyze methods for discussing hydration and nutrition options with terminally ill patients and their families.

This chapter begins with a discussion about artificial nutrition and hydration, comparing and contrasting the risks and benefits of this therapy for terminally ill persons. Alternate treatment options for artificial nutrition and hydration are discussed, including the appropriateness of this therapy for patients at the end of life. The chapter concludes with an analysis of the various ways that health care professionals may initiate and discuss artificial hydration and nutrition with terminally ill persons and their family members.

PRETEST

1. The health care delivery team has met the goal of working with the patient and family when they:
   1. Discuss the treatment options with other health care providers.
   2. Understand the basic concepts and options for the patient.
   3. Discuss the treatment options with the patient and family.
   4. Discuss the difference between artificial and natural hydration and nutrition with the patient and family.
2. A competent adult patient is given IV fluids on an emergency basis, but now has decided to forego artificial hydration. The nurse should: (Select all that apply.)
   1. Advocate for the patient and notify the physician of the patient's decision.
   2. Instruct the patient on the risks, benefits, and potential outcome of his or her decision.

   3. Provide support to the family and patient in this decision.
   4. Contact the family to persuade the patient to continue with IV fluids.
3. Advanced technology has allowed artificial nutrition and hydration interventions to become common practice. Therefore:
   1. It is important to know when artificial nutrition and hydration may be harmful versus beneficial.
   2. Artificial nutrition and hydration can be used in all areas of practice on all patients.
   3. Only families—not the patients—should be instructed on the benefits.
   4. Artificial nutrition and hydration should be considered as the option of choice at the end of life.

98

4. Many treatments are started because there is still a chance of recovery or improving comfort. In this case:
   1. It is easy to know when to stop this treatment.
   2. Artificial hydration and nutrition may become an issue for discussion.
   3. The family decides when to stop such treatments if the patient becomes terminal.
   4. Physicians often recognize when it is time to withdraw treatment.
5. Artificial hydration and nutrition can present potential conflicts for patients, families, or health care providers due to underlying social and cultural issues. Conflicts that might arise for nurses include:
   1. Separating the concept of nurturing from providing nourishment.
   2. Differentiating between holiday and special occasions where food is served.
   3. Discussing artificial hydration and nutrition with families.
   4. Separating a patient's need for social involvement from consuming food.

GLOSSARY

anorexia   Markedly reduced appetite or total aversion to food and fluids.

artificial hydration   Involves the non-oral route of delivering fluids through one of the following routes: intravenous (via a peripheral or central line), subcutaneous (also called hypodermoclysis), rectal (proctoclysis), or enteral, sometimes referred to as rehydration therapy.

artificial nutrition   Non-oral means of administering nutrition to a person, including enteral and intravenous delivery routes.

cachexia   Physical wasting or emaciation with loss of weight and muscle mass caused by disease.

enteral administration/feeding   Means of ingesting food so that it can be digested; routes of ingestion include the mouth (oral) or through tube feedings via several routes: a nasogastric, gastrostomy, jejunostomy, and/or esophagostomy tubes.

total parenteral nutrition (TPN)   Nutrition and hydration administered intravenously; generally called hyperalimentation.

xerostomia   Dry mouth, the condition of not having enough saliva to keep the mouth wet, resulting from thickened or reduced saliva flow.

SECTION ONE: Importance of Hydration and Nutrition

Eating and drinking are the two obvious means to accomplish obtaining the adequate ingestion of calories, nutrients, and water that are required in order to sustain life and to ease possible suffering associated with hunger, thirst, and decreased functional status. Both eating and drinking represent basic enjoyment in life and they are often associated with socialization and gathering activities. These activities of eating and drinking offer opportunities for nurturing and being nurtured. However, the general public as well as selected health care providers are often unaware that there are separate goals for these two activities. Eating and drinking may be solely for nourishment or may be solely for pleasure and socialization or may incorporate both nourishment and socialization. These distinctions often present dilemmas in end-of-life and palliative care, which then create significant distress to patients, family members, and health care providers alike (Hallenbeck, 2003).

Advances in technology have allowed **artificial nutrition and hydration** (ANH) to become a relatively common health care practice, while simultaneously creating some very controversial ethical concerns. A major dilemma occurs when determining when ANH is a benefit for the patient versus when it becomes detrimental to the overall well-being of the person. Merely because the technology exists to support ANH does not mean that this is an acceptable or advantageous practice. One must consistently weigh the potential benefit versus potential harm. Nurses must participate in identifying individual treatment goals and anticipated outcomes when patients are at the end of their lives. Many health care providers and patients alike believe that dehydration is very uncomfortable and that it is unethical to let someone "starve to death," though research data often contradict this assumption (Clay & Abernathy, 2008; Smith & Andrews, 2000; Whitworth, Whitworth, Holm, Shaffer, Makin, & Jayson, 2004).

The aging of the population along with increased chronic illnesses among this population potentially impacts the frequency with which palliative and hospice nurses face dilemmas involving hydration and nutrition in clinical settings. Increasingly more patients with limited oral intake will be assessed and offered ANH (Mion & O'Connell, 2003). In each of these cases, risks, benefits, and expected outcomes should be examined and thoroughly discussed.

Adequate nutritional intake is often difficult, if not impossible, for patients with a terminal illness. The health care team serves a vital role in providing timely, valid information and education to patients and their families regarding hydration and nutrition. Health care providers need to have knowledge and resources regarding these issues, specifically when it comes to end-of-life care. Patients, family members, and caregivers frequently struggle to continue providing food and fluids when a patient's disease states become more pronounced. Nutrition issues often need to be addressed by nurses, who should be prepared with the basic concepts and options to educate and counsel those involved in end-of-life and palliative care hydration and nutrition issues (Cline, 2006).

The health care delivery team works together with the patient and family in making the best decisions for the patient; team members must remain impartial in presenting the risks of hydration and nutritional options, as well as their benefits, burdens, and expected outcomes based on the status of the individual patient (American Dietetic Association [ADA], 2002; Pichard, Kyle, & Morabia, 2004).

What Is Feeding?

The meaning of feeding is often symbolic and cultural. Some of the first actions that occur after the birth of an infant involve human contact and feeding activities. Social events, most holidays, and special occasions involve the serving and consuming of food and drink. In many religions, food is part of sacred rituals, and in cultures throughout history the offering of food has been a sign of hospitality. Additionally, people enjoy eating with family and friends.

The concept of feeding is associated with caring, compassion, nurturance, and commitment (Koretz, 2007). Seen in this light, patients and health care providers alike have difficulties separating the concept of nurturing from the provision of and intake of food and fluids. Nurses understand feeding as part of basic caring; because caring is a characteristic central to the profession of nursing, assessing and managing the nutritional needs of patients from birth to death becomes a critical component for professional nurses (Slomka, 2003).

Many people may not want to eat and drink when they are physically ill, and loss of appetite may be distressing to family members. As the physical body ages and health problems begin to develop, elders usually eat less and need fewer nutrients. Similarly, terminally ill and dying patients often experience this decline in appetite. Thus efforts to ensure good nutrition may be unnecessary and can actually be inappropriate for individuals at the end of life (American Academy of Hospice and Palliative Medicine [AAHPM], 2002).

Health care providers should recognize that the inability to maintain nutrition through the oral route in conjunction with a chronic, life-limiting illness and declining function is usually a beginning marker of the dying process. This lack of oral consumption of food and drink should signal to the health care team that discussions regarding the overall end-of-life goals should be undertaken at this time if they have not previously been discussed.

With end-of-life and terminal conditions, weighing the risks and benefits of treatment options is essential. As organs in the body begin to cease their normal functioning, physical needs are less, and patients have reported being more comfortable without eating or drinking. Forcing food or liquids usually is not beneficial, especially if restraints, intravenous (IV) fluids, or hospitalization are required. Not forcing someone to eat or drink should not be confused with letting a patient "starve to death." For those who are dying, it may be more compassionate and caring to allow a natural dehydration to occur. Forcing enteral and/or **total parenteral nutrition** interventions on dying patients may make the last days of their lives more uncomfortable and intolerable (Cervo, Bryan, & Farber, 2006; Hospice and Palliative Nurses Association [HPNA], 2003; Koretz, 2007).

Often patients request that they not become dependent on extraordinary measures and life-sustaining machines at the end of life. Treatments may be initiated, especially if there is still the possibility of recovery or additional comfort. In that case, AHN may become an issue for discussion, despite the fact that the terminally ill person had requested not to implement such treatments when he or she became terminal. When it can be shown that the benefits of AHN outweigh its disadvantages, health care providers generally advise the initiation of AHN in this patient population (American Academy of Family Physicians [AAFP], 2001).

Finally, if the inability to eat and drink is associated with dysphagia (inability to swallow) the individual will be scheduled to undergo a swallowing evaluation rather than merely accepting the fact that the person is refusing food and/or liquids. If the patient's study is abnormal, an enteral tube, such as nasogastric (NG), percutaneous endoscopic gastrostomy (PEG), or gastrojejugostomy (GJ) tube may be recommended. Risks and benefits of these treatment modalities are discussed in further sections in this chapter.

SECTION ONE REVIEW

1. Eating and drinking are two obvious means to sustaining life. However:
   1. The meaning of feeding is consistent from person to person.
   2. Nourishment and nurturing are synonymous.
3. There may be separate goals for intake and socialization.
4. Dilemmas generally do not involve issues of hydration and nutrition.

2. Technology has provided artificial means for hydration and nutrition. This progress:
   1. Has resulted in the creation of new ethical dilemmas.
   2. Allows for easy choices and decisions.
   3. Always provides comfortable alternatives to oral nutrition and hydration.
   4. Provides an ethical means to prevent someone from starving to death.
3. The current aging population:
   1. Has fewer chronic health problems and thus the inability to eat or drink is generally not of great concern.
   2. Is frequently not offered newer technologies for artificial hydration or nutrition.
   3. Is well aware of their choices as well as the risks and burdens of these choices.

4. Should be part of the team when discussing their status and potential outcome for hydration and nutritional goals.
4. Often when a person's health is failing:
   1. They have increased appetite, just as in other illness episodes.
   2. Most family members are accepting of their loss of appetite.
   3. Natural anorexia and loss of appetite are common.
   4. Allowing natural dehydration is not an appropriate choice.
5. At the end of life, a patient may develop dysphagia. It is common:
   1. For the family to accept this.
   2. To evaluate this problem with a swallow study.
   3. To ignore the choices of tube insertion and use.
   4. To have good survival and outcomes with long-term use of feeding tubes at the end of life.

SECTION TWO: Artificial Interventions

Artificial versus Natural Nutrition and Hydration

AHN is not the same thing as eating and drinking naturally. Not only are AHN mechanical and unable to respond to an individual's feelings of hunger or thirst, they are often described as bothersome and uncomfortable. These treatment options are, in fact, medical procedures that do not allow for activities normally associated with eating, such as chewing, swallowing, or tasting. Perhaps Koretz (2007) described this distinction best when he noted that "tube feedings have no perception of feeling good. It is a cold process devoid of the sensation of nurturing" (p. 379).

When health care providers imply they are "feeding" patients, and discuss machines and tubes as if they were natural, the choice of language shapes the health care providers' thinking and insulates team members from the patients' experience. Thinking to ask patients, "Are you hungry or thirsty?" gives patients themselves control over the amount of hydration and nourishment they desire. This approach to meeting the needs of patients is often difficult for families to accept. However, the side effects and discomforts from lack of food and water, which are their primary concern, easily can be managed, as outlined later (Miller, 2004).

Early in the 1990s, the American Nurses Association (ANA) determined that nurses should distinguish the administration of AHN from the provision of food and water (1992). Even force feeding a patient with a spoon orally could be viewed as artificial nutrition. Artificially provided hydration and nutrition may or may not be justified. Additionally, ethical difficulties may arise for patients and families if they do not have a clear understanding of the benefits and risks associated with these medical interventions. Sometimes implementing aggressive treatments, including AHN, can be seen as causing harm to the patient. In extreme cases, AHN may be considered as abuse for selected patients and a greater harm than death itself (Karel, 2004).

Benefits and Burdens Associated with Nutrition and Hydration

Refusing food and drink is most often viewed as a sign of the last phase of terminal condition. Natural **anorexia** brings with it less nausea and vomiting, as well as less exertion to chew, swallow, and breathe. Patients express fewer complaints of hunger with the passage of time. Overall, the experience of anorexia and **cachexia** is not uncomfortable (Lynn & Harrold, 1999).

Terminal dehydration or natural loss of thirst is also reported as not being painful. Few people feel or complain of any thirst. There is less lung fluid and congestion, and a lessening of oral secretions and the need for suctioning (Cervo et al., 2006). If the person experiences pain from a cancerous tumor, terminal dehydration decreases this pressure and less pain is reported by the individual. Terminal dehydration may also decrease tumor pressure and lessen pain because of a decrease in circulating fluid. This decrease in circulating fluid may also lessen the potential for edema and decubiti (Koretz, 2007). According to some research, there is a natural release of the pain-relieving chemical endorphin, as the body dehydrates (Critchlow & Bauer-Wu, 2002).

A major complaint of patients as they experience less thirst and hunger is the lack of social and mealtime interaction (Koretz, 2007). Family members and visitors are often uncomfortable eating in front of someone who is not also eating, so they will avoid interactions during mealtime and social events requiring food. Additionally, when a patient does not eat, it may seem as if not feeding him or her demonstrates a lack of fundamental nurturing. This emotional reality has an important impact on the patient, family, and health care providers.

The state of anorexia will not provide adequate nutritional intake for sustenance and will decrease a patient's energy levels over time. The loss of control is one of the most challenging consequences of illness for many people. Food may have been an important aspect of the patient's life. It becomes difficult when a patient is unable to consume items that loved ones bring as gestures of caring. Patients sometimes feel they must eat something for the sake of their families and visitors, to the point of being uncomfortable or nauseated (Huang & Ahronheim, 2000).

The main burden associated with dehydration at the end of life is a dry mouth. **Xerostomia** can be easily treated with sips of favorite drinks, popsicles, ice chips, mouth swabs, suckers, peppermint or lemon drops and gum. Even for those individuals who do not chew gum, sports gum can be sliced and sucked on for relief of dry mouth (HPNA, 2003). However, there may be an increased risk of pulmonary embolism and deep vein thrombosis due to the decreased flow of fluids. End-stage dehydration is not generally accompanied by headache, delirium, nausea and vomiting, and/or abdominal cramps (Arinzon, Peisakhi, & Berner, 2008).

The Benefits and Burdens of Artificial Nutrition and/or Hydration

There is no question that artificial nutrition helps speed the recovery of many patients or allows them to live with illnesses that formerly would have led to death (Cervo et al., 2006). Often, stroke patients who are unable to swallow are provided adequate hydration and nutrition through NG or gastrostomy tubes, often learning to eat again, at which point the tube is removed. Likewise, **enteral administration** of nutrition is used with patients who have had throat cancer that left them unable to swallow. Enteral nutrition is also helpful in other cases, such as certain bowel obstructions or chemotherapies involving intestines. Some enteral tubes allow patients to continue to perform normal activities of daily living. Few would question whether artificial nutrition is appropriate in these types of conditions and diagnoses (Hallenbeck, 2003; Kudsk, 2007).

Medically, AHN may prolong life and prevent wasting, emaciation, or cachexia, as well as weight loss in stable patients. Some authors have noted that AHN may prevent aspiration pneumonia (Chang & Roberts, 2008; Serna & McCarthy, 2006; Scolapio, 2007). With added nutrition, independence and physical function may be maintained. Most importantly, allowing patients the option of deciding for or against AHN guarantees their basic human right of autonomy. This treatment choice also recognizes, acknowledges, and honors cultural and spiritual beliefs.

There are many cases where artificial hydration and nutrition are more of a burden to the patient than a benefit. Research has shown increased risk of aspiration with the possibility of tube displacement (Serna & McCarthy, 2006; Scolapio, 2008). There is the potential for increased fluid overload, though the lack of current research studies would indicate that this is not a major problem. Patients have reported increased pain with the necessary procedures that must be performed to place the tubes required to administer AHN. Finally, because of the necessity to continuously be attached to equipment and machines for delivery of AHN, there is decreased mobility (AAHPM, 2002, HPNA, 2003).

Misconceptions Associated with AHN

There are many misconceptions regarding enteral administration of AHN. The first of these misconceptions is that enteral nutrition prolongs life with calories and nutritional support. Data concerning this misconception are limited and there are no data to support significant improvement in survival rates (Cervo et al., 2006; Owen & Fang, 2007). An additional study found no survival advantage in patients with AHN and dementia (Hallenbeck, 2005).

A second misconception is that artificial hydration and nutrition may enhance quality of life or reduce suffering (van der Riet, Good, Higgins, & Sneesby, 2008). Where true hunger and thirst exist, quality of life may be enhanced. Most actively dying patients, however, do not experience hunger or thirst. Limited to only a few observational studies, research regarding palliative care (comfort care) and enteral nutrition found no studies demonstrating improved quality of life with this intervention. On the other hand, AHN may adversely affect quality of life through increased need for physical restraints, infections, pain, indignity, cost, and the denial of the pleasure of eating (ADA, 2002; Cline, 2006; Lynn, 1989).

SECTION TWO REVIEW

1. Natural nutrition and hydration:
   1. Provide the same effects as artificial nutrition and hydration.
   2. Give the patient control of his or her intake.
   3. Are frequently considered the only method of intake.
   4. Always provide adequate nutritional needs.

2. The nurse has just completed a teaching session with a family regarding the patient's natural loss of appetite and loss of thirst. The nurse recognizes the need for more teaching when the family member comments:
   1. "Will you be giving the patient medicine to decrease the hunger pains?"

2. "I am glad the patient is likely to have less nausea than when we force the patient to eat."
3. "The edema seems to be decreasing since the patient has been eating less."
4. "The patient's decrease in eating and drinking is one of the signs of the body slowing down."

3. Unlike dehydration from other causes, end stage dehydration:
   1. Often causes headache and abdominal cramps.
   2. Is usually not accompanied by other symptoms.
   3. Can be improved with IV fluids.
   4. Is always accompanied by xerostomia.

4. An example of a patient that might benefit the most from artificial nutrition and hydration is:
   1. A stroke patient who is unable to feed himself or herself and is not a candidate for rehabilitation.
   2. A terminally ill patient with end-stage renal disease.
   3. A stomach cancer patient who has had the stomach and intestines removed.
   4. A patient with tongue cancer who has had tongue surgery to remove a diseased portion of the tongue.

5. A nursing intervention for _____ includes having the patient suck on sports gum for relief.

SECTION THREE: Choices Regarding Nutrition and Hydration at the End of Life

The Choice to Stop Eating and Drinking

The cessation of natural eating and drinking allows one to die gradually and naturally. For the nurse, the patient's choice to stop eating and drinking is ethically and legally established (ANA, 1992) and is supported by the *Code of Ethics for Nurses* (ANA, 2001). Losing control is often a major issue for patients; thus, the choice to stop eating and drinking empowers the patient and needs to be honored. To voluntarily stop eating and drinking (VSED) can be an active and deliberate decision of a competent, informed, and physically capable individual. Often patients in the last stages of a terminal disease do not exhibit depression or other conditions that have affected their reasoning, nor are they suicidal in the usual sense of the word. These patients seem to conclude that the burden of living is greater than the act of dying (Stinson, Godkin, & Robinson, 2004).

The choice to stop eating and drinking is usually disturbing to family members as well as health care providers. When a patient makes such a choice, the family and caregivers do need to ensure that the patient is not suffering from depression or inadequate pain control. A patient may have emotional burdens, such as discord in the family or have problems that are spiritual in nature. If these conditions are being adequately managed and the terminally ill person's death will not place further burdens on family members, the patient may no longer want to delay death through the use of AHN. Health care providers should support these difficult decisions and continue to provide needed support and counsel to both the person and his or her family members (Quill, 2001). Additionally, a patient's valid advance directive may assist the family members in understanding the specific wishes of the patient and prevent disagreements if the patient should

become incompetent and no longer able to verbalize his or her desire not to institute AHN.

The health care provider's role in addressing emotional and spiritual issues as well as symptom management as the patient decides between continuing to receive nutrition and hydration or makes the decision to refuse to eat or drink is vital. This usually happens in the last days of the disease's progression. The competent patient's decision is binding on everyone involved in the patient's care. Death generally occurs in one to three weeks following the cessations of continuing nutrition and hydration, though the patient and family members should be informed that death may take longer (Hallenbeck, 2003; Koretz, 2007).

Treatment Trials

When doubt exists as to whether a treatment or therapy such as AHN will improve the terminally ill person's comfort and/or quality of life, a time-limited trial may be implemented. Such an implementation for a reasonable time frame allows everyone involved to see if there are benefits to be gained using the proposed treatment or therapy. To be considered a success, individuals involved in the time trial must know when the outcomes will be assessed and what benefits should occur or be evident (Robert, Kennerly, Keane, & George, 2003). Usually health care providers can reach a consensus as to how much time it will take to weigh the disadvantages versus the benefits of a treatment or therapy. Currently, there are no specific guidelines regarding the optimal solutions, amounts, or administration rates for AHN in terminally ill persons (American Society for Parenteral and Enteral Nutrition [ASPEN], 2007; Cervo et al., 2006). Thus each situation will vary and will be individually evaluated. Dunn (2001) suggested that the outcomes of a time-limited trial for AHN should involve the person's ultimate comfort, alertness, and energy levels.

Some patients and families have expressed the concern that once a treatment or therapy is begun, especially a time-limited trial for AHN, they will not be able to stop the AHN if there is no evidence of benefit to the patient. Additionally, they have expressed that discontinuing the AHN might be seen as "killing" their loved one or letting the patient "starve to death" (van der Riet et al., 2008). Like any other treatment modality, if there is no improvement in the person's condition and no clinical evidence that positively affects the person's comfort level or increase in quality of life measures, then there is no reason to continue the therapy. The natural progression of the disease is what prevents patients from eating or drinking normally and naturally. Stopping treatments that replace these natural functions only allows the disease to follow its natural course. Even if these treatments have been in place for months or years, it is permissible to stop them and allow death to occur (End of Life Nursing Consortium, 2008; Education for Physicians on End-of-life Care, 1999).

Making the Choice

Nutritional support frequently becomes an ethical and legal dilemma that health care providers must face when dealing with the elderly population of patients at the end of life in multiple clinical settings. Nurses have the responsibility to understand the issues and choices patients and their families make regarding AHN and assist them with their decisions from an unbiased, objective, and factual position.

The debate concerning the issue of nutritional support and the implications to terminate treatment can create fears and uncertainty in patients and family members. As with all medical treatments and therapies, the risks, benefits, burdens, and anticipated outcomes should be balanced when deciding whether or not to start or stop artificial hydration or nutrition. The burdens imposed by these artificial treatments should not be ignored merely because the treatments are a terminally ill person's sole means of remaining alive. Health care professionals must always consider patient and family wishes, emotions, beliefs, and understanding. The decision to accept or refuse food and fluids should always be respected and the person should continue to receive competent and caring nursing support, regardless of the person's decision to accept or not accept ANH (ANA, 1992; Arinzon et al., 2008; Owens & Fang, 2007).

Patients and their families must be given impartially presented and factual information. Timing and clarifying the understanding of patients and their families are critical. Health care providers should be sympathetic to the emotional aspects of this discussion. A family conference, allowing open discussion and utilizing the interdisciplinary team, may be the best method to present all the information needed for a person to make an educated decision. Having to make a choice and having limited control adds to the burden of the outcome.

Patients and families should understand and be able to weigh the benefits and burdens of natural dehydration and loss of appetite over the benefits and burdens of artificial hydration and nutrition. Nurses can assist by reviewing patient and family wishes with them and helping them understand the ramifications of these wishes. Ethically, it is essential that patients make their own decisions once they have the facts.

Health care providers continually provide high-quality care, minimize discomfort, and promote patient dignity. They must also demonstrate caring, and provide support and education. AHN should always be considered relative to patient's goals. Information regarding risks, benefits, and burdens should be explored when discussing the option of enteral nutrition. Alternative interventions such as spoon feeding or other comfort measures should be addressed at the same time that goals and possible invasive procedures are discussed. Only by facilitating these frank discussions can health care providers ensure that the patients and families are able to give truly informed consent prior to decisions regarding AHN.

Health care providers continuously consider the benefits and burdens that AHN present for the individual patient and family members and allow these individuals to reach decisions that they can implement. These decisions do not come easily and adequate time must be allowed in this process (Frederich, 2002; van der Riet et al., 2008).

Members of the health care team may be faced with implementing therapies, especially AHN, in patients who would not have allowed such therapies had they been competent to make their wishes known. For example, an issue that often arises concerns the implementation of AHN in a patient who did not complete an advance directive and who is now incompetent and near the last days of his or her life. Family members are reluctant to see their loved one denied hydration and nutrition, despite the fact that the health care members have discussed the benefits and burdens of initiating such therapy for the given patient. Nurses may be requested to initiate AHN, especially in the situation where the primary health care provider sees the need to "treat the family as well as the patient" and orders AHN.

Some of the proactive measures nurses can implement to prevent the preceding scenario include working with legal staff of the institution in developing guidelines for educating patients and family members about the benefits and burdens of AHN at the end of life. Discussions should be initiated when the patient is first admitted to hospice or other health care agencies, following the steps of the respectful death model as presented in Chapter 2. These discussions assist members of the health care team to more fully comprehend the concerns and goals of patients and family members before the patient becomes incompetent. For patients who are incompetent at admission, these conversations begin the dialogue early and assist family members to more fully comprehend the benefits and burdens of AHN as early as possible.

Other proactive measures that members of the health care team may employ include requesting that the ethics committee work with them to understand their values, concerns, and allow a vehicle for conversation. Being able to express one's concerns and values and know that others concur with these values does bring some peace of mind when confronting situations where team members feel that the best interventions are not being implemented. These situations are always difficult and nurses should also remember that the situation is equally difficult for the family of the terminally ill person. Table 6–1 enumerates some additional items that health care providers should consider when discussing hydration and nutrition in terminal care.

Remember, there are no right or wrong conclusions when assisting patients and family members to understand these issues. Each patient's circumstance must be evaluated and the patient allowed to make informed choices independently. Although decisions are individual, in the majority of reported hospice experiences, most patients do quite well

without hydration or nutrition in the advanced stages of the dying process (Hallenbeck, 2003).

TABLE 6–1 Considerations in Deciding Hydration and Nutrition at the End of Life

- The patient's choice to stop eating and drinking
- The patient's physical condition and prognosis
- Artificial versus natural hydration and nutrition
- Benefits and burdens of anorexia and terminal dehydration
- Benefits and burdens of artificial hydration and nutrition
- Trial and stopping of treatment

SECTION THREE REVIEW

1. A time-limited trial of artificial nutrition or hydration:
   1. Is illegal and unethical.
   2. Must have a designated end point for reassessment and evaluation as part of the treatment.
   3. May have different outcomes for individual patients.
   4. Has a set protocol that is followed for every eligible patient.
2. Artificial nutrition and hydration need to be considered in relationship to the patient's _____.
3. If the patient chooses to refuse nutrition and hydration, which interventions might be appropriate? (Select all that apply.)
   1. Discuss the patient's decision with the family and provide support.
   2. Assess the patient for depression and/or pain.
   3. Ask for a different nursing assignment.
   4. Encourage the family to go home and let the patient rest.
4. When determining if artificial nutrition and hydration are appropriate courses of action, the health care provider will need to take the following into consideration:
   1. The patient's underlying beliefs
   2. The patient's formal educational experience
   3. The patient's family history
   4. The legal consequences of potentially withdrawing artificial nutrition and hydration

---

CHAPTER SUMMARY

- Nutrition and hydration are essential to maintain life and are also associated with enjoyment and socialization.
- Advances in technology have allowed artificial nutrition and hydration to become a relatively common health care practice, while simultaneously creating some very controversial ethical concerns.
- With end-of-life and terminal conditions, weighing the risks and benefits of artificial hydration and nutrition options is essential.
- Refusing food and drink may be a sign of the last phases of a terminal condition.
- Misconceptions regarding enteral administration of hydration and nutrition include:
  ○ Enteral nutrition prolongs life with calories and nutritional support
  ○ Artificial hydration and nutrition may enhance quality of life or reduce suffering.

- The health care provider's role in addressing emotional and spiritual issues as well as symptom management as the patient decides between continuing to receive nutrition and hydration or makes the decision to refuse to eat or drink is vital.
- Treatment trials may be conducted to see if artificial hydration and nutrition enhance the terminally ill person's quality and quantity of life.
- Patients and their families must be given impartially presented and factual information regarding the benefits and burdens of artificial hydration and nutrition at the end of life.

CHAPTER REVIEW

Milton is an 89-year-old gentleman admitted to the hospital with increased weakness, loss of appetite, weight loss, and found to be anemic, hemoglobin of 3.7. During his hospital stay, Milton was diagnosed with leukemia. The oncologist explained a short prognosis of weeks. Milton, his wife, and his brother were not surprised. His son, who lives out of state, was notified by phone and was available to come to participate in further planning for his father.

During his hospitalization, Milton was offered nutritional supplements, which he refused. He consumed less than one-quarter of his meals and drank very little water or other beverages. He had no appetite or thirst and found no pleasure in consuming food or drink. He became more nauseated and short of breath whenever he tried. His wife and brother were concerned, but they saw the outcome of Milton's attempts.

Milton decided to stop eating and drinking altogether. He was offered IV fluids, but required furosemide (a diuretic) with every liter of fluid he was given. He told the doctors, nurses, and dietitian, "No more." He said he wanted to stop eating and allow "nature to take its course." He said he based his decision on his shortness of breath, his diminished appetite, and his desire to avoid prolonging his life. He asked the nurses to help explain his decision to his family. He also asked how much time he had left if he continued abstinence from food and fluid.

Questions

1. Should other options and choices be presented to Milton regarding hydration and nutrition?
2. Is it ethical for a patient to stop eating and drinking or is this a sign of depression, incompetence, or unrealistic goals?
3. Can a patient legally and ethically refuse fluids and food?
4. Who was it helping to have his family offer Milton hydration and nutrition?
5. If Milton was not capable of making the decision, who would?

Suggested Responses

All choices and options should be presented to Milton as well as his family. The risks, benefits, and burdens, along with expected outcomes should also be given to Milton and his family. They should be presented objectively, without bias. Even if asked what your choice would be, remember this is the patient and family's situation, beliefs, and understanding.

It is legal and ethical for patients to choose to stop eating or drinking, as long as they are deemed capable of making the decision, know and understand what the outcomes could entail, and are not suicidal. Depression and sadness is common at the end of life, but it is important to consider if this patient would be too depressed to sign a surgical consent or other form. Competency and degree of depression may need to be further examined.

Although it is often difficult to predict death with any certainty, the nurse talked with Milton and his family about the dying process, the role of food and fluid in the end-of-life stages, and the physical changes that he might experience before death. His wife, brother, and son had different perspectives about Milton's decisions; however, they agreed to carry out his wishes and not to force him, but only offer fluids or food periodically. Milton's wife feared that Milton was starving himself to hasten the dying process. His son, brother, and physicians did not object to Milton's withdrawal from food, feeling Milton was competent and capable to make the decision, not suicidal or depressed, and thinking Milton did understand the outcome of his decision.

It is uncertain who would benefit from having the family offer Milton hydration and nutrition. Milton did not want these options, but might have agreed to accept such interventions for the sake of his family and not for his own sake. If Milton was not capable of making the decision, his appointed health care agent would make the choice. If no health care agent is assigned, this decision is generally given to the next of kin, which in this scenario is his wife.

Milton was admitted to a nursing home with hospice services. He lived another four weeks with only mouth swabs and oral care, no measurable food or water, all the while maintaining his own oral care for xerostomia. He remained alert and oriented and, although weak, had less dyspnea than he did in the hospital. His children and wife convinced Milton to try a small amount of food and fluids, and ice chips and broth were reintroduced into his diet.

During his last weeks, Milton reported very little pain. He spent his time with his family, reminiscing about their lives together. The family continued to be supportive, reinforcing his decisions and his right to make the choices that he felt were best for him. He died with his family feeling that his self-directed medical decisions were honored throughout the course of his hospice care.

REFERENCES

American Academy of Family Physicians. (2001). *Artificial nutritional support at end-of-life: Is it justifiable?* Retrieved from http://www.aafp.org/afp/20010701/tips/6.html

American Academy of Hospice and Palliative Medicine (2002). *AAHPM Position statement on advanced hydration and nutrition.* Retrieved from http://www.aahpm.org/education/arthy.pdf

American Dietetic Association. (2002). Position of the American Dietetic Association: Ethical and legal issues in nutrition, hydration, and feeding. *Journal of the American Dietetic Association, 102*(5), 716–726.

American Nurses Association. (1992). *ANA position statement on foregoing nutrition and fluid.* Task Force on the Nurses Role in End-of-life Decisions. Retrieved from http://www.nursingworld.org/readroom/position/ethics/etnutr.htm

American Nurses Association. (2001). *Code of ethics for nurses with interpretive statements.* Washington, DC: Author.

American Society for Parenteral & Enteral Nutrition [ASPEN]. (2007). Statement on parenteral nutrition standardization. Retrieved from http://www.nutritioncare.org/profdev/stnds.html

Arinzon, Z., Peisakhi, A., & Berner, Y. N. (2008). Evaluation of the benefits of enteral nutrition in long-term care elderly patients. *Journal of the American Medical Directors Association, 9*(9), 657–662.

Cervo, F. A., Bryan, L., & Farber, S. (2006). To PEG or not to PEG: A review of evidence for placing feeding tubes in advanced dementia and the decision-making process. *Geriatrics, 61*(6), 30–35.

Chang, C.-C., & Roberts, B. L. (2008). Feeding difficulties in older adults with dementia. *Journal of Clinical Nursing, 17*(17), 2266–2274.

Clay, A. S., & Abernathy, A. P. (2008). Total parenteral nutrition for patients with advanced life-limiting cancer: Decision making in the face of conflicting evidence. *Progress in Palliative Care, 16*(2), 69–77.

Cline, D. (2006). Nutrition issues and tools for palliative care. *Home Healthcare Nurse, 24*(1), 54–57.

Critchlow, J., & Bauer-Wu, S. (2002). Dehydration in terminally ill patients: Perceptions of long-term care nurses. *Journal of Gerontological Nursing 28*(12), 31–39.

Dunn, H. (2001). Artificial hydration and nutrition. In *Hard choices for loving people* (4th ed.). Herndon, VA: A&A Publishers.

Education for Physicians on End-of-life Care Project, Robert Wood Johnson Foundation. (1999). Considerations in initiating, withholding or withdrawing artificial hydration and nutrition. Education for Physicians on End-of-Life Care Trainer's Guide, Module 11. In L. L. Emanuel, C. J. von Gunten, & F. D. Ferris, *Education for physicians on end-of-life care: Institute for Ethics at the American Medical Association.* Chicago: EPEC Project, Robert Wood Johnson Foundation. Retrieved from http://www.epec.net/EPEC/Media/ph/module11.pdf

End of Life Nursing Consortium. (2008). *Advanced end of life nursing care: ELNEC supercore training program 2008.* Washington, DC: American Association of Colleges of Nursing.

Frederich, M. E. (2002). Artificial hydration and nutrition in the terminally ill. *AAHPM Bulletin,* 8–9, 13.

Hallenbeck, J. (2003). Chapter 6: Hydration, Nutrition, and Antibiotics in End-of-Life Care. In *Palliative Care Perspectives.* New York: Oxford University Press.

Hallenbeck, J. (2005). Fast facts and concepts #11: To feed or not to feed (2nd ed.). *End-of-Life Palliative Education Resource Center.* Retrieved from http://www.eperc.mcw.edu/fastFact/ff_010.htm

Hospice and Palliative Nurses Association (HPNA). (2003). HPNA position paper: Artificial nutrition and hydration in end-of-life care. *Journal of Hospice and Palliative Nursing, 5*(4), 231–234.

Huang, Z., & Ahronheim, J. (2000). Nutrition and hydration in terminally ill patients: An update. *Clinical Geriatric Medicine, 16*(2), 313–325.

Karel, J. (2004). The ethics of tube feeding at the end-of-life. *Colorado Health Ethics Forum,* 1–7.

Koretz, L. (2007). Should patients with cancer be offered nutritional support: Does the benefit outweigh the burden? *European Journal of Gastroenterology and Hepatology, 19*(5), 379–382.

Kudsk, K. A. (2007). Beneficial effect of enteral nutrition. *Gastrointestinal Endoscopy Clinics of North America, 17*(4), 647–662.

Lynn, J. (Ed.) (1989). *By no extraordinary means: The choice to forgo life-sustaining food and water.* Bloomington, IN: Indiana University Press.

Lynn, J., & Harrold, J. (1999). Tube feeding (fluids and food). In *Handbook for mortals: Guidance for people facing serious illness.* Retrieved from http://www.mywhatever.com/cifwriter/library/mortals/mor11105.html

Miller, E. (2004). Chapter 12: Nutrition. In J. Panke & P. Coyne (Eds.) *Conversations in palliative care.* Pittsburgh, PA: Hospice and Palliative Nurses Association.

Mion, L., & O'Connell, A. (2003) Parenteral hydration and nutrition in the geriatric patient: Clinical and ethical issues. *Journal of Infusion Nursing, 26*(3), 144–152.

Owen, C., & Fang, J. C. (2007). Decisions to be made when initiating enteral nutrition. *Gastrointestinal Endoscopy Clinics of North America, 17*(4), 687–702.

Pichard, C., Kyle, U. G., & Morabia, A. (2004). Nutritional assessment: Lean body mass depletion at hospital admission is associated with increased length of stay. *American Journal of Clinical Nutrition, 79,* 613–618.

Quill, T. (2001). *Caring for patients at the end-of-life: Facing an uncertain future together.* New York: Oxford University Press.

Robert, S. R., Kennerly, D. A., Keane, D., & George, C. (2003). Nutrition support in the intensive care unit: Adequacy, timeliness, and outcomes. *Critical Care Nurse, 23*(1), 49–57.

Scolapio, J. S. (2007). Decreasing aspiration risk with enteral feeding. *Gastrointestinal Endoscopy Clinics of North America, 17*(4), 711–716.

Serna, E., & McCarthy, M. S. (2006). Heads up to prevent aspiration during enteral feeding. *Nursing 2006, 36*(1), 76–77.

Slomka, J. (2003). Withholding nutrition at the end-of-life: Clinical and ethical issues. *Cleveland Clinic Journal of Medicine, 70*(6), 548–552.

Smith, S. A., & Andrews, M. (2000). Artificial nutrition and hydration at the end-of-life. *Medical-Surgical Nursing 9*(5), 233–247.

Stinson, C., Godkin, J., & Robinson, R. (2004). Ethical dilemma: Voluntarily stopping eating and drinking. *Dimensions of Critical Care Nursing, 23*(1), 38–43.

van der Riet, P., Good, P., Higgins, I., & Sneesby, L. (2008). Palliative care professionals' perceptions of nutrition and hydration at the end of life. *International Journal of Palliative Nursing, 14*(3), 145–151.

Whitworth, M. K., Whitworth, A., Holm, S., Makin, W., Shaffer, J., & Jayson, G. C. (2004). Doctor, does this mean I'm going to starve to death? *Journal of Clinical Oncology, 22*(1), 199–201.

Caring for End-of-Life Patients Across the Life Span

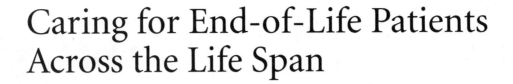

OBJECTIVES   Following completion of this chapter, the learner will be able to:

7.1. Discuss the impact of death and dying as it affects the family structure.

7.2. Describe the nursing care of patients at the end of life across the life span, including nursing care that is unique to the developmental stage of the dying individual.

7.3. Describe nursing interventions that family caregivers can implement to assist with end-of-life care for their loved ones.

7.4. Explore challenges in caring for patients at the end of life across the age continuum.

In this chapter the care of the dying person is examined using a developmental stage framework that explores the impact of death across the life span. Ages that are addressed include the infant, toddler, adolescent, young adult, middle-age adult, and older adult. Important concepts that are described include nursing challenges that are unique to the developmental stage of the dying individual and acknowledging how death and dying affects the entire family structure. Understanding how family caregivers can contribute to the care of the dying individual is addressed. The chapter concludes by exploring multiple end-of-life challenges facing nurses, patients, and family members and suggests the need for continuing research concerning the perceptions of patients as they die.

PRETEST

1. One of the greatest benefits for the family of a dying individual is for the health care workers to:
   1. Be about the same age as the terminally ill patient.
   2. Communicate with the family, to listen to their expressions of grieving, and assist with understanding that grieving is a normal process.
   3. Be present in the patient's room at all times so that the patient is not left alone.
   4. Be cost conscious and focus on the patient's physical care.
2. Because patients in the last hours of their lives generally require more skilled nursing care, these patients should be cared for in settings that are:
   1. Located within acute care hospitals and institutions.
   2. Located within the person's home environment.

3. Conducive to meeting the privacy needs of the person.
   4. Easiest for relatives and caregivers to access.
3. When making decisions for neonates, the standard of decision making should be the:
   1. Paternalistic model for decision making.
   2. Substituted judgment standard for decision making.
   3. Best interest standard of decision making.
   4. Decision-making model with which the health care practitioner is most familiar.
4. Parents who have a dying child need the following interventions: (Select all that apply.)
   1. Someone to listen to their thoughts and concerns.
   2. Information about the child's illness, prognosis, and treatment plans.

3. Others to assist them when they are not available because of treatment schedules and appointments.
4. Assistance with making decisions.
5. The grieving process of denial often lasts longer in the terminally ill young adult because the young adult:
   1. Is not capable of moving through the grief stages.

2. Is dealing with the grieving process from the loss of a parent.
3. Does not anticipate death.
4. Is not concerned with anything other than work.

GLOSSARY

Erickson's Eight Stages of Development   Published in 1959, Erickson depicted eight stages that individuals accomplish as they age from birth to old age, including infancy, early childhood, mid-childhood, school age, adolescent, young adulthood, middle adulthood, and late adulthood; understanding of these stages of development assists in providing expert care of the dying individual across the life span.

SECTION ONE: Impact of Death and Dying within the Family

The past century has seen a dramatic shift in how and where Americans die. In the early 1900s, the life expectancy was less than 50 years of age and death came fairly quickly (Centers for Disease Control [CDC], 2001 and 2002). The majority of individuals died due to infections, including pneumonia, tuberculosis, and diarrhea and enteritis (United States Department of Health and Human Services, 2003). The time from onset of disease to death was measured in days or weeks rather than months and years, and most individuals died at home with family members serving as caregivers.

Today, the life expectancy is approximately 77.8 years for all races, with women living slightly longer (80.4 years) than men (75.2 years) in all categories (CDC, 2007). This increased longevity has impacted the care needs at the end of life and the three most common trajectories of care needs are depicted in Box 7–1.

This trajectory for end-of-life care has produced three distinct care patterns. The first trajectory requires expert medical and nursing care over the long period of competent functioning, augmented with supportive palliative and hospice care for the patient and family members. The second trajectory requires expert medical and nursing care so that the periods of rapid exacerbation do not result in additional loss of functioning for as great a time period as possible. This trajectory also requires expert care planning and instructions for family members so that appropriate medical and nursing interventions can be initiated during the sudden, serious exacerbations of the patient's underlying condition. These timely interventions may prevent more serious complications and allow the terminally ill person additional quality of life. With the third trajectory, supportive medical and nursing care is required over multiple years, with ever-increasing assistance with activities of daily living, housing, and comfort (Lynn, 2005).

Many Americans, regardless of the final trajectory of illness, live out their final days in acute care facilities and caregivers tend to be paid professionals rather than family members (Kring, 2006; Lynn, 2005). This has added a new dimension to caring for individuals at the end of life, requiring that educational programs and continuing education offerings provide those individuals who deliver health care the information they need to expertly care for individuals at the end of life. Additionally, because family members are uniquely important to the care of their loved ones, health care providers have an added responsibility to ensure that these family members are competent to expertly care for the loved one at the end of life (Weman & Fagerberg, 2006).

Traditionally, the concept of family meant two parents, a mother and a father, and either one child or children living together as a unit. Sometimes, there were additional members of the family, such as a grandparent or aunt or uncle, within the family unit. The defining characteristic was that all were related and lived as a unit. Today, family has come to incorporate single-parent households, unmarried couples with children from previous marriages of either or both parents, couples who are of one gender, couples with no children, and households where children

---

BOX 7–1   Trajectories of Care Needs at the End of Life

- Long-term maintenance of adequate physical and mental functioning despite a terminal diagnosis
- Slow decline in physical capacities interspersed with serious exacerbations, with death often coming very suddenly when it does occur
- Long-term loss of physical and mental functioning, requiring more and more personal care as the individual becomes more incapacitated (Lynn, 2005)

from previous and current marriages are "blended" into a family unit (Allender & Spradley, 2005). In using the term *family* in this chapter, the reader is reminded to consider the family group in its broadest configuration. Whatever the specific family configuration, health care providers are reminded that illness and death affects all persons within the family (Hutchings, 2007).

Research has shown that the loss of a family member is one of the most traumatic and emotionally distressing events in a person's life (Brazil, Bedard, & Willison, 2002). Thus, family interactions and communication styles are important areas to assess when working with persons at the end of life. Healthy families generally value both internal and external relationships; that is, there are close ties within the family group and community engagement is equally valued. A healthy family relationship can be seen in that the members respect each other, are able to discuss difficult topics with the same honesty and openness that occurs when discussing humorous happenings and more lighthearted topics, and are able to set mutual goals. Characteristics of healthy communications include that family members appear interested in what each other has to say, listen when other family members are speaking, avoid drawing snap conclusions, attempt to see each other's point of view, and avoid being critical of other's views and thoughts (Allender & Spradley, 2005).

Interventions that can assist with family dynamics at the end of life include understanding that the patient and family members may be at various stages of the grief process (Brazil et al., 2002). Often, family members are not at the same stage of the grief process as the patient. Health care providers should thus remember to listen and initiate communications with individual members of the family, including the patient, in order to understand how each person is experiencing the grief process. Encourage the patient to verbalize his or her feelings, addressing these concerns openly and honestly. Help the patient to understand emotions, fears, and expectations and why family members' concerns and desires may not be the same as his or her concerns and desires. Encourage the patient to talk openly with family members, making them aware of the patient's perceptions and concerns. If needed, health care providers may be present during these conversations (End of Life Nursing Consortium [ELNEC], 2008).

Health care providers also affect family communications by encouraging the various family members to express their feelings and desires for the dying person (ELNEC, 2008). Help family members understand that they have lives of their own, encouraging them to balance care and visits with the dying person with their own responsibilities and duties. Help family members and the dying person to utilize resources appropriately, remembering that there will be times when all family members cannot be present and/or an active part of the person's care. There will be unique challenges for family members and these are discussed individually in the following sections.

SECTION ONE REVIEW

1. The shift over the last century in how and where Americans die has changed the way health care is delivered. Which of the following helps to explain the differences?
   1. Americans die slower, more lingering deaths with care provided by paid caregivers. The health care setting is more often in an acute care facility.
   2. Americans die faster with illnesses being more chronic. Care is equally provided by family and paid caregivers. The health care setting is more often in an acute care setting.
   3. Americans die slower with illnesses being more acute. Mostly family or friends provide care. The health care setting is more often in a long-term care facility.
   4. Americans die younger with illnesses being more lingering with care provided mostly by paid caregivers. The health care setting is more often in a long-term care facility.
2. Families continue to be a vital part of a patient's care. However, the definition of "family" has changed over the last century. Why is it important for the nurse to recognize the individual(s) that the patient considers family?

   1. The family member may be able to provide care when the nurse is unavailable.
   2. The loss of a family member is a very personal and traumatic event.
   3. The family member needs to be watched to prevent taking advantage of the patient.
   4. The family member should be listed as next of kin on the facility admission papers.
3. When the nurse is assessing the family dynamics, which one of the following scenarios might indicate a healthy family relationship?
   1. All family members gathered around the patient, everyone talking at once about what they think should be done with the patient.
   2. One family member at the bedside of the patient, arguing with the patient about the patient's choice of care options.
   3. Some family members gathered outside the patient's room with one of the members talking negatively about another member who isn't present.
   4. All family members gathered around the patient, with one person talking at a time, discussing alternatives to the patient's care.

Case Study 1

Judy, age 56, has been diagnosed with terminal colon cancer, which has now metastasized to her bones. She has been admitted to an in-patient hospice unit for terminal care. Her husband, John, and their three children, ages 26, 18, and 16, all visit on a regular basis. You note that their conversation tends to be confrontational and that there is great disagreement about what should be done for Judy. The children openly argue in front of Judy as though she is not present or should have any input into her own care. Individual members of the family also find fault with the care Judy is receiving, including that she still has some continual pain. The latest argument among the four family members concerned how to announce her death, with two of the family members noting that, as they have no outside friends in the community, they need not put an expensive obituary notice in the local newspaper.

Questions

How does this family group differ from what could be described as a healthy family? What can you, as the nurse assigned to Judy, begin to do so that Judy is as comfortable as possible during her final hours?

Suggested Responses

The more obvious distinctions are that family members have not developed internal or external relationships. Each of the family members appears to be more concerned about his or her individual needs. Two of the family members note that they have not developed external relationships, as there are no community persons for whom an obituary notice is required. Additionally, nothing is mentioned of marital partners for the three children, although it is possible that there are significant relationships that are not mentioned in the scenario. No mutual goals are being set, as each member seems to have different wants and desires for Judy.

You could begin by helping the family members know that the grieving process is a normal process that accompanies death and dying. This would seem to be a central theme about which there could perhaps be some agreement. You might also begin with the pain that Judy is experiencing and give the family some answers about potential causes for the continuing pain, possible variations in medications for the pain, or other measures that the family could do to assist with relieving her pain, such as diversion techniques. You could speak individually with the family members one-on-one, addressing each family member's specific questions and concerns. If these concerns overlapped between family members, you could perhaps initiate a family meeting. If there is a family meeting, Judy should be present and encouraged to voice her concerns and needs, as she is the central individual about whom the family meeting was initiated.

Finally, you may initiate conversations about how the family members will support each other after Judy's death. Each of the members will need support and bereavement measures in order to make a healthy transition after Judy dies.

SECTION TWO: Developmental Stages

To fully appreciate the needs of persons at the end of life, there must be a framework to guide understanding and information. One framework that addresses the various stages of persons across the life continuum includes a model addressing developmental stages, such as **Erickson's Eight Developmental Stages**. Realizing that this is an older model and recognizing that other models could also be chosen as the unifying framework for the development of end-of-life nursing care across the life span, Erickson's model was selected as it aids understanding of this content. Health care providers can use these stages to promote better insight and appreciation for appropriate interventions and communications with terminally ill persons, family members, and others involved in the care of the patient. Additionally, understanding the developmental stage of the family members gives needed insight into the behaviors and reactions of family members and those close to the terminally ill person.

The reader is cautioned to remember that although these ages and developmental stages are appropriate for the majority of persons, there may be some variation. Factors that influence variation within the stages include negative experiences in previous stages, cultural considerations, and environmental issues. Children who have experienced losses in early life often have greater challenges in negotiating later stages of development. For example, children who were not cuddled and held as infants often are unable to fully trust in later life (Erickson, 1963). The influence of culture and environment on the developmental stages is seen from the perspective that humans place on emphasis on external events and happenings as they grow and develop (Rogoff, 2003). Without these external forces, stages of development can greatly be slowed. Erickson's (1959) stages of development are outlined in the following sections and a general overview of the stages of development is found in Table 7–1.

Infancy

Infancy, from birth to approximately 18 months, is essentially synonymous with Erickson's Oral Sensory Stage. The major emphasis of this stage is on the parent's, particularly the mother's, positive and loving care for the child. Close contact, especially touch, is required if the infant is to pass successfully through this stage and develop trust and have confidence in the future. Erickson described this stage as trust versus mistrust, with the basic strengths being drive and hope (1959).

TABLE 7–1 Overview of Erickson's Eight Stages of Development

DEVELOPMENTAL STAGE	DESCRIPTION OF CHARACTERISTICS	BASIC STRENGTH(S)
Infancy, age to approximately 18 months	Trust versus mistrust	Drive and hope
Early childhood, 18 months to 3 years of age	Autonomy versus shame	Self-control, courage, and will
Mid-childhood, 3–5 years of age	Initiative versus guilt	Purpose
School age, 6–12 years of age	Industry versus inferiority	Method and competency
Adolescence, 12–18 years of age	Identity versus role confusion	Devotion and fidelity
Young adulthood, 18–35 years of age	Intimacy and solidarity versus isolation	Affiliation and love
Middle adulthood, ages to approximately 65	Generativity versus stagnation	Production and care
Late adulthood, the years beyond 65	Integrity versus despair	Wisdom

Source: Adapted from E. H. Erickson (1959). Identity and the Life Cycle. New York: International Universities Publishers.

Early Childhood

Early childhood, from 18 months to approximately 3 years of age, is the stage where the child learns to master skills for himself or herself. Fine motor development is emphasized and the child learns to walk, talk, and self-feed. Significant relationships remain with the parents, and the child has the opportunity to develop self-esteem and autonomy. Basic strengths at this stage include self-control, courage, and will. This is the stage of autonomy versus shame and, if not successfully mastered, the child is left with doubt concerning his or her capabilities.

Mid-Childhood

Mid-childhood, sometimes termed the "play age," generally covers the years between 3 and 5. During this stage, the child begins taking initiative in creative play and begins to imitate adults. Children at this age can be seen creating multiple stories about their toys and imaginary playmates, experimenting with what they perceive it means to be an adult. The most significant relationships are with the family group. Erickson termed this the stage of initiative versus guilt, with the basic strength being that of purpose.

School Age

School age, generally seen as the years between 6 and 12, is the developmental stage where the child develops a sense of industry, learning, creating, and accomplishing numerous new skills. This is a very social age, with the child expanding his or her relationships to include children at school and throughout the neighborhood. Parents no longer are the sole authority, though they are still very important to the child. Erickson saw this stage as industry versus inferiority, with the basic strengths those of

method and competency. Failure to develop adequate relationships with peers often results in feelings of incompetency and low self-esteem later in life.

Adolescence

Adolescence covers the teen years of 12 to 18. During these years, the person begins to develop a philosophy of life, thinking in terms of ideals rather than reality. Accomplishments of the individual have a greater impact than events that are occurring around the individual. A person's identity begins to more fully emerge, guided by social interactions and moral issues, and the peer group is much more significant than the family group. This is the stage of identity versus role confusion, with the basic strengths being those of devotion and fidelity.

Young Adulthood

Young adulthood occurs between the ages of 18 and 35. This is the stage of intimacy and solidarity versus isolation, with the basic strengths being affiliation and love. During this stage, the person generally seeks one or more close companions, attempting to find a mutually satisfying relationship, often with the goal of marriage and beginning a family. If negotiation of this stage is successful, intimacy on a deeper level is attained. If the stage is not negotiated successfully, isolation and distancing from others occurs.

Sometimes, within this isolation, the person develops a superiority complex as a means of accepting a lack of intimacy and love. Significant relationships are with marital partners and friends. Today, it is not uncommon to see marriage and beginning one's family moved toward the upper ends of this stage as opposed to occurring in the early twenties (Allender & Spradley, 2005).

Middle Adulthood

Occurring between the ages of 35 and approximately 65, middle adulthood is the stage of generativity versus stagnation, with the basic strengths being production and care. Work is essential in this stage and most of the middle adulthood stage is occupied with creative and meaningful work and with issues surrounding family. A significant task is to transmit values of culture to our children. Erickson called this generativity, meaning that individuals are contributing to the betterment of society (1959). Fears at this stage include that one will be inactive or that life will be meaningless. Significant relationships are with the family and groups within the workplace and community.

Late Adulthood

Seen as the years beyond 65, late adulthood encompasses the stage of integrity versus despair, with the basic strength being wisdom. Life has had great meaning and adults at this stage are able to reflect on a happy and useful life. Strength comes from the perception of wisdom that the world is vast and that they have truly made a difference in that world.

SECTION TWO REVIEW

1. If the adolescent is unable to integrate his or her many roles and develop self-esteem, he or she is likely to develop a sense of:
   1. Isolation later in life.
   2. Role confusion later in life.
   3. Inferiority later in life.
   4. Shame later in life.
2. Trust, which is necessary for the nurse-patient relationship to be fully effective, develops in:
   1. Infancy.
   2. Early childhood.
   3. Middle childhood.
   4. School-age child.
3. The stage at which the person develops more social skills and begins to rely more on friends than on close family ties is:
   1. Adolescence.
   2. Infancy.

3. Young adult.
4. School-age child.

4. An understanding of the developmental stages of the person assists the nurse in more effectively caring for the person at the end of life by: (Select all that apply.)
   1. Giving the nurse a fuller appreciation for the emotions that the person may be experiencing.
   2. Helping the nurse understand the emotions that family members may be portraying.
   3. Creating better communication between nursing and other health care providers.
   4. Assisting the nurse in planning more appropriate nursing interventions.

SECTION THREE: Children and End-of-Life Issues

For the calendar year 2003, approximately 30,000 children died during their first year of life, with two-thirds of these infant deaths occurring during the first 28 days of life. Additionally, another 25,000 children over the age of 1 and below the age of 10 died during the same calendar year (CDC, 2007).

When discussing children and end-of-life issues, the reader is cautioned to remember that the death of a child is but one aspect of concern. The other aspect is how children who are part of the family structure deal with the death of family members and other loved ones, primarily grandparents, parents, aunts, and uncles. Children may also be faced with the death of a sibling or close childhood relative, such as a cousin. Knowing how children grieve can begin to assist parents and health care deliverers in providing the appropriate and effective guidance that children need to deal with their grief in a positive manner.

Grieving Children

It is generally understood that children grieve differently than do adults (Goldman, 2000; Huntley, 2002). Generally, children are not continuously consumed with the death or impending death, but are able to put their feelings aside and return to normal activities of life, such as play activities. For some children, their grief is confined to times when they are alone, such as at naptime or bedtime, leaving parents and others to remark that the child is not grieving, but is "his or her normal self." Conversely, some children, unable to understand that they are grieving, repeatedly ask about the deceased person and seem not to be satisfied with answers as given. Younger children are often unable to express their grief orally, but act out their grief through temper tantrums, verbal outbursts, and sudden changes in mood and behaviors (Huntley, 2002).

Remember, children do not have the coping skills of adolescents and adults, so they are much less able to express exactly what they are experiencing. Like adults, children dealing with death and separation may have difficulty in completing tasks, may withdraw from social activities, and become withdrawn or overly dependent (Currier, Holland, & Neimeyer, 2007). Depending on the child's stage of development, the grief process may prevent the child from achieving developmental skills. Eventually, like adults and older children, the grief that the child experiences will begin to decline and more "typical" activities and moods will be displayed.

The developmental stage of the child who is experiencing the death of a family member assists the caregiver in more effectively working with these children and their parents. Though infants are unable to appreciate the events around them, parents and caregivers need to remember that this is the stage where trust is developed and that extra touch and cuddling of the infant is crucial. Nurses working with these parents and caregivers need to particularly observe or question the parents about the infant's care to ensure that adequate periods of time are being spent with the infant. If the parents are unable to spend this time providing closeness with the infant, other adults and/or older children need to step into this role (Goldman, 2000).

During the stage of early childhood, children are developing their sense of autonomy and are very reliant on the family group, especially parents and older siblings, to assist in developing the beginning skills of walking, talking, and self-feeding. Parents are again encouraged to spend quality time with children at this stage of development or arrange for another to serve in this role. Parents should ensure that familiar routines are maintained and that the child knows that he or she is loved. Simple explanations and allowing the child to ask questions, even if already answered, assist the child in working through his or her grieving.

Children in the mid-childhood stage of development are beginning to imitate adults and are developing initiative and creativity. During these years, the child is less able to appreciate the fact that the person who is at the end of life will not return (Rosof, 1995). Once he or she accepts the fact that the person is truly gone, the child may begin to question how soon the family group will be reinstituted and may question if the remaining parent will soon find another mate. If the death of a parent has occurred because of violence, the child may voice fears that the perpetrator will also harm him or her. These fears may be seen in the form of nightmares, bed-wetting, or the constant need to be with the remaining parent (Carpenito, 2007). Additionally, the child at this developmental stage may question who will care for him or her in the future. Nurses can help the parents and older children in the family understand that this is a common occurrence at this stage of development, so that they are not surprised by the child's request or questions (ELNEC, 2008).

School-age children are beginning to fully develop relationships outside the family group. Younger school-age children may feel that they have somehow caused the death and need to be reassured that they are not at fault. Children at the opposite end of this age spectrum comprehend fully the fact that this person will soon die and, therefore, parents are urged to answer their questions as completely as possible. This will assist the child coming to closure more quickly (Christ, 2000). The younger adolescent, as he or she becomes more involved with a peer group, is becoming more autonomous and may express anger and/or fear with the death of a parent. Remember, this is a time when the adolescent thinks in terms of ideas rather than reality and the full impact of the fact that he or she is still supported by the remaining parent may not be evident.

The older adolescent reacts much as adults do to the loss of a loved one, though the period of grieving may not be as long as that of an adult. Peer groups generally assist in preventing a long mourning period, as this is a very active time in their lives and the adolescent quickly moves back into his or her normal activities (Christ, 2000). Throughout all of these stages of development, the nurse answers questions as directly and completely as possible, giving answers that are appropriate for the child's age and stage of development, and including the parents and other caregivers in these discussions (ELNEC, 2008). Box 7–2 enumerates some appropriate interventions for children who are grieving the death of another person.

Caring for the Dying Child

Despite the best efforts to prevent death among children, they do die and the impact on the family is immense (Rini & Loriz, 2007). Unfortunately, palliative care has never been fully implemented for infants and very young children, yet the need to provide such care for parents and their infants is vitally needed. In older age groups, palliative care is better utilized, though improvements still need to be made (Romesberg, 2007).

The Committee on Palliative Care and End-of-Life Care for Children and Their Families clearly states, "We can and should do more than we are currently doing to prevent and relieve the physical and emotional suffering of dying children and the psychic pain of their families . . . and to allow all who are affected by a child's death the opportunity to address their feelings and concerns" (Institute of Medicine of the National Academies, 2003, p. xv).

One means of achieving this end is by the development and implementation of palliative care programs for neonates and children. Such a palliative care program consists of three essential components: comfort care; end-of-life decision making; and bereavement support measures for remaining family members. Comfort care focuses on discomfort and pain with the ultimate goals to maximize the infant's or child's comfort and provide emotional support to the family so that the potential for later regrets is lessened. Traditional models that deliver solely comfort care measures are not generally appropriate for children who die of non-oncology diseases and illnesses. There are multiple short-term uncertainties in children that most often mandate

---

BOX 7-2 **Appropriate Interventions for Children Grieving the Loss of Another**

- Spend extra time with the child who has experienced another's death, remembering that children often grieve during times when they are alone, such as nap time or bedtime.
- Continue to promote familiar routines and ensure that the child knows that he or she is continually loved and that the family group is stable.
- Remember that younger children act out their grief through temper tantrums, verbal outbursts, and sudden changes in mood and behaviors, and thus require additional understanding and support when these behaviors are exhibited.
- Be alert for indications, such as nightmares, bedwetting, or the need to be continuously with another person, that the child fears that he or she will also die, and give appropriate reassurance.
- Children may require additional support, asking the same question repeatedly and needing continued assurance and attention; simple answers and recognition that the questions are important serve to reassure the grieving child.
- Observe the child for difficulty in completing tasks or behavior that is overly dependent or isolated; these may be signs that the child is grieving.
- School-age children may need assurance that they did not cause the death.
- Answers to the child's questions should be as complete as possible, remembering to frame answers appropriate to the child's age and stage of development.

---

the hospitalization of the child. Thus, the comfort care component of palliative care in children is often interwoven with more technologically advanced care measures (Tuffrey, Finlay, & Lewis, 2007, Rosof, 1995).

End-of-life decision making concerns deciding when, where, and how the infant or child will die. This type of decision making is an area that is generally considered to be foreign to most parents and families and requires learning new and often complex information, emotional integration of a tragic situation, and communication on multiple levels (Swigart, Lidz, Butterworth, & Arnold, 1996). Health care providers may find themselves reinforcing the parent's and family's decision to withdraw life-saving measures and face the task of choosing which day their child will die. This component may involve the implementation of ethics committee meetings to better support the family in decision making. Always, this component involves the active advocacy of all members of the health care team in reassuring the parents and family members that the best decisions are being made for the child (Swigart et al., 1996).

Decision making for the dying child warrants helping parents see that the standard for such decision making is the best

interest standard. Best interest mandates that the decision makers truly examine what is in the best interest of the child and not rely on what may be called the paternalistic decision-making model. Such a paternalistic model has its basis solely in what the parent desires and may not be in the best interest of the child. The best interest standard truly requires acting for another's good, irrespective of the parent's wishes or desires in the matter (Spence, 2000). As can be expected, such a standard is not easy for parents, and health care providers must be able to help the parents do what is in their child's best interest as opposed to their best interests (Keesee, Currier, & Neimeyer, 2008).

Bereavement support measures are an equally important component of palliative care. Bereavement follow-up programs enable supportive relationships to continue after the death of the child. Most parents, in a study by Davies and Connaughty (2002), expressed that they greatly appreciated the follow-up care from a familiar staff member. The abrupt end to relationships and what had become familiar routines was very disconcerting to parents and families (Institute of Medicine of the National Academies, 2003) and these study participants expressed a need for continual support from those members of the health care team that they knew and trusted (Davies & Connaughty, 2002). Additionally, parents do not always return home to friends and other family members who are supportive and understanding, thus requiring the need for this continued relationship with health care providers (Ruden, 1996).

Keesee and colleagues (2008) studied the predictors of grieving following the death of a child and concluded that the majority of parents were more able to accept their child's death if they could find a sense of meaning to the death. One-hundred-and-fifty-seven parents completed two inventories designed to measure the significance of their grief following the death of a child. Factors that emerged that most influenced their grief included the age of the child, the cause of death, and length of time of bereavement. The authors concluded that additional studies were needed to assist care providers with exploring how health care professionals may assist parents to find the sense of meaning in the death of a child and that the parents need to move beyond their grief. Bereavement support programs may begin to help these parents.

Bereavement support programs may also be designed for staff members and offer the emotional support that staff members need. Formal or informal conversations among the health care team members allow these individuals to express their feelings of grief after the death of a child in a supportive environment. Additionally, these discussions may center on the ethics and emotions surrounding the event, allowing the health care team members to come to terms with their feelings and thoughts.

Davies and Connaughty (2002) studied parental responses to a survey designed to enable parents to document details related to their experience of the death of a child. Forty-five parents responded to the survey. Areas where the parents expressed greatest concern was the need for continual communication, especially to be told the truth about their child's condition and what to expect in the final hours. Parents suggested that staff should anticipate the need for such information and offer information accordingly. Parents noted that the staff must be sensitive to the need to know such information and acknowledged that not all parents want the same depth of information. Thus, staff must be able to read the parents' cues for when and how much information is acceptable.

Parents wanted staff members who were compassionate and could provide emotional support. Many of the parents in the study perceived that the staff members were too focused on the curative aspects of care to be able to effectively interact or support the grieving parents. Parents also recommended that one or two staff members be assigned to follow each family through the course of the child's illness, as this was seen as one means to provide parents with consistency in care. Parents noted that they desired to be with the child for as much time as possible, holding the child, and caring for their child in as many ways as they could. Privacy, especially when phoning friends and other family members, was greatly appreciated and desired. Finally, parents appreciated all the "small acts of human kindness" that the health care members bestowed on them and their child (Davies & Connaughty, 2002).

Rushton (2005) supported these parental concerns when she recommended that it is the model of "being with doing" that provides the development of quality care practices for dying children and their parents. Strategies that integrate "being with doing" palliative pediatric care include "listening, fostering respect for the child and parents across the organization, nurturing collaborative connections . . . making peace with conflict, and committing to self care" (Rushton, 2005, p. 311).

Finally, Rini and Loriz (2007) noted that though children do die, these children are often more generally focused on cure and continuing life, while their parents are more cognizant of the fact that death will be the eventual outcome of a terminal illness or condition. This contradicts findings that children, especially adolescents who are acutely focused on the future, are aware of the brevity of the time that they have left (Beale, Baile, & Aaron, 2005). Whether children are aware of the limited time that is left to them or not, Rani and Loriz (2007) concluded that allowing and helping parents to express their grief in an anticipatory rather than reactive manner assisted the parents in

accepting the death and shortened the bereavement time following the death of the child. Means of assisting parents with anticipatory grieving include ensuring that they are fully knowledgeable about the disease and its natural course and that health care providers allow parents to openly express their feelings, fears, and concerns. Box 7–3 summarizes some of the more appropriate interventions for children at the end of life.

BOX 7–3   Appropriate Interventions for Children at the End of Life

- Initiate palliative care programs for dying children, remembering the three essential components of palliative care: comfort, end-of-life decision making, and bereavement support measures for family members.
- The best interest standard for decision making should be incorporated into the child's care and mandates that one truly acts and promotes actions that are best for the child.
- Provide open and continued communication with the parents and family members, especially regarding the truth of the child's condition and what to expect as the child nears death.
- Remember that supportive care to the child, parents, and family members may be equally or more important in the eyes of the parents than the actual physical care given the child.
- Allow parents to spend as much uninterrupted time as possible with the child and allow them to be as fully involved in the physical care as possible.
- Provide privacy as needed.
- Allow parents and family members time for anticipatory grieving, through honest communication and allowing parents to openly express their fears, feelings, and concerns.
- Help the parents and family members to find meaning in the child's death, remembering that studies have shown that finding meaning does assist in acceptance of the child's death.

SECTION THREE REVIEW

1. When a 2-year-old child experiences the loss of a loved one, the nurse should educate the family on which of the following?
   1. The child may turn quickly to peers for comfort.
   2. The child may have occasional temper tantrums.
   3. The child may need an earlier bedtime.
   4. The child needs familiar routines and simple explanations.

2. The nurse is seeing a patient who has recently experienced the death of a parent due to violence. The patient is having nightmares and cries when left alone in a room. The nurse recognizes which age group to be most likely to have these issues?
   1. School-age children
   2. Mid-childhood–stage children
   3. Adolescents
   4. Young adults

3. Palliative care is critical to nursing care, especially for children and infants. The nurse knows that which of the following interventions are included in the concept of palliative care? (Select all that apply.)
   1. Pain control
   2. Emotional support
   3. Reassurance to the family regarding withdrawal of life-support measures
   4. Follow-up care for families
4. A pediatric patient is dying from a terminal disease. The supportive family has just been told by the physician that the patient has less than a week to live. The family members are gathered around the patient. The nurse overhears the family members arguing with each other and blaming the patient's physician for not providing adequate care and an earlier diagnosis. A possible nursing diagnosis might be:
   1. Failure to thrive
   2. Compromised family coping
   3. Disturbed thought process
   4. Knowledge deficit

Case Study 2

Judy, 3 years of age, was diagnosed with a brain tumor at age 1. She has had several surgeries for the tumor, both with an attempt to remove the tumor and to alleviate her recurring symptoms. She has also undergone two rounds of radiation therapy and her parents have now been told that there is little more that can be done for her. Judy has been hospitalized for the past two weeks, primarily to perform yet one more surgery, which has helped to alleviate her intense headaches. Judy is currently being managed with pain medications, steroid therapy, and antibiotics. Her parent's desire is that she be allowed to die at home and they are requesting assistance in how to best ensure that Judy can be discharged from the hospital. They are also asking for assistance with her care once she returns home.

Question

As Judy's primary nursing provider, how do you begin to work with Judy and her parents?

Suggested Answer

Her parents need to be supported in this decision, as they have come to the realization that Judy will not survive this diagnosis and are striving to do what is best for Judy and the family group. If they have not yet been exposed to hospice care, this is the ideal time to teach them about the benefits of hospice care, including the fact that hospice personnel will work with them at home, ensuring that Judy is comfortable and that she will receive quality nursing interventions. The parents need to know that they, too, will be supported in caring for Judy during her dying and after she has died. They also need to know that the hospice team will keep them informed about Judy's trajectory of illness, including what to expect and what subtle changes in her condition mean. If there are other children in the family, hospice personnel will work with them in the same caring manner that they are working with Judy's parents.

Judy is at the developmental stage of early childhood, where she is beginning to assert her autonomy while remaining very dependent on her parents. Because she has been ill since her first birthday, she may still be developing some of the skills more typically performed by younger children, especially physical skills. Her parents should encourage her continual development as much as appropriate, as this encouragement will allow Judy to have as much quality of life as possible. The parents also need to know, though, that Judy should be allowed to dictate what she can do or not do on a daily basis.

Judy's parents should be encouraged to treat her honestly, helping her to understand that they will be there to comfort and care for her. The parents can help Judy to understand that the time has come when she will not need to be in the hospital, that there will not be as many treatments as before, and that the family will be spending more time with her. A storybook, appropriate for Judy's age, which addresses the issue of dying and the afterlife, may be suggested to her parents. In the alternative, you might suggest that Judy's parents work with their religious advisor to begin to speak honestly with Judy about her dying.

SECTION FOUR: Young Adults and End-of-Life Issues

Young adults, according to Erickson (1959), are those between the ages of 18 and 35. Developmentally, this age is defined as intimacy versus isolation, where the individual is learning to make commitments to others, primarily marital partners and significant others. The task at this stage of life is in developing lasting relationships that require accepting independence, responsibility, and the ability to trust (Erickson, 1963). Sexuality is an important component of this developmental stage.

Young adulthood is frequently seen as a time of vigor, health, and well-being. Today's young adult may often be found working out at health care facilities, playing games of basketball or touch football with friends, or stopping after work hours to relax with friends and colleagues. Health promotion centers on good eating habits, routine exercise, and adequate periods of sleep and relaxation. Childhood diseases and illness and the threat of the upcoming chronic illness of more aged persons are far removed from the mind of this typical young adult.

Approximately 60,500 young adults died in 2004, with the leading causes of death intentional self-harm, accidents, assaults and homicides, neoplasms, and acquired immunodeficiency syndrome (AIDS) (CDC, 2007). Most of these causes are preventable, which has influenced how society experiences the death of a young individual. There is generally some aspect of blame, though often there is no one to blame, as the person has now died. Thus acceptance and closure become more difficult, which may extend the grieving process of those close to the individual (Carpenito, 2007).

Because death is not anticipated by the younger person, denial is not only their first reaction, but this stage of grieving persists much longer in the young adult. Typical reactions to terminal conditions are that a mistake has been made in the diagnosis or that the individual will be able to overcome the illness. Denial generally acquiesces to acceptance of the fact that the individual will die (Zimmermann, 2004). As this acceptance occurs, anger is most often the next reaction. This anger may be directed at a variety of aspects of one's life, such as why he or she had worked so hard to save for the future rather than enjoying each day as it came, to wishing that he or she had made better financial arrangements for a spouse and children. Anger may also be directed to the fact that the person will not be able to see his or her children grow, and fear that children are too young to be able to remember the parent.

At the same time, family members of the dying young adult deal with multiple issues. The spouse or significant other may fear the loss of intimacy, especially if death will follow a lingering and debilitating illness. Abandonment and fear of isolation may also consume the spouse or significant other. Additionally, the fear that he or she may not be able to raise young children without the assistance of a loved one is often expressed. Parents of the dying young adult express their grief in multiple ways, from being very stoic and resilient to expressing grief that it is the end of their family lineage (Corless, Germino, & Pittman, 2006). Siblings and peers are generally in the same young adult category and the death of their loved one may raise questions about their lives, leaving the sibling or peer with feelings of guilt that it is someone else who is dying and not themselves. Siblings may feel the need to take responsibility for their nieces and nephews, especially if the nieces and nephews are younger (Huntley, 2002).

Palliative care and hospice care revolves around the same three components that were presented earlier in this chapter in the discussion about children and end-of-life issues. Comfort measures, assistance with decision making, and bereavement support measures are also important in the care of the young adult at the end of life. Care is provided for the person who is dying as well as family members. The dying individual takes an active role in decision making, as this person most often is cognitively able to make decisions and give valid informed consent. If ethics committee meetings are initiated to assist with decision making, the dying individual should be invited to attend or the committee may meet in the patient's hospital room or at the person's home.

Nurses continue to be instrumental in assisting terminally ill persons and their spouses to attain hope in the face of impending death. Syren and colleagues (2006) reported that nurse-initiated conversations provided couples the opportunity to discuss hope and suffering, strengthening the couple's relationship and allowing them to unburden themselves through open and frank conversations. These conversations allowed them to find strategies for managing life following the death of the terminally ill person.

Since the underlying cause of death for many young adults is related to homicides, self-inflicted injuries, and accidents, there may be very little time between the terminal condition and the death of the person. Thus bereavement measures may be the most important aspect for the family that remains after the young adult dies (Syren, Savemen, & Benzein, 2006).

Each person's life is unique and there is no one way to address the needs of the dying young adult or the family of that young adult. Health care providers must "read" the cues that the dying individual and family members express both orally and nonverbally and respond appropriately. Health care providers may also benefit from formal and informal discussions following the death of a young adult, for these deaths are frequently the more difficult for health care providers to overcome. One reason for this is the perception that young people are not supposed to die, but live to become older individuals. Another reason is that the health care providers may relate with the dying individual and see themselves in the family members' places, thus engendering multiple emotions in those who care professionally for dying persons.

SECTION FOUR REVIEW

1. Knowing that the most common causes of death in the young adult are most often preventable, the nurse can anticipate possible interventions for the grieving family as:
   1. Assisting with the family's acceptance and closure of the death.

2. Discussing the possible causes of who might be to blame for the death.
3. Encouraging health promotion.
4. Forgoing bereavement measures since the family has usually already come to terms with the death.

2. Difficulties that health care providers have in overcoming the death of a young person include:
   1. Guilt that such a young person has been allowed to die.
   2. Fear that something else could have been done to save the person.
   3. The fact that young people are not supposed to die.
   4. Inability to adequately express condolences to the young person's family and friends.
3. One's peer group may avoid contact with the dying younger adult because:
   1. They do not know how to express sympathy and thus choose to avoid contact altogether.
   2. They are closest in age to the dying younger adult and feel threatened by this person's death.
   3. They have busy lives themselves and fail to make time to spend with the dying individual.

4. Because of their lack of previous experiences with death, they fail to appreciate the severity of the diagnosis.
4. Bereavement measures may be the most important aspect of palliative care with a young adult because:
   1. These deaths may be sudden and family members are first approached after the person has died.
   2. Acceptance of the death of a younger adult extends for a greater time period than does acceptance of the death of an older person.
   3. Family members do not have time to grieve, thus bereavement services are needed for a longer period of time.
   4. Family members often deny that the younger adult has died and thus family members need support to accept the death.

SECTION FIVE: End-of-Life Issues During Mid- and Late-Adulthood

Though death is inevitable, it is generally better accepted in later adulthood rather than in a person in the 35–65 age range. Americans are living healthier and longer lives and many experience relatively good health through their 70s and 80s. The Centers for Disease Control reported that approximately 500,000 middle-age adults and 1,120,000 older adults died during in 2004, with the leading causes of death in both categories being heart disease, neoplasms, strokes, chronic respiratory disease, injury, and complications of type 1 or type 2 diabetes mellitus (2007). These diseases tend to be chronic, with death coming long after the individual is first diagnosed with the illness. These diseases also tend to be concurring conditions and caring for these individuals entails expert physical, psychosocial, cultural, and spiritual care. Caring for these individuals also restructures how one thinks about palliative care, as more chronically ill elderly individuals require both expert palliative care and intermittent curative care aimed at treating symptoms and exacerbations as they arise (Nakashima & Canda, 2005).

Individuals in Erickson's (1959) mid-adulthood stage of development are actively pursuing the more productive years of their lives or are anticipating retirement. Family, the workplace, and community are all important and generally the individual is busy in all three spheres. The availability of family members to assist with the care of the dying middle-age adult generally varies greatly. Children may be away at school and reluctant to interrupt their studies for extended periods of time. Children may be unable to assist with a dying parent because of their own family obligations, especially if they have young children of their own. Parents are more elderly and may be experiencing health care issues themselves that limit their ability to be caregivers. Spouses may have demanding careers of their own and be unable to take long absences from their employment.

Kressler, Peters, Lee, and Parr (2005) noted that caregivers for persons who were in this stage of development desired realistic information regarding the person's disease and expected to be present when the individual died. These caregivers readily shared decision making with the dying individual and reported much less anxiety when they were actively involved in a decision-making role. As expected, the caregivers who trusted their health care providers reported less anxiety, noting that the following factors were important in developing this trust: continuity of care; clear information and advice; a planned course of care; and rapid response in times of crises. Interestingly, most of the caregivers reported feeling safer having their loved one in the hospital rather than at home. This contrasts with the results of a study that found that terminally ill individuals prefer home care as opposed to hospitalized care (Brumley et al., 2007).

These research studies point to the challenges facing health care providers in working with this population. Issues such as determining the greater importance of needs and desires weighted with the extent of required interventions are concerns facing health care professionals today. Research studies also point to the enormity of differences in care expectations that exist from the perspective of the person at the end of his or her life and the individual's family members (Gott, Small, Barnes, Payne, & Seamark, 2008; Nelson et al., 2006; Rosenfeld, Roth, Gandhi, & Penson, 2004).

Individuals in this age range frequently note that they have many life goals that have yet to be attained. Among these goals may be the fact that they want to see their children or grandchildren grow up and become successful citizens and have families of their own. Others may express the need to be remembered by their younger children and grandchildren and query how this is possible (Corless et al., 2006; Cicirelli, 2006). One means of achieving this goal is to have the dying individual record messages for the child or grandchild, either using a written medium such as a diary or letter approach or by taping messages that the child or grandchild can play after the person dies. Some individuals have left letters to be opened at critical times in the child's or grandchild's life, such as upon graduation from high school or college, as he or she turns 21, or on other special occasions.

Family resources may not yet be secured and the dying individual may request assistance with setting up trust funds or other means of financial support for the family. Health care providers can assist with these types of requests by ensuring that financial planners consult with the patient early in the terminal illness. Alternatively, business partners or associates may be able to assist the dying individual in planning for long-term financial support for the family.

The late adulthood's developmental stage concerns reviewing life accomplishments, dealing with loss, and preparing for death. This may be a very turbulent time for individuals who perceive that they have not accomplished much in their lives or that their accomplishments would be much greater if given more time to attain these desired accomplishments. Thus, depression and a sense of failure may need to be addressed by health care providers (Grassi, Malacarne, Maestri, & Ramelli, 1997). As the person's peer group grows smaller, there may be additional feelings of depression, complicating the care of these individuals. The person and his or her spouse may benefit from consultation with social workers and religious personnel (ELNEC, 2008).

Many of the issues facing this population concern family caregivers who themselves are more apt to be elderly and have health issues of their own. Care for the individual in this age group may also be more time consuming and the amount of physical care required much greater than when the individual was younger; thus the older caregiver's health status may decline as he or she attempts to care for the dying individual. Care needs to focus on supporting family caregivers and meeting the everyday needs of both the dying individual as well as the family caregiver (Merck Institute of Aging and Health and the Gerontology Society of America, 2002). Meals on wheels, legal aid services, and family respite may be required to assist this person and his or her family caregiver. Alternate arrangements, such as assisted living, adult day care centers, and residential nursing home, may also need to be addressed. Finally, the care system must be structured to accommodate progression of the person's prognosis and care needs, changing family situations, decline in capacities, and either a sudden or lingering death trajectory.

Mid-adulthood or late adulthood individuals generally have additional chronic health conditions as well as a primary terminal disease, thus prompting the need for both palliative and curative treatment measures. Appropriate care measures for middle and older-age individuals at the end of life are depicted in Box 7–4.

BOX 7–4   Appropriate Interventions for Individuals in Mid- and Late-Adulthood

- Building advanced care planning into treatment as early as possible, adapting the plan of care as appropriate, and including planning that provides advance directives
- Providing palliative care for symptoms and rehabilitation for disabilities throughout the course of the person's illness
- Teaching the dying person and family members the essentials of disease management, especially the recognition of symptoms and prevention of continuing deterioration
- Continuing to provide some aggressive therapies throughout the terminal illness, as these more aggressive therapies can enhance quality of life
- Attending to the multiple needs of family members, including their needs to be physical caregivers for their loved ones
- Easing the transition across care setting, dependent upon the physical, psychosocial, and spiritual needs of the patient in tandem with the needs of the family caregivers
- Providing needed education, financial support, and respite for family caregivers

---

SECTION FIVE REVIEW

1. The mid-adulthood and late-adulthood terminally ill patient poses unique challenges for nursing. Because of these unique needs, it is especially important to include which of the following during an initial assessment? (Select all that apply.)
   1. Other comorbidities
   2. Age
   3. Availability of family caregivers
   4. Financial concerns

2. A nursing intervention to include for the mid-adulthood and late-adulthood terminally ill patient is:
   1. Assessing for elderly abuse.
   2. Attending to the financial affairs of the patient.
   3. Teaching the patient and family members to recognize symptoms that might be treatable.
   4. Teaching the patient and family members the essentials of bathing the patient.

3. Barriers to planning care for a mid-adulthood, terminally ill patient might include: (Select all that apply.)
   1. No family available to assist with care.
   2. Patient's desire for realistic information regarding his or her disease.
   3. Family's desire for patient's hospitalization.
   4. Patient's request for financial support.
4. The patient in the late-adulthood developmental stage is concerned with reviewing life accomplishments,

reflecting upon a happy and useful life with gained wisdom. Because of these developmental tasks, this patient is at higher risk for which problem?
   1. Skin disorders
   2. Cancer
   3. Depression
   4. Suicide

Case Study 3

Maria Chen is an 82-year-old woman with metastatic breast cancer who receives care at home provided by her 58-year-old daughter with the assistance of a home hospice program. Maria developed aspiration pneumonia and was treated with aggressive antibiotic therapy for 4 days in an acute care facility. She is now back at home. She is adamantly opposed to further hospitalization and has refused to be readmitted if the oral antibiotics are not effective against her pneumonia. Maria states that she has "had a good life" and that she is "ready to go at any time." Her daughter, who also suffers from high blood pressure, osteoarthritis of both knees, and bouts of depression, is unsure if she can care for her mother in the final stages of Maria's illness.

Question

How do you begin, as the hospice nurse caring for Maria, to address the needs of Maria and her family?

Answer

Begin by educating Maria and her daughter about the implications that this newest diagnosis has on Maria, including the possibility that oral antibiotics may not be effective against the aspiration pneumonia. Additional education is needed to prevent further aspiration and the daughter should be taught, along with Maria, how to prevent such aspiration in the future. Alert Maria and her daughter about the signs and symptoms that may herald Maria's demise due to the pneumonia, including measures that can be taken to make her more comfortable in her final hours. Assure them that these measures, including medications, can be made available as they are needed.

Assess the status of Maria's daughter as a caregiver for Maria. Is additional assistance needed to help the daughter care for Maria? Would having a home health aide assist in the more physical care of Maria? Does the daughter require additional medical attention for her arthritis or her depression? Though the scenario does not indicate that there are additional family members who could also assist at this time, the nurse may want to explore this possibility with Maria. Perhaps respite care for the daughter is required.

Help the daughter accept the fact that Maria is in control of her life and dying and the importance of Maria not being readmitted to the hospital. If the daughter is aware of subtle changes in her mother's condition and understands the need for Maria to die in a familiar setting, then she is less apt to panic when her mother's condition worsens and call for assistance, especially for emergency 911 assistance. Remember to reinforce the fact that bereavement services are also a part of hospice care, so that the daughter knows that there will be someone there for her when her mother dies, whether from this bout of pneumonia or from the primary disease.

SECTION SIX: Research Concerning Resolving Difficult Situations

Caring competently for individuals at the end of life requires knowledge about how these individuals perceive their final time on this earth. Research conducted that begins to address the meaning of experiences of persons who are nearing the end of life is relatively recent. As early as 1998, Corner reviewed published literature and noted that there was a lack of studies on the human experiences of persons living their dying process. His work led to the determination that a single paradigm is unlikely to capture the multiple and diverse range of issues that arise in the area of palliative care. Additionally, his work supports the wholeness that is central to nursing care (Hutchings, 2007).

Research is beginning to explore studies that attempt to understand the process of dying and how it is interpreted by individuals (Carter, MacLeod, Brander, & McPherson, 2004; Grumann & Spiegel, 2003; McKechnie, MacLoed, & Keeling, 2007). In one of the more recent studies in this arena, Hutchings (2007) describes a descriptive study that involved personal interviews of eight patients who were in the final stages of their lives. The three themes that emerged from these interviews are found in Box 7–5.

The first theme supported the notion that dying persons' views of themselves intensify in complexity and diversity. The individuals in the study were able to articulate the fact that they had much to be thankful for in their lives and that they remain integrated and "whole" in their thoughts. This stands in contrast to the idea that dying persons gradually lose contact with reality or become progressively less corporeal and more ethereal as they move closer to death (Hutchings, 2007).

The second theme contradicts the more popular idea that terminal illness is riddled with unpredictability amidst periods of stability. The patients in this study sought answers to questions such as what to expect, what the dying process would be like, and how long they had yet to live. Seeking answers to these questions directed the patients to seek further clarifications from health care professionals, to join support groups, and to read more extensively about their illnesses. Persons in this study expressed a trust in the uncertain, as exemplified by such statements as, "I do not know what it will be like, but I'm not worried" (Hutchings, 2007, p. 36).

The third theme revealed the ability of these patients to remain steady and unwavering despite hardships imposed by their illnesses, such as reduced energy, seemingly endless treatment regimens, and leaving their loved ones. In this study, such perseverance was noted as the desire to die at home, to maintain independence as long as possible, and to be remembered by loved ones. Individuals in the study created videotapes for their grandchildren so that they would be remembered positively, attempted to make amends for broken relationships, and attempted to remain happy during visits with loved ones (Hutchings, 2007).

Findings from this study and other studies that explore meaning and perceptions from the dying persons' perspectives will begin to assist health care providers in developing and implementing realistic plans of care for these patients and their families. These findings will also help educate nurses so that more meaningful nursing interventions can be explored with these persons and their family members.

SECTION SIX REVIEW

1. Based upon recent research, a patient is best served during their last days by the nurse answering questions such as:
   1. "How long will I have to live?"
   2. "What will my family do without me?"
   3. "Do you know if I can travel to Mexico without any problems?"
   4. "Why did this happen to me?"
2. One of the lessons learned from recent research involves opportunities for more meaningful interventions for the terminally ill patient by the nursing staff. For the terminally ill patient, which of the following interventions could provide lasting memories for the family members after the patient's death?
   1. Family discussions with the patient
   2. Family portrait
   3. A videotape from the patient
   4. A will discussing distribution of belongings

Case Study 4

Reread the scenario involving Juan, presented in Chapter 2. Juan, a 19-year-old individual rejected further therapy and hospitalization for his cancer. He has "made his peace with God" and does not desire to undergo further therapies or rounds of chemotherapy for a condition he now fully comprehends as incurable.

Question

How does Juan "fit" the three themes as described in Hutchings research study about terminally ill patients' perceptions of their dying?

Suggested Response

Juan's case can be viewed as vividly bringing to life the three themes described in the Hutchings' research study and the need for health care providers to recognize these perceptions. Juan insists that he remain at home during the final stages of his life, however brief it may be. Though he does not express that he has come to the realization that he has had a "good life," he does express the fact that he is at peace and understands that his life will conclude soon. Perhaps he is questioning what the final stages will be or how much longer he will have in this life. His desire to remain at home with the parents he has come to love and treasure can be seen as the thankfulness that he appreciates. This could also be seen as his need to be remembered in the context of his living, rather than in a hospital setting with multiple tubes and other invasions of his personhood. He takes measures to remain calm, tranquil, and in control as he passes from this life to the next. Though the need to seek ways to ensure that he will be remembered are not obvious, he does convey the way in which he wants to be remembered—at home and at peace.

CHAPTER SUMMARY

- The loss of a family member is one of the most traumatic and emotionally distressing events in a person's life.
- Families today have multiple structures, including the more traditional structure with a father, mother, and children, and a variety of structures that include single-parent households, extended families, couples without children, and households where children from previous and current marriages are blended into the family unit.
- One way of approaching issues concerning end of life care is through the incorporation of a developmental stages model, such as Erickson's Eight Developmental Stages.

- When addressing children and end-of-life issues, two sets of needs and perceptions are important to address, those of the terminally ill child and those of the children who remain after the death of a family member.
- Essential components of palliative care programs regardless of the age of the terminally ill person are comfort care, end-of-life decision making, and bereavement support measures.
- Though death is inevitable, it is generally better accepted in later adulthood than in earlier age groupings.
- Caring competently for individuals at the end of life requires knowledge about how these individuals perceive their final time on this earth.

CHAPTER REVIEW

Henry Applewood, age 52, was at the height of his career as a chemical engineer for a major company when he was diagnosed with a rare but rapidly progressive form of lung cancer. He received radiation therapy and chemotherapy for the tumor, which was so far advanced when diagnosed that surgery was not an option. He was treated at a tertiary cancer center for the past several weeks, and is now at home. Because of the poor prognosis and the age of his family, Henry has elected home hospice care for his final days. Henry married later in life and his family consists of a teenage son, a daughter aged 11, and twin 5-year-old boys. Until his illness, his wife worked as the dean of the business school at a large university. She is on leave from that position so that she can assist with Henry's care and be with him until he dies.

Question

How do Erickson's stages of development give direction to the hospice team when working with Henry and his family?

Suggested Response

The stages of development as developed by Erickson assist members of the team in addressing issues specific to members of the family in various age groups. Henry is at the mid-adulthood stage of development and may be experiencing ambivalence with not being able to continue in the work world, especially as he is at the height of his career. He is also dealing with not being able to continue as a companion to his wife and seeing his children grow and develop into adults. Fears that he may have include the idea that his children will forget him, especially the younger boys. Though many individuals who face death at this stage of development also fear lack of financial stability for their families, this would appear not to be a factor in Henry's life.

Mrs. Applewood, who must be younger than her husband, is presumably at the upper edges of young adulthood or the earlier stages of mid-adulthood. Fears that she may experience include raising four children as a single mother who has great demands placed on her time as the dean of the business college. She may also fear being able to support the family if she resigns this position so that she can spend more time with her children. She may fear the lack of intimacy, as part of her developmental stage is intimacy and love.

The teenage son is at the developmental stage of adolescence, a time when his identity is truly beginning to emerge and expressions of grief are difficult. His parents should be informed that expressions of grief at this stage of development may be expressed in multiple ways, from withdrawing emotionally to escaping totally into his peer group, leaving the family to feel that he has no feelings for what is happening. Rebellious behavior may also be manifested as he begins to fully appreciate the gravity of the situation and that his father will soon die. Clinical depression may be a factor and Mrs. Applewood may need assistance in getting him into counseling and how to set limits in his behavior.

The 11-year-old daughter is at the developmental stage of school age—a social age and a time when the individual escapes into activities to avoid facing the issue that her parent is dying and will soon be away on a permanent basis. She may also be expressing her feelings in multiple ways, from being angry to intense sadness. Her mother should be aware that this death may affect her school work for months after the actual death. Interventions that may assist the daughter include encouraging her to assist with her father's care, giving honest and realistic information to her about her father's condition, encouraging her to be involved with after-school events, and ensuring that family activities are structured and have routines.

The 5-year-old twins are at the developmental stage of mid-childhood. Generally, these children do not fully appreciate the significance of a terminal illness, as they cannot fully comprehend that death is not reversible. They may, after their father's death, continue to inquire about his return; thus, their mother needs to be informed that such requests are normal developmentally. Means of helping them include using simple explanations and answering their questions honestly, using play therapy to help them express their feelings, reminding Mrs. Applewood that the twins will feel the need to stay close to her after their father's death, and helping her to prepare for the twins' need to talk and ask questions after Mr. Applewood dies.

REFERENCES

Allender, J. A., & Spradley, B. W. (2005). Assessment of families. In *Community health nursing: Promoting and protecting the public's health* (pp. 515–538). St. Louis: Lippincott Williams & Wilkins.

Beale, E. A., Baile, W. F., & Aaron, J. (2005). Silence is not golden: Communicating with children dying from cancer. *Journal of Clinical Oncology, 23*(15), 3629–3631.

Brazil, K., Bedard, M., & Willison, K. (2002). Correlates of health status for family caregivers in bereavement. *Journal of Palliative Medicine, 5*(6), 849–855.

Brumley, R., Enguidanos, S., Jamison, R., Seitz, R., Morgenstern, N., Saito, S., McIlwane, J., Hillary, K., & Genzalez, J. (2007). Increased satisfaction with care and lower costs: Results of a randomized trial of in-home palliative care. *Journal of the American Geriatric Society, 55*(7), 993–1000.

Carpenito, L. (2007). *Nursing diagnosis: Application to clinical practice* (12th ed.). Philadelphia: Lippincott Williams & Wilkins.

Carter, H., MacLeod, R., Brander, P., & McPherson, K. (2004). Living with a terminal illness: Patients' priorities. *Journal of Advanced Nursing, 45*(6), 611–620.

Centers for Disease Control, National Center for Health Statistics. (2001). Deaths: Preliminary data for 2000. *National Vital Statistics Report, 49*(12), 2011–2120.

Centers for Disease Control, National Center for Health Statistics. (2002). United States Life Tables. *National Vital Statistics Report, 50*(6), 2002–2120.

Centers for Disease Control, National Center for Health Statistics. (2007). Health, United States, 2007. *National Vital Statistics Report, 55*(19), 2007–2120.

Christ, C. H. (2000). *Healing children's grief.* New York: Oxford University Press.

Cicirelli, V. G. (2006). *Older adults views on death.* St. Louis: Springer.

Corless, I., Germino, B. B., & Pittman, M. A. (Eds.) *Death, dying, and bereavement: A challenge for living* (2nd ed.). (2004). St. Louis: Springer.

Corner, J. (1998). Is there a research paradigm for palliative care? *Palliative Medicine, 10*, 201–208.

Currier, J. M., Holland, J. M., & Neimeyer, R. A. (2007). The effectiveness of bereavement interventions with children: A meta-analytic review of controlled outcome research. *Journal of Clinical Child and Adolescent Psychology, 36*, 1–7.

Davies, B., & Connaughty, S. (2002). Pediatric end-of-life care: Lessons learned from parents. *Journal of Nursing Administration, 32*(1), 2–6.

End of Life Nursing Consortium. (2008). *Advanced end of life nursing care: ELNEC supercore training program 2008.* Washington, DC: American Association of Colleges of Nursing.

Erickson, E. H. (1959). *Identity and the life cycle.* New York: International Universities Publishers.

Erickson, E. H. (1963). *Childhood and society* (2nd ed.). New York: W. W. Norton.

Goldman, L. (2000). *Life and loss: A guide to help grieving children* (2nd ed.). Philadelphia: Accelerated Development.

Gott, M., Small, N., Barnes, S., Payne, S., & Seamark, D. (2008). Older people's views of a good death in heart failure: Implications for palliative care provision. *Social Science and Medicine, 67*, 1113–1121.

Grassi, L., Malacarne, P., Maestri, A., & Ramelli, E. (1997). Depression, psychosocial variables, and occurrence of life events among patients with cancer. *Journal of Affective Disorders, 44*(1), 21–30.

Grumann, M. M., & Spiegel, D. (2003). Living in the face of death: Interviews with 12 terminally ill women on home hospice care. *Palliative and Supportive Care, 1*(1), 23–32.

Huntley, T. (2002). *Helping children grieve: When someone they love dies.* Minneapolis: Augsburg Books.

Hutchings, D. (2007). Struggling in change at the end of life: A nursing inquiry. *Palliative and Supportive Care, 5*(1), 31–39.

Institute of Medicine of the National Academies, Committee on Palliative and End-of-Life Care for Children and their Families. (2003). In M. J. Field & R. E. Behrman (Eds.) *When children die: Improving palliative and end-of-life care for children and their families.* Washington, DC: National Academies Press.

Keesee, N. G., Currier, J. M., & Neimeyer, R. A. (2008). Predictors of grief following the death of one's child: The contribution of finding meaning. *Journal of Clinical Psychology, 64*(10), 1145–1163.

Kressler, D., Peters, T. J., Lee, L., & Parr, S. (2005). Social class and access to specialist palliative care services. *Palliative Medicine, 19*, 105–110.

Kring, D. L. (2006). An exploration of the good death. *Advances in Nursing Science, 29*(3), E12–E24.

Lynn, J. (2005). Living long in fragile health: The new demographics shape end of life care. Improving end of life care: Why has it been so difficult? *Hastings Center Report Special Report, 35*(6), S14–S18.

McKechnie, R., MacLoed, R., & Kelling, S. (2007). Facing uncertainty: The lived experience of palliative care. *Palliative and Supportive Care, 5*(3), 255–264.

Merck Institute of Aging and Health and the Gerontology Society of America. (2002). *The state of aging and health in America.* Washington, DC: Authors.

Nakashima, M., & Canda, E. R. (2005). Positive dying and resiliency in later life: A qualitative study. *Journal of Aging Studies, 19*, 109–125.

Nelson, J. E., Angus, D., Weissfeld, L. A., Puntillp, K. A., Danis, M., Deal, D., Levy, M. M., & Cook, D. J. (2006). End-of-life care for the critically ill: A national intensive care survey. *Critical Care Medicine, 34*(10), 2547–2553.

Rini, A., & Loriz, L. (2007). Anticipatory grieving in parents with a child who dies while hospitalized. *Journal of Pediatric Nursing, 22*(4), 272–282.

Rogoff, B. (2003). *The cultural nature of human development.* New York: Oxford Press.

Romesberg, T. (2007). Building a case for neonatal palliative care. *Neonatal Network, 26* (2), 111–115.

Rosenfeld, B., Roth, A. J., Gandhi, S., & Penson, D. (2004). Differences in health-related quality of life of prostate cancer patients based on stage of cancer. *Psycho-Oncology, 13*, 800–807.

Rosof, B. (1995). *The worst loss: How families heal from the death of a child.* New York: Macmillan.

Ruden, B. M. (1996). Bereavement follow-up: An opportunity to extend nursing care. *Journal of Pediatric Oncology Nursing, 13*, 219–225.

Rushton, C. (2005). A framework for integrating pediatric palliative care: Being with dying. *Journal of Pediatric Nursing, 20*(5), 311–325.

Spence, K. (2000). The best interest principle as a standard for decision making in the care of neonates. *Journal of Advanced Nursing, 31*(6), 1286–1292.

Swigart, V., Lidz, C., Butterworth, V., & Arnold, R., (1996). Letting go: Family willingness to forgo life support. *Heart and Lung, 25*, 483–494.

Syren, S. M., Saveman, B.-I., & Benzein, E. G. (2006). Being a family in the midst of living and dying. *International Journal of Palliative Care, 22*(1), 26–32.

Tuffrey, C., Finlay, F., & Lewis, M. (2007). The needs of children and their families at end of life: An analysis of community nursing practice. *International Journal of Palliative Nursing, 13*(1), 64–71.

United States Department of Health and Human Services, Office of Disease Prevention and Health Promotion. (2003). *Healthy People 2010: Objectives for Improving Health, Part A.* Retrieved from http://www.healthypeople.gov/Document/tableofcontents.htm#parta

Weman, K., & Fagerberg, I. (2006). Registered nurses working together with family members of older people. *Journal of Clinical Nursing, 15*(3), 281.

Zimmermann, C. (2004). Denial of impending death: A discourse analysis of the palliative care literature. *Social Science and Medicine, 59*(8), 1769–1780.

Communication at the End of Life

8

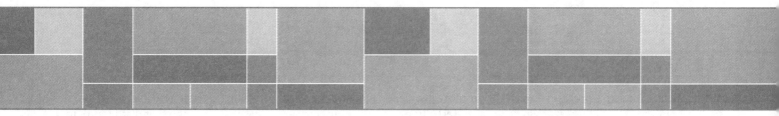

OBJECTIVES Following completion of this chapter, the learner will be able to:

8.1. Describe the importance of communication at the end of life.

8.2. Identify steps toward gaining comfort and competence in end-of-life communication.

8.3. Discuss the role of active listening, sensitivity, and presence.

8.4. Identify facilitators and barriers to communication.

8.5. Discuss the importance of self-awareness related to end-of-life issues.

8.6. Identify issues related to conflict resolution, including mediation.

8.7. Describe the role of storytelling at the end of life.

This chapter is devoted to the effectiveness of communication with persons at the end of life, their family members/caregivers, and professional interdisciplinary health care team members. The importance of developing comfort and competence in communication is discussed, as well as ways to increase competence. The need for self-awareness related to

end-of-life issues is addressed. Challenges to communication are discussed, as well as ways to facilitate communication, and it is assumed that the learner possesses knowledge of basic verbal and nonverbal communication skills. The chapter concludes with a discussion of the importance of storytelling.

PRETEST

1. A nurse has been caring for a patient for three years. The nurse has just learned that the patient died. How should the nurse deal with the death?
   1. It is important for the nurse to work through the grief related to the patient's death as with other losses in the nurse's life.
   2. The nurse could send a card to the family, but should not have any further contact with them, in order to maintain a professional distance.
   3. It would be in the nurse's best interest to try not to think about the death, as death is a part of the nursing profession.
   4. If the nurse feels the need to cry, it would be best to do so only when alone. Otherwise the nurse's professionalism may be questioned.

2. Nurses are often the primary communicators with patients and families regarding end-of-life issues. What is the rationale to support this practice?
   1. Nurses typically receive the best end-of-life communication education of all the health disciplines.
   2. The role of patient advocate requires that the nurse be the sole source of end-of-life information.
   3. The nurse is often the one who spends the most time with patients and their families. This allows for development of a trust relationship, as well as early identification of communication issues.
   4. It is mandated by the nurse practice act in most states.

3. A nurse who works in a hospice program begins to feel burned out, as a result of dealing with some very intensely

emotional situations in recent months. What should the nurse do? (Select all that apply.)
1. Examine his or her coping abilities and feelings about death
2. Discuss frustrations with patients and family members
3. Evaluate his or her support system
4. Seek professional counseling as needed

4. What are the benefits of open communication between patient, family, and health care team? (Select all that apply.)
1. Increased staff independent decision making
2. Informed decision making
3. Economic benefits related to decrease in unwanted and unnecessary treatments
4. Decreased anxiety on the part of the patient and family

GLOSSARY

communication   An active process between two or more people that involves sending and receiving messages verbally or nonverbally.

empathy   A quest to understand the situation as experienced by another.

presence   The act of making oneself available, either physically or in spirit, often in silence, to express empathy and support.

SECTION ONE: Nursing Professionals and Communication

The importance of communication is increasingly evident as more research is being done in areas related to end-of-life issues. The benefits of openly discussing end-of-life issues include reduction of anxiety, clarity in decision making, and confronting fears in the light of factual information. Open and clear communication also has an economic impact, often helping to eliminate unnecessary and unwanted treatments, as well as reducing length of stay in acute care units such as the intensive care unit (Ahrens, Yancy, & Kollef, 2003). Reduction in costs related to human suffering is also a benefit of ongoing communication (McDonald et al., 2003).

Since nurses are the ones who routinely spend the most time with patients and families, they are often the ones who take the lead in facilitating end-of-life discussions (Griffie, Nelson-Marten, & Muchka, 2004). Even though communication has been identified as a key issue in end-of-life care, it is often difficult to accomplish (Boyle, Miller, & Forbes-Thompson, 2005). In desiring to improve quality of care at the end of life, communication issues have been specified as a primary target area by organizations such as the American Association of Colleges of Nursing and the American Medical Association (Norton, Tilden, Tolle, Nelson, & Eggman, 2003).

In order to provide appropriate information, however, it is important that nurses be aware of the issues that are involved. Many nurses may feel uncomfortable in dealing with end-of-life issues, and may therefore not communicate optimally with patients and their families. Nurses must search their own hearts to examine their level of comfort with discussing death and to identify areas where improvement is needed (Boyle et al., 2005). An important first step in gaining comfort with addressing end-of-life issues is to first address one's own mortality (Clayton, Butow, Psych, & Tattersall, 2005).

Nurses must also be cognizant of their own experiences with loss of those to whom they have been close (Moore, 2005). It is not uncommon for nurses to become attached to patients and families with whom they have spent many hours, days, or months. Providing end-of-life care will give rise to deep emotions in patients, families, and nurses alike. It is of utmost importance that nurses be aware of their own feelings, reactions, and interactions with others.

It should be considered normal for nurses to suffer grief when they lose someone that is close to them. This includes the death of a patient. It is important for the nurse to acknowledge the grief and work through it as with any other loss that may occur (Radziewicz, 2001). In a study by De Araujo, Silva, and Francisco (2004), it was learned that nurses who care for patients at end of life would benefit from psychological as well as emotional support. Nurses should avail themselves of the opportunity to attend support groups or seek counseling, as needed, and to pursue balance in their personal lives and careers.

Nurses who work with patients at end of life may be especially prone to stress and burnout if their own support needs are not met (Holmberg, 2006), and denial of their emotions will cause further complications (Moore, 2005). Inability to cope on a personal level may also lead to avoiding end-of-life communication, resulting in distancing oneself from the patient (De Araujo, Silva, & Silva, 2004).

Patients and families are quick to pick up on areas that cause stress or tension for the nurse. If a nurse does not respond to end-of-life issues in a manner that opens the door to discussion, end-of-life issues will be considered off limits, no matter how urgently they need to be addressed (Griffie et al., 2004).

Many nurses who deal with end-of-life issues have expressed a desire to learn more effective ways to communicate with patients and families at end of life (Meraviglia, McGuire, & Chelsey, 2003; Zapka, Hennessy, Carter, & Amella, 2006). Undergraduate nursing programs have unparalleled opportunity to provide training to students in the area of end-of-life communication skills. Continuing education courses also offer resources for seasoned nurses to develop and improve their expertise in this area.

The most important thing that a nurse can do to improve end-of-life communication techniques is to take the first step. Observation of a more experienced staff member may help to increase the learner's knowledge and level of comfort (Forest, 2004). Visiting with end-of-life caregivers, role playing, reviewing literature, and attending end-of-life conferences may be other possibilities.

SECTION ONE REVIEW

1. A nurse has just transferred from the Labor and Delivery Unit to the inpatient Hospice unit. The nurse identifies a self-learning need for improving end-of-life communication skills. Which of the following will best meet this need?
   1. Refer end-of-life communication issues to others who are more experienced.
   2. Use a script when talking with patients and families to ensure that information is consistent.
   3. Explain to patients and families that the nurse is learning, and ask them for tips about what communication techniques work best.
   4. Identify the learning need, have a desire to learn, and take action to pursue learning.

2. A nurse with experience caring for patients with terminal illnesses is precepting a new graduate nurse to the unit. The experienced nurse observes that the new nurse avoids discussing end-of-life issues with patients. Which of the following would be the best initial course of action by the preceptor?
   1. Share the observations with the new nurse and ask the nurse to assess her own feelings about death, considering her personal experiences.
   2. Report these observations to the manager and ask that the new nurse be transferred to another unit.
   3. Facilitate more frequent opportunities for the nurse to communicate with patients diagnosed with terminal illnesses.
   4. Instruct the nurse to enroll in a continuing education course that includes curriculum on end-of-life issues.

3. Following the death of a patient that a nurse had particularly enjoyed caring for, the nurse finds it difficult to come to work, or even to get involved with friends. The nurse cries frequently, wants to sleep more than usual, and does not want to talk with patients or their family members. What is the most important action the nurse should take?
   1. Begin an exercise program and review eating habits for a healthier lifestyle.
   2. Make an appointment with the supervisor to seek feedback for performance improvement.
   3. Attend a support group or seek individual counseling.
   4. Take a leave of absence.

SECTION TWO: Communication with Patients and Families

Patients are not the only ones who are affected by a terminal illness. The family will also be significantly impacted (Holmberg, 2006). Family members will be especially affected by the quality of **communication** at the end of life (Royak-Schaler et al., 2006). Issues such as the need for education about the disease process, options for end-of-life care, and assistance with making decisions are of great importance to the families of dying patients. The information must be presented in a timely manner, and it needs to be accurate and consistent throughout the caregiving team. If there is dissonance between members of the health care team, it will have a negative impact on families, eroding trust and affecting the family's ability to remain informed and empowered in the decision-making process (Boyle et al., 2005).

Because of this, regular interdisciplinary meetings, often daily, are conducted by many agencies that are in place to serve the needs of the dying and their families. Discussions may center around disease state, plan of care, family concerns, etc. Inconsistent information received by family members will decrease satisfaction with care, and will also compromise the way that the family deals with care decisions (Royak-Schaler et al., 2006). Specifically, it is the language that is used by caregivers, the timing of discussions, the content of the messages, and the perceived sensitivity of communication that are important to family members. Communication that takes into account each of these areas will be of prime importance to patients and families who are dealing with difficult decisions.

Patients and families who are dealing with a terminal illness will often shift very quickly from aggressive treatment of the illness to transitioning into hospice or palliative care (Norton et al., 2003). This may result in a significant need for information and guidance in decision making. The family may be left feeling confused or conflicted, or they may wonder if the significant change in the plan of care meant that the communication received up to that point had been inaccurate or incomplete. Box 8–1 enumerates ways that nurses can encourage communications.

Need for Information

Patients and families desire to have information related to the patient's condition provided in a timely manner (London & Lundstedt, 2007). They also desire information that is in language that they understand (Clayton, Butow, Arnold, & Tattersall, 2005). Conferences scheduled periodically with patients and families will allow for timely discussion of significant issues.

It is important, however, to first ascertain the current level of understanding, and to clarify how much the patient and family really want to know (Clayton, Butow, Psych, & Tattersall, 2005). Families should therefore be allowed opportunity to express their needs and desires related to end-of-life issues (London & Lundstedt, 2006). In some cultures, diagnosis and prognosis are rarely discussed with patients and their families (Bruera, Neumann, Mazzocato, & Stiefel, 2000). People from some cultures even believe that the very act of discussing death will serve to hasten it (Curtis & Patrick, 1997). Because of the many

variations in values, beliefs, and traditions, it is of prime importance that the health care professional take the time to really learn about the patient and family. Without truly knowing them, it will not be possible to adequately assess their learning needs, thus leading to conflict or avoidance of important issues.

The use of open-ended questions regarding the needs and desires of patient and family will contribute toward maximizing the information obtained. Referring to feelings or emotions (such as saying "that must be a scary feeling") will give permission to further discuss those issues (Griffie et al., 2004). Summarizing what the patient and family have said may also help to clarify and solidify important points (Moore, 2005). Assessments of this nature should be conducted periodically, beginning early in the treatment process (Forest, 2004), and the frequency of this type of communication will often increase as the patient's condition changes.

In a study of communication needs at end of life (Norton et al., 2003), it was found that families desired information that was timely, honest, and clear. Although it may be difficult to predict the specific course of illness, Norton and her fellow researchers found that honesty about the prognosis was of great importance to families. Acknowledging that there is uncertainty related to the prognosis is acceptable, and may serve to open further discussion (Griffie et al., 2004). Difficulties related to developing an accurate prognosis, therefore, should be relayed to family members, thus allowing them to understand the possibilities related to end-of-life issues for their loved one. They will then be able to hold out realistic hope for the positive possibilities, while understanding that there may also be more negative turns of events. Discussing these issues at various points in the timeline of care may help to ease the difficulty of making decisions as the end of life approaches. Toward the end of life, frequent meetings with family will contribute greatly to the communication process (Boyle et al., 2005).

Written Communication

Provision of written materials has also been found to be an effective communication strategy. Lautrette et al. (2007) studied families of patients dying in intensive care units. Families assigned to an intervention group received a brochure about bereavement and spent an average of 10 extra minutes in an end-of-life conference where they had opportunity to discuss their feelings and emotions. Three months after the death of their loved one, the families in the intervention group were found to exhibit fewer symptoms of anxiety and depression than those in the control group. Another study found that providing written material, a question prompt list, to patients and their families enhanced communication during conferences with physicians (Clayton et al., 2007).

Another written communication tool that has been very helpful for nursing home patients is a one-page medical order form that was developed in Oregon (Tilden, Nelson, Dunn, Donius, & Tolle, 2000). A product of collaboration between

---

BOX 8–1	Ways for the Nurse to Encourage Communication

- Maintain a calm, unhurried presence. Don't be afraid of silence.
- Position self to keep eyes level with the patient/family member's eyes.
- Listening attentively.
- Ask open-ended questions such as "Tell me more about that" or "What was your interpretation of the information you heard this morning?"
- Encourage communication at the feeling level with statements such as "You seem quiet today" or "That must have been a disappointment for you."
- Be sensitive to cues. Some patients or family members may prefer to discuss their feelings when alone with the nurse. Provide for those opportunities as needed.
- Respect the patient/family's right to privacy. Accept that there may be those who appreciate your concern, but may choose not to verbalize their feelings.

disciplines, it is known as the POLST (Physician Orders for Life-Sustaining Treatment). This simple form opens the door to communication with the patient/family regarding wishes for treatment. It addresses basic issues such as desire for resuscitation, aggressiveness of treatment, use of antibiotics, and artificially administered nutrition. It should be noted that there may be variations in the form between states, and some states do not yet endorse the use of the POLST form. See Chapter 3 for a more complete review of the POLST.

Since it is a signed order form, the bright pink POLST is easily found in the patient's chart, and eliminates the need to search for advance directives, which may not have accompanied the patient when transferring to the hospital. The patient's wishes, therefore, can be known and followed from the time of entrance into the hospital. Ensuring that the wishes of the patient are followed can be done only through maintaining communication as a top priority (Tilden et al., 2000). Whatever means can be found to facilitate such communication are well worth investigating.

Successful communication with patients and families will lead to empowerment on an individual and group basis. It must be remembered that keeping control over decision making is a key concept at end of life, and the ability to maintain control may be related to maintenance of hope (Holmberg, 2006). Often a patient will choose to relinquish decision-making power to family or to health care providers. Even by making this choice, however, the patient's right to choose remains central.

Communication between patient and family will also be facilitated as they are kept informed about the current situation and prognosis. They will have opportunity to make informed choices related to completing matters that are important to them such as putting finances in order, making peace with God, and arranging final conversations to resolve conflicts and say goodbye to friends and family (Keeley, 2007; Steinhauser, Christakis, Clipp, McNeilley, McIntyre, & Tulsky, 2000).

Toward the end of life, curative treatment options may have been exhausted. It may be that the only decisions left to be made relate to palliative treatment options. A patient, for example, may choose to limit the use of medications that alter cognitive function, deciding rather to endure some level of discomfort in order to have a clear thought process when saying final goodbyes to family and friends. Patients and families may be highly vulnerable during these times, but should never feel that their sense of hope or power has been taken from them.

Sensitivity

Life-threatening health issues, especially those requiring significant treatment decisions, will be a source of fear and anxiety (Zapka et al., 2006). Although responses such as fear, stress, and anxiety may be considered normal, they will have a definite impact on communication (Norton et al., 2003). It may be difficult for families to listen to or absorb information about their loved one's condition or prognosis. Information will often need to be clarified or repeated at a later time in order to facilitate comprehension, and this responsibility will often be fulfilled by the nurse.

With the patient's permission, it may also be helpful to have a support person in the room when difficult issues are discussed. A trusted friend, family member, pastor, or social worker may be of great support. This will facilitate later family discussion (Griffie et al., 2004). Unless communication problems are addressed and resolved as they arise, it will be very difficult to arrive at end-of-life care decisions with which patients, families, and health care providers all agree (Norton et al., 2003).

The patient and family need to be treated with care, dignity, and compassion (London & Lundstedt, 2007). Royak-Schaler et al. (2006) found that availability of information that was accurate and thorough, when relayed to the family with compassion, helped to increase the family's comfort level with decision making, as well as their comfort with the care that was given.

The manner in which information is offered to the family, along with accurate appraisal of the readiness of family members to receive information, is crucial to successful end-of-life communication (Holmberg, 2006). The circumstances surrounding the final days of the patient will live on in the memories of family members for many years (Griffie et al., 2004). Investing in treatment of the patient that emphasizes respect and dignity will facilitate not only open communication, but will build meaningful memories as well.

Active Listening/Presence

Active listening by nurses will also contribute greatly to the communication process with patient and family. The nurse should take the time to listen to questions and concerns, conveying a feeling of being unhurried and sincerely caring. It is important that distractions and interruptions be minimized, giving the impression that the nurse is fully present and genuinely interested in hearing what is to be said (Moore, 2005). It has been suggested that **empathy,** along with a silent **presence,** may offer more support than any words could ever bring (Penson, Partidge, Shah, Giansiracusa, Chabner, & Lynch, 2005). Indeed, there may be times of such intense emotion that a sense of presence is the greatest therapy that can be offered by the nurse (Forest, 2004).

In discussing nursing care at end of life, the following statement is especially meaningful:

> The ways that nurses communicate their willingness to bear witness to suffering and offer their presence are often perceived by patients and families as the most important of all interventions. Taking the time to listen actively and process not only words and facts, but also meanings and feelings, is the quintessential task of communication at the end of life. (Matzo, Sherman, Sheehan, Ferrell, & Penn, 2003, p.183)

It is also import to be aware of body language. Nodding or acknowledging statements by patients and families will convey continued interest, as well as maintaining appropriate eye contact, though appropriate eye contact will vary between different cultures and situations. There are times when physical touch, such as a touch on the shoulder or holding a hand, may also be appreciated by the patient (Steinhauser, Christakis et al., 2000).

A system for facilitating communication that emphasizes the importance of listening, as well as encouraging patient/family involvement in discussion, was developed for use in end-of-life discussions in the intensive care unit (Curtis, Patrick, Shannon, Treece, Engelberg, & Rubenfeld, 2001). The mnemonic for this system is VALUE, and it includes:

Valuing the issues communicated by patients/families
Acknowledging their feelings and emotions
Listening to what is said
Understanding and respecting the individuality of the patient
Eliciting questions

A study by Clayton, Butow, Psych, and Tattersall (2005) revealed that health care professionals are not necessarily expected to be able to provide answers to all questions. A greater need, rather, may be met just by listening and providing support with warmth and sincerity. The study revealed that the use of humor may be appreciated as well.

Negotiating Death

In these times of modern technology, it has become more common for patients to be able to negotiate circumstances related to their death (Bowman, 2000). They may request withdrawal of specific treatments, or addition of others. It is also becoming more common for patients to request measures that may hasten death. The importance of active listening becomes especially crucial in circumstances such as these. The values and beliefs of the patient and family, as well as those of the nurse and other members of the health care team, must be respected as such crucial information is discussed (Volker, 2001).

With so many variables and possibilities during these modern times, conflicts may arise that involve family members, patients, and health care personnel. If the patient is no longer able to communicate end-of-life care wishes, the family may not be able to agree on treatment options. It is the ultimate responsibility of the health care provider to facilitate productive communication and to resolve conflict. If an amicable agreement cannot be reached, it may be necessary to involve a neutral third party as a mediator (Bowman, 2000), but every effort should be made to resolve issues before they get to that point.

Advance directives should also be used as a springboard to discussion about patients' wishes. It is possible that patients' wishes may have changed if several years have passed since advance directives were prepared. Wishes may also change as the patient's condition changes, so an advance directive should always be used as a means to open communication with the patient. Some patients believe that preparation of an advance directive means that further discussion is inappropriate or unnecessary, so the existence of such documentation may potentially be perceived by the patient as a barrier to communication, rather than a facilitator (Curtis & Patrick, 1997). Some barriers to communication at end of life are listed in Box 8–2 and facilitators to communication at the end of life are listed in Box 8–3.

BOX 8–2   Barriers to Communication

Patient/Family Barriers

- Discomfort with death and the issues related to it
- Fearing that withholding treatment will hasten death or add suffering
- Resistance/denial
- Distrust of health care providers
- Rapidly changing status of patient's health
- Lack of availability of family members
- Failure to designate specific family contact person/s
- Movement among different health care settings
- Belief that the caregiver should initiate conversation
- Family wanting to protect the patient from bad news
- Inability to process information due to stress
- Fear of bothering or upsetting the health care professional

Health Care Professional Barriers

- Discomfort with death and the issues related to it
- Discomfort with withholding treatment
- Viewing death as a treatment failure
- Fear that discussing prognostic possibilities will scare the patient/family
- Lack of experience in dealing with end-of-life issues
- Lack of communication skills
- Use of health care jargon
- Failure to listen to patient/family needs
- Belief that the patient/family should initiate conversation
- Lack of collaboration between caregivers
- Discontinuity of care (often due to inconsistent patient assignments)
- Minimal time available
- Heavy patient assignment load
- Lack of availability of physician or other health care professionals
- Thought that patient or family will not be able to handle the truth
- Disrespect for patient/family values and beliefs
- Personal biases
- Struggling to balance hope with delivery of bad news

BOX 8–3   Facilitators to Communication

- Trusting relationship
- Mutual respect
- Previous experiences with end-of-life care that had positive outcomes
- Increased comfort level of health care professionals
- Patient perception that health care professionals truly care
- Viewing death as a natural part of life
- Use of lay terminology
- Self-awareness of health care professionals related to personal feelings and biases
- Patient/family support system
- Honesty
- Full disclosure of information (to level desired by patient/family)
- Continuity of care
- Multidisciplinary care
- Clear understanding about scheduling of conferences
- Clear understanding about availability/how to contact if needed
- Active listening in a relaxed environment
- Permission for patient/family to verbalize feelings

SECTION TWO REVIEW

1. During report a nurse states that family members for an actively dying patient have been demanding and making irrational requests. The nurse believes this is a reflection of unmet communication needs. Which of the following should be added to the family plan of care? (Select all that apply.)
   1. Schedule periodic meetings with the patient and family.
   2. Practice active listening during all interactions.
   3. Assess level of understanding and desire for information.
   4. Refer family to the nurse manager for all requests.

2. A patient is admitted with a terminal diagnosis and states that she has an advance directive on file. What considerations should be given for the plan of care regarding the advance directives?
   1. It is not necessary to discuss the patient's wishes again once they have been put into writing.
   2. They should not be discussed again until death appears to be imminent.
   3. The patient's wishes should be discussed periodically to maintain open communication about end of life.
   4. They should be discussed only when there is a change in health status.

3. A patient with a terminal diagnosis and a life expectancy of about two months asks to speak with the nurse privately. The patient expresses the desire to stop nasogastric feedings to relieve bloating, swelling, and nausea. Which of the following would be appropriate actions by the nurse? (Select all that apply.)
   1. Actively listen to the patient, asking open-ended questions about the patient's symptoms and the request.
   2. Assess the patient's understanding of the situation and ensure the patient is making an informed decision.
   3. Explain that the family will not understand or support the decision and avoid discontinuation of nasogastric feedings to prevent added anxiety.
   4. Discuss with the patient the need to communicate the decision with the family, and offer staff support, such as an interdisciplinary care meeting.

4. An experienced nurse observes a nurse new to the Hospice unit during a patient interaction. The patient and family are asking questions about the plan of care and voicing a desire to make significant changes. The new nurse continues to hang the intravenous medication, measure urine output, and administer oral medications as the

family speaks. The nurse then leaves the room without discussing the issues mentioned by the family. Which of the following concepts should the experienced nurse discuss with the new nurse? (Select all that apply.)

1. Therapeutic communication includes active listening, conveying a feeling of being unhurried and sincerely caring.

2. Therapeutic communication includes supportive body language, such as maintaining eye contact, nodding, and touch.

3. Patients and families may change the overall plan of care at any point, and may withdraw treatments or add others.

4. Communication with patients and family members is a priority in the delivery of end-of-life care.

Case Study 1

Grace Clark, age 63, was admitted to the hospital with a broken hip. She came through surgery without incident, and was recovering well for the first week. Her family has just come in after receiving a 2 a.m. call telling them that she is having difficulty breathing, and that she is being transferred to the intensive care unit. When they arrive, they find her intubated and unresponsive. Her family demands to know what has happened, and they ask why this wasn't predicted. They state that it is obvious they have not been receiving accurate information. The on-call physician tells them that "she probably threw a PE" and asks what should be done if she "codes," then he is paged for an emergency in another area.

Question

As the nurse, what is your evaluation of the situation?

Suggested Response

You realize that the rapid deterioration in Mrs. Clark's status is overwhelming for the family. They are confused and angry. They don't know what a "PE" is, or what "code" means. They do not know the physician on call, and state they do not trust him. You take the time to listen to their concerns, answer their questions, and clarify information. You ask if they have a support person that you could call and offer the services of the hospital chaplain. You explain the equipment in the patient's room and assure them that she is comfortable. Having answered their questions, you get them coffee and offer to let them use the small conference room to try to process the information that they have received. You leave them with the chaplain, tell them that you will be just across the hall at the nurse's station, and state that you will be back to check on them in a few minutes. By your course of action, you have defused the situation. You have also begun to build trust, which will be a key factor in the decision-making process that they face.

SECTION THREE: Storytelling

Families in the process of losing a loved one to death will often use storytelling as a means for coping throughout their time of vulnerability and loss. Storytelling is defined as an account of an event to create a memorable picture in the mind of the listener (Kirkpatrick, Ford, & Castelloe, 1997). Stories may entertain, teach lessons, relieve tension, pass on traditions, or communicate a message. Stories about another person, such as the stories told by the families of the dying, help other people to relate to the dying person. Even though the dying person may no longer be able to communicate, the family wishes to help their loved one's story to continue, so that others who may become involved will appreciate the uniqueness and character of the person who is nearing the end of life.

The suffering that is encountered by families at the end of life causes people to struggle with assignment of meaning to the experience of death and loss. Storytelling may be used to assign meaning in suffering, to illuminate an inner struggle, to instill hope, and to offer distraction from pain.

Brody (1987) contends that human lives are, in a sense, stories. The story of each individual involves a sense of self that includes the story of past, present, and future. At the time of death, the person's story becomes a legacy left for the world. Individuals may struggle with adjustment in bringing their story to a close, but families also struggle with the fact that their loved one's story is reaching a conclusion. The suffering that occurs often leaves them feeling vulnerable and helpless. One of the things that helps to bring comfort and meaning to their suffering is the attempt to assist their loved one's story to live on. Storytelling at end of life may be helpful to families as they search for meaning and purpose in what they are experiencing (Heiney, 1993).

Believing that family members will be shaped by the death experience of their loved one, Finlay (2003) recommended that the stories of each individual in the family should be heard. Even children need to discuss their thoughts and questions with those who are caring for their loved one. If no one appears to take an interest in the family, family members believe that no one actually cares about them or their loved one, leaving them feeling isolated and often powerless. Once in a situation of feeling isolated and powerless, anger on the part of the family will often follow. Anger leads to the possibility of being viewed as difficult, which could result in further isolation (Durham, 1998).

A health care system in which the caregivers are frequently changing also causes frustration, as there is lack of relationship with caregivers and the need to retell the patient's story over and over, while believing that no one is really listening (Finlay, 2003). Such inconsistency among caregivers contributes to the vulnerability of patients and their families by increasing the potential for negative feelings, thus making coping or adaptation more difficult. For this reason, continuity of care among nursing caregivers is a very important aspect of care at the end of life.

The suffering that is experienced by family, and the family's need to relate stories about the patient, are outward signs of an inner struggle to attach meaning to the patient's life and death. Byock (1996) described the end of life as a loss of meaning that results in suffering. The usual sources of meaning are often lost as families face the loss of a loved one. New sources of meaning must be found, and often that new source of meaning is found in sharing the dying person's story.

Storytelling may also reveal the struggle that patients or family members are experiencing (Kirkpatrick et al., 1997). Stories shared by families shed light on the unseen forces that are battling within. Nurses who are able to listen carefully to the stories being told by family members will find that they are able to gain insight that will help them to prioritize and optimize their care.

When working with the dying, a large percentage of the nurse's time will be spent in care of the family. Taking the time to listen to the family is one of the major issues that will decide the course of patient care. Unless a nurse understands the family's unique struggles and concerns, it will not be possible to provide appropriate nursing care. The family's needs, therefore, could remain unmet simply because no one listened to their story.

Instillation of hope is another benefit that may be attributed to storytelling. Mayers (1995) described the importance of storytelling, explaining that sharing stories about problematic issues may transform a sense of powerlessness into a sense of hope. As family members share stories about their loved one, the atmosphere in the room will often become a brighter place. Tears may turn to smiles and laughter as the family discusses enjoyable moments from the patient's past.

Distraction may also be attributed to storytelling (Chelf, Deshler, Hillman, & Durazo-Arvizu, 2000). Because pain is one of the most significant fears faced by the dying and their families, distraction is an important part of pain management therapy (Steinhauser, Clipp, et al., 2000). Engaging the patient or family member in storytelling is a valuable method, along with other appropriate pain management techniques, for taking one's thoughts away from the painful reality at hand. Talking about pleasant memories takes thoughts away from the bedside of the dying, mentally carrying each person away to a more pleasant place and time.

Such retelling of an experience is a therapeutic technique recommended in literature (Leske, 1998). Family members are encouraged to talk through the events that have occurred through the time of diagnosis, treatment, and death. They should discuss the impact that the events have had on them, along with their feelings about the future. Storytelling such as this will help family members to mourn for the person that they knew, while allowing them to express feelings of guilt or anger that are often involved at the time of death. Being able to discuss the story of each event, along with their feelings about it, will help to legitimize the intense emotions that they are experiencing and help them to find hope for the future.

Nurses who care for the dying and their families will develop the skills needed to encourage the use of storytelling. Asking questions about the patient's past experiences or about the family's caregiving role will often be all that is needed to start the healing therapy of storytelling in motion.

SECTION THREE REVIEW

1. Why is storytelling important at end of life? Storytelling: (Select all that apply.)
   1. Helps to keep the memory of the patient alive, even as death approaches.
   2. Allows the family to share the individuality of the patient when the patient is no longer able to communicate.
   3. Helps to build a relationship of respect and trust.
   4. Isolates the family from the nurse/patient relationship and should be discouraged.
2. When evaluating pain control interventions for a patient, a nurse providing end-of-life care finds that the patient is able to go an additional 30 minutes without pain medication when the nurses plan time for storytelling. What is the likely rationale for this finding?
   1. The patient is taking more pain medication than actually needed.
   2. The nurses are not meeting the patient's pain control needs.
   3. Storytelling serves as a distraction for the patient.
   4. There is inaccurate documentation of medication administration.
3. A family member begins to tell the nurse a story about a trip the family took prior to the patient's diagnosis. The nurse needs to administer pain medication to

another patient down the hall. What is an appropriate response by the nurse?

1. "I am sorry, but I do not have time right now to hear your story. Perhaps another time."
2. "I would really like to hear about your trip, however, I need to give another patient pain medication. Once I give the medication, I will come back and would like to hear more."
3. "Go ahead and talk about the memories of your trip without me, I have another patient who needs my care at this moment."
4. "I think there are more important things for us to discuss at this point. You have some important decisions to make."

4. The wife of a dying patient tells the nurse, "I do not know why I keep telling you about our life prior to this illness. It is not very interesting and does not help him now." What is the best response by the nurse?

1. "If you do not think it helps, then do not feel like you have to do it."
2. "Ask your husband if he enjoys listening to the stories or not."
3. "Talking about the past will only make him grieve more deeply and make his remaining time poor quality."
4. "Telling your story is part of coping with illness and death. It may bring you and your husband comfort to talk about your experiences."

Case Study 2

Aleen, a patient in a palliative care unit, was a woman who was just nearing the age where she had been thinking about retiring from teaching. Her husband, who kept vigil at her bedside, was already retired. He had been looking forward to the time when they could enjoy more quality time together in their golden years. Her sons, both in their 30s, spent most of their time in her room also. Amidst sobs, the family members would smile as they shared stories about her. They spoke of her classroom full of third-graders, where she had taught for 38 years and was still under contract. They told how she made sugar cookies with her granddaughter, how she took a walk every morning with her canine companion, how she visited sick people for her church, and how she had filled the freezer with her husband's favorite meals so that he wouldn't be hungry when she was no longer there to cook for him. They created a mental picture of her at the dance where she met her husband, and laughed as they told how she would not let anyone else work in her garden (where she believed men were not qualified to set foot).

Question

What is being accomplished by the stories that Aleen's family are telling?

Suggested Response

The family is searching for meaning in their suffering, revealing their inner struggle, searching for hope, and seeking distraction from their pain. Through sharing stories about Aleen, they are also keeping her story alive and helping others to know that their loved one is special and unique.

CHAPTER SUMMARY

- The benefits of openly discussing end-of-life issues include reduction of anxiety, clarity in decision making, and confronting fears in the light of factual information.
- Many nurses who deal with end-of-life issues have expressed a desire to learn more effective ways to communicate with patients and families at end of life.
- Family members as well as the terminally ill individual will be especially affected by the quality of communications at the end of life.
- Patients and families who are dealing with a terminal illness will often shift very quickly from aggressive treatment of the illness to transitioning into hospice or palliative care, necessitating a significant need for information and guidance in decision making.
- The use of open-ended questions regarding the needs and desires of patient and family will contribute toward maximizing the information

obtained and the health care team's ability to assist with decision making at the end of life.
- Provision of written materials has also been found to be an effective communication strategy.
- Unless communication problems are addressed and resolved as they arise, it will be very difficult to arrive at end-of-life care decisions with which patients, families, and health care providers all agree.
- A system for facilitating communication that emphasizes the importance of active listening is the VALUE system.
- Families in the process of losing a loved one to death will often use storytelling as a means for coping throughout their time of vulnerability and loss.
- Storytelling may also reveal the struggle that patients or family members are experiencing.

CHAPTER REVIEW

A 41-year-old patient has recently been admitted to the hospice program, and you have just conducted a home visit. The patient, who is just eight years older than you, is aware of her diagnosis of breast cancer with metastasis to liver and bone. Although she has consented to admission to hospice, she states that she does not wish to talk about her illness. She asks that you just give her whatever she needs for medications and then leave because she wants to watch her favorite afternoon television show. You notice that she tears up and looks away from you when she pets her dog. When you leave her house, you feel sad and empty. You begin to cry as you plan your next visit to her home.

Questions

1. What factors may influence your interaction with this patient?
2. How will you plan for the next visit?

Suggested Response

It is important for you, as the nurse, to determine why this patient is affecting you so deeply. Is it because she is so close to your age? Are there mortality issues that you need to address in yourself? Your search for self-awareness will be a key factor in this relationship.

Regarding the next visit, you determine to try a different strategy to communicate with the patient. A relationship of trust has not yet been built. You may decide to ask about her dog or other things that seem to interest her, hoping that initiating conversation will lead to open discussion related to her situation. You also plan to assess her support system, and will explore the possibility of having another family member there for future visits, if that is acceptable to the patient. You will look for and respond to clues that may lead to trust-building as well as more effective communication.

REFERENCES

Ahrens, T., Yancey, V., & Kollef, M. (2003). Improving family communications at the end of life: Implications for length of stay in the intensive care unit and resource use. *American Journal of Critical Care, 12*(4), 317–323.

Bowman, K. (2000). Communication, negotiation, and mediation: Dealing with conflict in end-of-life decisions. *Journal of Palliative Care, 16*, S17–S23.

Boyle, D., Miller, P., & Forbes-Thompson, S. (2005). Communication and end-of-life care in the intensive care unit: Patient, family, and clinician outcomes. *Critical Care Nursing Quarterly, 28*(4), 302–316.

Brody, H. (1987). Stories of sickness. New York: Yale University Press.

Bruera, E., Neumann, C., Mazzocato, C., & Stiefel, F. (2000). Attitudes and beliefs of palliative care physicians regarding communication with terminally ill cancer patients. *Palliative Medicine, 14*, 287–298.

Byock, I. (1996). The nature of suffering and the nature of opportunity and the end of life. *Clinical Geriatric Medicine, 12*, 237–252.

Chelf, J., Deshler, A., Hillman, S., & Durazo-Arvizu, R. (2000). Storytelling: A strategy for living and coping with cancer. *Cancer Nursing, 23*(1), 1–5.

Clayton, J., Butow, P., Arnold, R., & Tattersall, M. (2005). Discussing end-of-life issues with terminally ill cancer patients and their careers: A qualitative study. *Supportive Care in Cancer, 13*, 589–599.

Clayton, J., Butow, P., Psych, M., & Tattersall, M. (2005). When and how to initiate discussion about prognosis and end-of-life issues with terminally ill patients. *Journal of Pain and Symptom Management, 30*(2), 132–144.

Clayton, J., Butow, P., Tattersall, M., Devine, R., Simpson, J., Aggarwal, G., et al. (2007). Randomized controlled trial of a prompt list to help advanced cancer patients and their caregivers to ask questions about prognosis and end-of-life care. *Journal of Clinical Oncology, 25*(6), 715–723.

Curtis, J., & Patrick, D. (1997). Barriers to communication about end-of-life care in AIDS patients, *Journal of General Internal Medicine, 12*, 736–741.

Curtis, J., Patrick, D., Shannon, S., Treece, P., Engelberg, R., & Rubenfeld, G. (2001). The family conference as a focus to improve communication about end-of-life care in the intensive care unit: Opportunities for improvement. *Critical Care Medicine, 29*, N26–N33.

De Araujo, T., Silva, P., & Francisco, B. (2004). Nursing the dying: Essential elements in the care of terminally ill patients. *International Nursing Review, 51*(3), 149–158.

De Araujo, T., Silva, P., & Silva, G. (2004). Communication with dying patients: Perception of intensive care unit nurses in Brazil. *Journal of Clinical Nursing, 13*(2), 143–149.

Durham, E. (1998). Caring for Cody. *American Journal of Nursing, 98*(4), 42–44.

Finlay, I. (2003). Dying with dignity. *Clinical Medicine, 3*(2), 102–103.

Forest, P. (2004). Being there: The essence of end-of-life care. *Urologic Nursing, 24*(4), 270–279.

Griffie, J., Nelson-Marten, P., & Muchka, S. (2004). Acknowledging the 'elephant': Communication in palliative care. *American Journal of Nursing, 104*(1), 48–57.

Heiney, S. (1993). The healing power of story. *Oncology Nursing Forum, 22*(6), 899–904.

Holmberg, L. (2006). Communication in palliative home care: A dying son and his mother. *Journal of Hospice and Palliative Nursing, 8*(1), 15–24.

Keeley, M. (2007). 'Turning toward death together': The functions of messages during final conversations in close relationships. *Journal of Social and Personal Relationships, 24*(2), 225–253.

Kirkpatrick, M., Ford, S., & Castelloe, B. (1997). Storytelling: An approach to client-centered care. *Nurse Educator, 22*(2), 38–40.

Lautrette, A., Darmon, M., Megarbane, B., Joly, L., Chevret, S., Adrie, C., et al. (2007). A communication strategy and brochure for relatives of patients dying in the ICU. *New England Journal of Medicine, 356*(5), 469–478.

Leske, J. (1998). Treatment for family members in crisis after critical injury. *AACN Clinical Issues: Advanced Practice in Acute Critical Care, 9*(1), 129–139.

London, M., & Lundstedt, J. (2007). Families speak about inpatient end-of-life care. *Journal of Nursing Care Quality, 22*(2), 152–158.

Matzo, M., Sherman, D., Sheehan, D., Ferrell, B., & Penn, B. (2003). Communication skills for end-of-life nursing care: Teaching strategies from the ELNEC curriculum. *Nursing Education Perspectives, 24*(4), 176–183.

Mayers, K. (1995). Storytelling: A method to increase discussion, facilitate rapport with residents, and share knowledge among long-term care staff. *Journal of Continuing Education in Nursing, 26*(6), 280–282.

McDonald, D., Deloge, J., Joslin, N., Petow, W., Severson, J., Votino, R., et al. (2003). Communicating end-of-life preferences. *Western Journal of Nursing Research, 25*(6), 652–666.

Meraviglia, M., McGuire, C., & Chelsey, D. (2003). Nurses' needs for education on cancer and end-of-life care. *Journal of Continuing Education in Nursing, 34*, 122–127.

Moore, C. (2005). Communication issues and advance care planning. *Seminars in Oncology Nursing, 21*(1), 11–19.

Norton, S., Tilden, V., Tolle, S., Nelson, C., & Eggman, S. (2003). Life support withdrawal: Communication and conflict. *American Journal of Critical Care, 12*(6), 548–555.

Penson, R., Partidge, R., Shah, M., Giansiracusa, D., Chabner, D., & Lynch, T. (2005). Fear of death. *The Oncologist, 10,* 160–169.

Radziewicz, R. (2001). Self-care for the caregiver. *Nursing Clinics of North America, 36*(4), 855–869.

Royak-Schaler, R., Gadalla, S., Lemkau, J., Ross, D., Alexander, C., & Scott, D. (2006). Family perspectives on communication with healthcare providers during end-of-life cancer care. *Oncology Nursing Forum, 33*(4), 753–760.

Steinhauser, K., Christakis, N., Clipp, E., McNeilly, M., McIntyre, L., & Tulsky, J. (2000). Factors considered important at the end of life by patients, family, physicians, and other care providers. *Journal of the American Medical Association, 284*(19), 2476–2482.

Steinhauser, K., Clipp, E., McNeilly, M., Christakis, N., McIntyre, L., & Tulsky, J. (2000). In search of a good death: Observations of patients, families, and providers. *Annals of Internal Medicine, 132*(10), 825–832.

Tilden, V., Nelson, C., Dunn, P., Donius, M., & Tolle, S. (2000). Nursing's perspective on improving communication about nursing home residents' preferences for medical treatments at end of life. *Nursing Outlook, 48*(3), 109–115.

Volker, D. (2001). Oncology nurses' experiences with requests for assisted dying from terminally ill patients with cancer. *Oncology Nursing Forum, 28*(1), 39–49.

Zapka, J., Hennessy, W., Carter, R., & Amella, E. (2006). End-of-life communication and hospital nurses: An educational pilot. *Journal of Cardiovascular Nursing, 21*(3), 223–231.

Psychosocial Issues at End of Life

Following completion of this chapter, the learner will be able to:

9.1. Describe the nurse's role in facilitating positive coping strategies.

9.2. Identify ways to address family/significant other issues.

9.3. Discuss issues related to grief and mourning.

9.4. Describe the nurse's role in providing after-death care.

9.5. Address special considerations that may arise when caring for patients in different stages of life.

9.6. Incorporate ways to promote caregiver well-being into practice.

9.7. Discuss the nurse's role in offering counsel.

This chapter examines psychosocial issues related to end-of-life care for patients and families. Coping and adaptation are discussed, as well as the nurse's role in dealing with caregiver and family issues. Aspects of grief and mourning are addressed from both the family and the caregiver's perspectives. Suggestions for providing after-death care are offered, and special considerations in caring for patients across the lifespan are discussed. Emphasis is placed on the fact that the nurse does not need to be the sole provider when it comes to addressing psychosocial issues. Appropriate resources should be utilized to meet the needs of patients and families, remembering that the nurse is a part of the multidisciplinary health care delivery team.

PRETEST

1. What is the nurse's role in providing care after the death of a patient? (Select all that apply.)
   1. The nurse should provide opportunity for the family to spend time with the body in a quiet place.
   2. The body should be cleaned and positioned to allow the patient to look as natural as possible.
   3. Excess equipment should be cleared from the room, decreasing clutter to create a more peaceful environment.
   4. All lines, tubes, and monitoring devices should be discontinued and removed so the family can view the body in a more natural state.

2. Why is positive coping important when it comes to end-of-life issues? Positive coping:
   1. Makes it easier to care for patients, as they tend to have less anger in facing death.

   2. Eliminates the psychosocial issues that would normally arise at end of life.
   3. Will result in better outcomes for the patient and family.
   4. Eliminates stressors for the family.

3. What is the responsibility of the nurse when it comes to offering counsel? The nurse:
   1. Will be able to counsel in any situation.
   2. Should refer all requests for counsel to other appropriate professionals.
   3. Should not offer counsel, as this may decrease the patient's confidence level.
   4. Is free to counsel in areas of expertise, but should refer to other professionals as appropriate.

GLOSSARY

bereavement   The state of experiencing desolation or sadness as a result of a significant loss.

coping   Response and adaptation to a situation.

grief   Sorrow or distress related to loss.

mourning   The experience or manifestations of grief; it may be perceptible (such as crying or expressing feelings) or difficult to discern (such as unexpressed feelings).

significant other   A life partner or nonrelative who has an intimate relationship with a person outside of marriage.

SECTION ONE: Coping, Grief, and Mourning

End-of-life care is a challenge that will be faced by nurses in many areas of practice. Nurses who work in hospice or palliative care are expected to be accustomed to working with the dying, but those who work in intensive care units, emergency rooms, home care, clinics, and many other settings will also be dealing with patients and families who are facing end-of-life issues. Although dealing with physical aspects of death and dying is an important focus, addressing psychosocial issues is equally important and may present an even greater challenge.

Nursing, as defined by Andrews and Roy (1986), is a discipline that uses special knowledge to help promote and restore health. Historically, health was defined in terms of the absence or presence of disease (Kozier, Erb, Berman, & Burke, 2000). Dubos (1978), however, proposed that health is a creative process, suggesting that individuals are in a constant state of striving to adapt to their environment. Assisting patients and families to adapt in the face of illness and death is an important part of the nurse's role.

Coping: Dealing with Loss

Human response to a situation, in essence, is measured by how a person copes. Research has indicated that inability to cope or adapt to life circumstances, along with a lack of hope, can be very detrimental to quality of life (Wonghongkul, Moore, Musil, Schneider, & Deimling, 2000). Hope, a key factor in the ability to cope, may be hindered by multiple losses, feelings of loneliness, and physical health concerns (Holtslander & Duggleby, 2008). Because of the variety of opportunities for service within the profession of nursing, nurses may assist patients and families with adjustment, coping, and fostering hope throughout various stages of health and illness.

Coping and adaptation may be especially challenging for the dying and their families. Facing the end of life is something that everyone is destined to encounter on a personal level at some point, but families of the dying are also challenged with trying to adjust to the loss of their loved one. Issues such as fear, anger, guilt, and denial will often be faced by the person who is approaching death, as well as by family members. Depending on the specific situation, there may also be changes in relationships, intimacy issues, and changes in body image. The trauma of loss may leave those affected with feelings of chaos or confusion (Dennis, 2008). Assisting the patient and family to cope is a challenge that nurses will face as they provide end-of-life care.

Coping has been defined as a persistent state of adaptation that is influenced by each individual's perception of the situation (Kim, Yeom, Seo, Kim, and Yoo, 2002). This state of adaptation could be either positive or negative. A positive coping style may be characterized by a spirit of inner strength. A negative coping style may be identified by helplessness or hopelessness, which may lead to more negative outcomes in dealing with life circumstances (Petticrew, Bell, & Hunter, 2002).

Nurses have a unique opportunity to assist patients and families at end of life. Religion and spirituality have been found to be powerful factors involved in coping with health-related issues (Baldree, Murphy, & Powers, 1982; Narayanasamy, 2003). Additionally, there are many coping mechanisms that may emerge and these coping mechanisms may be either positive or negative. A patient or family member may use negative coping mechanisms such as blaming, denial, or withdrawal. Previous negative habits may also become exacerbated during times of stress such as an impending loss. Family members, for instance, may overuse alcohol or begin to smoke more.

It is within the realm of the nurse's role to assist individuals in identifying their negative coping mechanisms, while encouraging the positive ones. Family members, for example, may be assisted to cope through having opportunity to attend support groups, becoming involved in an exercise program, or making use of artistic abilities.

Keeping patients and families informed about the current situation may also assist in building coping power. Explaining, for example, why the skin has a mottled appearance will help to demystify the dying process, thus contributing to positive coping.

Sharing information with the patient and family will also increase opportunities for communication, as well as for realistic planning for end-of-life care (Surkan, Dickman, Steineck, Onelov, & Kreicbergs, 2006).

Families in the process of losing a loved one to death will often use storytelling as another means of coping. This concept may be found in further detail in Chapter 8.

Grief and Mourning

Grief is the process of experiencing and reacting to the loss of a loved one, while mourning involves the integration of the loss into daily life (Rando, 1993). **Bereavement** involves a significant loss, but the experience of loss may or may not be accompanied by grief (Fulton & Metress, 1995).

Family members must go through the grief experience in order to adapt to loss. Each person will experience the grief process in a different way, and it is important that ongoing nursing support reflect individuality in the grief plan of care.

The process of grief and **mourning** typically involves four phases through which a person must move (Hockenberry & Wilson, 2007). There will at first be disbelief, or a feeling of numbness, after which a person moves into the second phase when there is a desperate longing to be with the deceased. The third phase involves a sense of disorganization and despair.

The person in this phase may become depressed or isolated, believing that life is meaningless without the person who has died. The fourth phase is reorganization, when the person begins to again find meaning in life, integrating the loss of the loved one into a renewed sense of normalcy. There may be movement forward and backward through the phases, and it is important that the family not be expected to get past the loss entirely. The nurse must offer reassurance that it is normal to feel a continued sense of loss related to the death of a loved one. Living with the loss and enjoying positive memories will be an expected part of adaptation.

The time required to move through the grief process will be different for each person. The majority of people will be able to move through the intense feelings of loss with the support of their friends and family (McChrystal, 2008). Those who are unable to move into the reorganization phase by the end of 12 months are considered to have a complicated grief reaction. A referral for professional help should be considered at that time.

When there is awareness that death will be approaching, there may also be anticipatory grief. Even though this may allow a person to begin to work through some aspects related to grief prior to the actual death, it does not mean that death will be any easier. The family who has been anticipating the death of a loved one for months will often move into the first stage, experiencing numbness and disbelief at the actual time of loss.

SECTION ONE REVIEW

1. When should family members be expected to be back to normal after the death of a loved one?
   1. At the 12-month anniversary of the death.
   2. It depends on how much time they had for anticipatory grieving.
   3. If the family is intact, 6 months after the death.
   4. The family should not be expected to be "back to normal." Adapting to the death will bring the family to a new sense of normalcy, as the loss is integrated into their day-to-day lives.

2. A patient has cancer and is dying. Her son has been her caregiver for several years, and there is no other family in the area. The nurse who is caring for the patient in the hospital notices that her son has been drinking heavily two or three times a week, which is out of the ordinary for him. What is the responsibility of the nurse related to the patient's son?
   1. The activity of the son should not be a concern of the nurse, since he is able to make his own decisions and care for himself.

   2. The nurse should tell him that his actions are reprehensible, and that he is causing his mother heartache during her last days.
   3. The nurse should assess the situation to be sure that the safety of the patient is not in jeopardy. She should then address the negative coping mechanism that she has identified in the patient's son, and offer to assist him with appropriate referrals.
   4. The son should be restricted from visiting his mother in the hospital.

3. What is an appropriate way to address a mother's recent loss of a child?
   1. Explain that the parent is still young enough to have another child.
   2. Tell the parent that a support group might help, as the people there would know exactly how she feels.
   3. Express sympathy for the loss of the child and inquire as to the well-being of the mother and family.
   4. Avoid discussing the loss of the child, as discussing it may give rise to painful memories.

SECTION TWO: Nursing Role Related to Patient/Family Issues

Remembering the Caregiver

Many family members have been caring for dying loved ones for several months at home, where they have been dealing with increasingly complex physical and psychological issues. As the patient's condition worsens, family caregivers often tend to resist offers of help for themselves. Their own needs are ignored as they focus on the needs of the dying family member, thus increasing their risks of developing physical or psychological disorders (Walsh & Schmidt, 2003). Research has found that family caregivers of the dying are especially prone to depression as a result of isolation and loss of relationships within the family (Black, 1998). Black describes depression as being caused by feelings of helplessness, fear, guilt, loss of self-confidence, and perceived inability to cope. The concept of care for the family caregiver is discussed in greater depth in Chapter 11.

Professional caregivers, such as nurses, may become overwhelmed by the experience of death that patients and families are facing as well. There may be situations where the patient is the same age as the nurse, or as the nurse's child, and it may cause deep psychological or emotional pain as the situation seems to be very close to the nurse's heart. Nurses may use defense mechanisms to allay their personal discomfort, including focusing only on the physical care needs of the patients, rather than caring for the whole person. Evading emotionally sensitive conversations with families, offering minimal verbalization, and talking only about topics that are comfortable to them are some of the defense mechanisms that may be used by nurses. These behaviors result in emotional distancing, avoidance, and withdrawal from the dying patients and their families, increasing vulnerability of the patient and family at a time when interaction with the professional is most needed (Matzo, Sherman, Lo, Egan, Grant, & Rhome, 2003). Being present for the patients and families, listening to their stories, and offering stories of their own, will help nurses to process their feelings about the end-of-life experience. This increased self-awareness will result in increased ability to provide the nursing care needed as patient and family face an end-of-life situation.

Dealing with Families/Significant Others

Families are defined in literature as a unique social group with generational ties, permanence, mutual concern, and a nurturing function (Leske, 1998). Family members may include a spouse, children, a life partner of the same or opposite sex, blended families (including stepparents or children), extended families (including multiple generations), or any number of other possibilities (Allender & Spradley, 2005).

Because of the complexity involved with families, situations may arise that call for creativity in navigating through the sea of family dynamics (*End-of-Life: A Nurse's Guide to Compassionate Care*, 2007). There may be a father who has been ostracized by the family, a sibling in another state who tries to override the decision making of other family members, or a life partner who does not get along with other family members.

A life partner who has been a **significant other** in the life of the patient for many years may wish to be at the bedside in the days or hours prior to death. It may be the significant other who has the best understanding of what the patient's wishes are, and he or she may be the one who will bring the greatest comfort to the patient at the end of life. The family, however, may ask that the significant other not be allowed to visit, not have a part in decision making, or not be involved in care conferences. Although it is possible that the legal rights of the significant other may be in question in these situations, the nurse may need to serve as an advocate. Attempting to bring family members and significant others to an understanding may be difficult, but will be in the best interest of the patient. Emphasizing the importance of keeping the focus on the patient may help to bring harmony to the situation (Berzoff & Silverman, 2004). If a peaceful environment cannot be achieved, it may be necessary to propose an agreement in which both sides will agree to specific terms. An example of this may be separate visiting hours for the life partner. If the patient is able to weigh in on the topic, the patient's wishes should be given top priority.

Whatever the situation, it is important to remember that the significant other will often be struggling with the impending loss of a partner. The nurse should make every attempt to assist the significant other in coping with the illness and death of a loved one (Corless, Germino, & Pittman, 2006).

Whatever the makeup of the family, learning to cope with an impending death is a daunting task for each member of the dying person's family. Following all of the family's leads will allow the nurse to play an integral part in helping family members to adapt to the loss of their loved one.

There may also be times when family members do not have the best interests of the patient at heart. Family decisions may be made that are inconsiderate or self-serving. It is often the nurse who must intervene in such a situation. For example, a patient's wife could make a decision to withhold nutrition from her terminally ill husband, stating that she does not want to prolong his suffering. Then, to everyone's surprise, his condition improves, he awakens, and begins to ask for food. It may be left to the nurse to explain to the patient's wife that the patient is now the decision maker related to his nutrition status and to help her come to terms with the fact that she still believes that nutrition should still be withheld since she had already come to terms with his impending death.

A second example of how nurses intervene in difficult family situations is in the case of a hospice patient, hours from death while his son stood on the mattress by his father's chest. The young man was removing a family picture from the wall at the head of the bed. An argument among the siblings ensued about who should be the rightful owner of the picture. In this situation, as in the previous one, it was the nurse who served as an advocate for the patient. The rights and dignity of the patient must not be overshadowed by thoughtless decisions of family members, and the nurse will often be the one who stands in the gap (Berzoff & Silverman, 2004).

End-of-Life Care Across the Lifespan

There are special considerations that come into play when working with patients and families at different stages in life. With over 50,000 children dying each year in the United States (Vats & Reynolds, 2006), many nurses will be called upon to provide care for dying pediatric patients and their families. The needs of children and their families will vary greatly. Children who are facing death may be fearful of separation from parents, sad that they have created a burden for parents, or guilt-ridden, believing that the illness is a punishment for evil deeds. For the very young, there may be little understanding of the concept of death, and parents will struggle with the helpless feeling that they are unable to alleviate the suffering associated with impending death. There may also be issues with parental feelings of guilt that the illness was not identified earlier. Siblings may feel isolated and unimportant because of the focus on the dying child (Huntley, 2002).

In order to provide nursing care, it is imperative that the nurse have an understanding of each family member's feelings and perceptions related to the impending death. Families need continued education and support throughout the time surrounding a child's death (Corless et al., 2006). Resources such as counseling, support groups, and community support (respite care providing someone to come in to stay with the patient, help with house cleaning, provision of meals and baked goods, etc.) can be among those considered very helpful for the family.

Working with young adult patients who are dying will also present challenging opportunities for nursing care. Issues related to loss of a valued career, inability to fulfill expectations as a parent, and impaired intimacy with a spouse may take a huge toll on the patient. As with other age groups, it is extremely important to do a thorough nursing assessment related to the patient and the family. The psychosocial issues that will be identified in the young adult patient may be exceptionally burdensome (Huntley, 2002). An understanding of the patient's situation will provide a solid foundation on which to build the plan of care, and will result in nursing interventions that are beneficial to the patient.

Care of the geriatric patient may give rise to an entirely different set of psychosocial concerns. There may be adult children or grandchildren who are struggling with the impending loss. It may be that the dying patient is all alone, having outlived spouse and children. The elderly patient may also have been the caregiver for an ailing spouse, and concern for the spouse's well-being is a heavy burden. The patient may be concerned about what legacy is being left, and whether there had really been meaning and significance in life (Cicirelli, 2006). For example, one elderly patient who was dying of cancer spent her last few weeks baking a variety of cookies. She put them in the freezer for her husband to eat in the weeks after her death, explaining that she knew he would be lonely and she wanted to leave him a tangible reminder

of her love for him. Review Chapter 7 for a more complete description of end-of-life care across the lifespan.

Offering Counsel

Often, nurses will be called upon to offer counsel to those dealing with end-of-life issues. Patients and families may turn to the nurse as a resource person, seeking support with decision making, information related to end of life, encouragement during difficult times, spiritual guidance, and much more. The more that a nurse is involved with end-of-life care, the more growth there will be in levels of experience and comfort in dealing with such issues. It must be remembered, however, that the nurse is a part of the health care team, and is not an island when it comes to counseling patients. If the nurse believes that the situation requires referral to a professional counselor, or if there is a need to seek advice from someone more experienced in a particular area, this should be explained to the patient. Then, with the patient's permission, appropriate inquiries and referrals should be made.

After-Death Care

Nursing care will be especially important during the time immediately after death. Often, the nurse will have had opportunity to discuss this time with family members prior to the occurrence of death. It is important to follow the wishes of the patient and family as much as possible during this time (Berzoff & Silverman, 2004).

The family will often want to spend time with the body after death. In the case of an infant or child, the parents may wish to hold or rock the child for an extended period. In preparation for the family's time with the body, the room should be straightened as much as possible, reducing unnecessary clutter around the patient. The patient's gown and bed linens should be clean, and equipment such as oxygen tubing, IV lines, etc. should be removed. Hospital policy, though, may require that invasive lines remain in place if an autopsy is scheduled. The need for any equipment left in place should be explained to the family. The patient's head should be elevated on a pillow, and positioning should allow for the mouth and eyes to be closed. Dentures should be placed in the mouth, if able. If the patient normally wears glasses, they may be put on as well. Boxes of tissue should be placed beside the bed.

The family may request that clergy be present in the room with them. If it is agreeable to family, the nurse who has been caring for the patient should also remain in the room, respectfully maintaining a presence. There may be family members who are overcome with grief and will require nursing assistance. The nurse should not be ashamed to shed tears with the family at the bedside. Shedding tears may be not only an emotional release for the nurse, but also an affirmation to the family that their loved one was important to those who were providing care.

After the family has spent the time desired with the body, arrangements should be made according to policy for transfer of the body. It can be very helpful to the family to discuss what actually happens to the body after they leave, such as explaining where the body will be held, how it will be transported to the funeral home, etc. (Clayton, Butow, Arnold, & Tattersall, 2005).

If the patient has passed away in an institution, valuables should be sent home with the family. They may ask that personal care items be disposed of by the institution's staff. The family may also ask that glasses and dentures be sent to the funeral home with the body. Accurate documentation of after-death care, as well as disbursement of personal items, is essential.

Nursing care during the time period after death will depend on the individual situation. If a nurse has been quite close to the patient and family, it is appropriate to attend the memorial service. Follow-up calls to assess movement through the grief process will often be appreciated. Cards sent on special days such as the deceased's birthday, the wedding anniversary date, and holidays may also be especially meaningful.

SECTION TWO REVIEW

1. A terminally ill elderly patient is admitted to the nurse's medical-surgical unit. The patient's spouse accompanies her. He has been the primary caregiver for months. The patient is confused, incontinent, needs to be fed, and does not sleep well. The husband is unkempt, pale, and has dark circles under his eyes. What action should the nurse take to address these caregiver issues?
   1. Speak with the husband about his well-being and assess how he is coping. If indicated, ask if he would like to speak with a social worker, counselor, or chaplain.
   2. Provide the husband with a list of inpatient Hospice units and nursing homes and suggest he place his wife where they can provide better care.
   3. Tell the husband to go home and rest while the wife is in the hospital and others can care for her.
   4. Call the adult children in this family and tell them to help care for the patient after discharge.
2. A nurse assesses a change in a colleague's interaction with patients. The colleague has become quiet, withdrawn, and avoids conversations with patients and family members. This change occurred following the deaths of two patients with whom the nurse had developed close relationships. What is the most appropriate first action for the concerned nurse to take?
   1. Ask the chaplain to talk with the nurse about her coping skills.

2. Ask the nurse if she is aware of the change in her interactions with patients and family members.
3. Report the change to the Nurse Manager so that she can follow up.
4. Encourage the charge nurse not to assign that nurse to dying patients.

3. The nurse is caring for a dying 10-year-old child who is exhibiting signs of poor coping and is acting out. What are some of the beliefs or feelings experienced by terminally ill children that the nurse may want to explore with this child? The child: (Select all that apply.)
   1. May be fearing separation from his parents.
   2. May believe that his illness is punishment for bad behaviors.
   3. Will talk only to his parents about his feelings.
   4. May have siblings who feel isolated and treat him differently.
4. What is the nurse's role in dealing with a life partner to whom the patient was never married?
   1. The nurse should ask the family to address any issues related to the life partner.
   2. The life partner should be allowed to visit only if the patient is alert enough to request it.
   3. The nurse has no responsibility in dealing with the life partner.
   4. The nurse should facilitate positive interaction between the patient's family and the life partner, keeping the patient's wishes and best interests in mind.

Case Study 1

Three-year-old Jeffrey has been diagnosed with leukemia, and is close to death. His mother is tearful at times, and also exhibits anger frequently, but she rarely converses with the nursing staff. Her husband states that the child's illness has been difficult for her, and says that Jeffrey had not been feeling well for "a long time" before he was diagnosed. He has expressed concern about his wife, and says that he would like to help her, but does not know what to do.

Questions

1. As a nurse, what is your assessment of Jeffrey's mother's lack of desire to communicate?
2. What nursing interventions would be appropriate?

Suggested Response

You realize that Jeffrey's mother may be struggling with guilt, since he was exhibiting symptoms of illness for a significant time before he was diagnosed. You decide that you will try to visit with her about the course of his illness, and also discuss her support system. You also decide that you will discuss the availability of a psychologist who may be able to help her with sorting through her emotions and to assist her with coping issues. Her husband has offered to accompany her to see the psychologist if she so desires.

CHAPTER SUMMARY

- Nurses who work in hospice or palliative care are expected to be accustomed to working with the dying, but those who work in intensive care units, emergency rooms, home care, clinics, and many other settings will also be dealing with patients and families who are facing end-of-life issues.
- Facing the end of life is something that everyone is destined to encounter on a personal level at some point, but families of the dying are also challenged with trying to adjust to the loss of their loved one.
- Grief is the process of experiencing and reacting to the loss of a loved one, while mourning involves the integration of the loss into daily life.
- Bereavement involves a significant loss, but the experience of loss may or may not be accompanied by grief.
- Assisting individuals toward positive coping mechanisms is a crucial part of the nursing role.
- Caregivers, whether family caregivers or professional caregivers, are frequently overwhelmed by the experience of death and use multiple defense mechanisms to allay their personal discomfort.
- Whatever the makeup of the family, learning to cope with an impending death is a daunting task for each member of the dying person's family.
- In order to provide nursing care, it is imperative that the nurse have an understanding of each family member's feelings and perceptions related to the impending death and assist each family member in coping with the death of the loved one.

CHAPTER REVIEW

Alice Greeley is a 72-year-old widow. You were the nurse who was caring for her husband when he died after a long battle with cancer two years ago. You have visited with Alice two or three times since her husband passed away, and today you see her in the supermarket. She appears to be disheveled and states that she misses her husband more now than she ever has. She says that she has stopped going to church, and she rarely visits her family, as it just isn't the same without her husband. She states that she is in a hurry to get home, as she and her husband always watched the six o'clock news together and she never misses it.

Questions

1. As a nurse, what is your assessment of Alice Greeley's situation?
2. What nursing interventions would be appropriate?

Suggested Response

Alice Greeley is dealing with complicated grief. She has been unable to move into the reorganization phase of grieving two years after her husband's death. She has an intense emptiness without her husband that has affected her ability for self-care. You decide that you will follow up with Mrs. Greeley and offer assistance in making arrangements for her to see a professional grief counselor.

REFERENCES

Allender, J. A., & Spradley, B. W. (2005). Assessment of families. In *Community health nursing: Promoting and protecting the public's health.* (pp. 515–538). St. Louis: Lippincott Williams & Wilkins.

Andrews, H., & Roy, C. (1986). *Essentials of the Roy adaptation model.* East Norwalk, CT: Appleton-Century-Crofts.

Baldree, K., Murphy, S., & Powers, M. (1982). Stress identification and coping patterns in patients on hemodialysis. *Nursing Research, (31),* 107–110.

Berzoff, J., & Silverman, P. R. (2004). *Living with dying: A handbook for end of life healthcare practitioners.* New York: Columbia University Press.

Black, D. (1998). Coping with loss: The dying child. *British Medical Journal, 316*(7141), 1376–1378.

Cicirelli, V. G. (2006). *Older adults views on death.* St. Louis: Springer.

Clayton, J., Butow, P., Arnold, R., & Tattersall, M. (2005). Discussing end-of-life issues with terminally ill cancer patients and their careers: A qualitative study. *Supportive Care in Cancer, 13,* 589–599.

Corless, I., Germino, B. B., & Pittman, M. A. (Eds.) (2006). *Death, dying, and bereavement: A challenge for living* (2nd ed.). St. Louis: Springer.

Dennis, M. (2008). The grief account: Dimensions of a contemporary bereavement genre. *Death Studies, 32,* 801–836.

Dubos, R. (1978). Health and creative adaptation, *Human Nature, 74*(1), 3–14.

End-of-Life: A nurse's guide to compassionate care. (2007). St Louis: Lippincott Williams & Wilkins.

Fulton, G., & Metress, E. (1995). *Perspectives on death and dying.* Boston: Jones & Bartlett.

Hockenberry, M., & Wilson, D. (2007). *Wong's nursing care of infants and children.* St. Louis: Mosby Elsevier.

Holtslander, L., & Duggleby, W. (2008). An inner struggle for hope: Insights from the diaries of bereaved family caregivers. *International Journal of Palliative Nursing, 14*(10), 478–484.

Huntley, T. (2002). *Helping children grieve: When someone they love dies.* Minneapolis: Augsburg Books.

Kim, H., Yeom, H., Seo, Y., Kim, N., & Yoo, Y. (2002). Stress and coping strategies of patients with cancer: A Korean study. *Cancer Nursing, 25*(6), 425–431.

Kozier, B., Erb, G., Berman, A., & Burke, K. (2000). *Fundamentals of nursing: Concepts, process, and practice.* Upper Saddle River, NJ: Prentice-Hall.

Leske, J. (1998). Treatment for family members in crisis after critical injury. *AACN Clinical Issues: Advanced Practice in Acute Critical Care, 9*(1), 129–139.

Matzo, M., Sherman, D., Lo, K., Egan, K., Grant, M., & Rhome, A. (2003). Strategies for teaching loss, grief, and bereavement. *Nurse Educator, 28*(2), 71–76.

McChrystal, J. (2008). The psychological impact of bereavement on insecurely attached adults in a primary care setting. *Counselling and Psychotherapy Research, 8*(4), 231–238.

Narayanasamy, A. (2003). Spiritual coping mechanisms in chronically ill patients. *British Journal of Nursing, 11*(22), 1461–1470.

Petticrew, M., Bell, R., & Hunter, D. (2002). Influence of psychological coping on survival and recurrence in people with cancer: Systematic review. *British Medical Journal, 325*(7372), 1066.

Rando, T. (1993). *Treatment of complicated mourning.* Champaign, IL: Research Press.

Surkan, P., Dickman, P., Steineck, G., Onelov, E., & Kreicbergs, U. (2006). Home care of a child dying of a malignancy and parental awareness of a child's impending death. *Palliative Medicine, 20,* 161–169.

Vats, T., & Reynolds, P. (2006). Pediatric hospital dying trajectories: What we learned and can share. *Pediatric Nursing, 32*(4), 386–392.

Walsh, S., & Schmidt, L. (2003). Telephone support for caregivers of patients with cancer. *Cancer Nursing, 26*(6), 448–453.

Wonghongkul, T., Moore, S., Musil, C., Schneider, S., & Deimling, G. (2000). The influence of uncertainty in illness, stress appraisal, and hope on coping in survivors of breast cancer. *Cancer Nursing, 23*(6), 422–429.

Cultural and Spiritual Care at End of Life

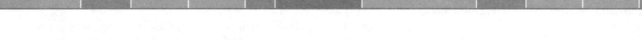

OBJECTIVES   Following completion of this chapter, the learner will be able to:

10.1. Describe culturally appropriate care.

10.2. Identify steps toward becoming more culturally competent.

10.3. Incorporate cultural competence into practice at the end of life.

10.4. Describe the nurse's role in providing spiritual care at the end of life.

10.5. Identify reasons for making spiritual care a priority.

10.6. Discuss the importance of spiritual self-awareness.

10.7. Identify nursing interventions related to spiritual care.

This chapter examines cultural competence and spiritual care as they relate to end-of-life nursing care. The importance of developing cultural competence is discussed, as well as ways to enhance competence and incorporate it into practice. The importance of spiritual care is also discussed. The need for spiritual self-awareness is addressed, as well as practical ways to incorporate spiritual assessment into nursing care. Emphasis is placed on the fact that the nurse does not need to be the sole provider when it comes to spiritual and cultural matters. Appropriate resources should be utilized to meet the needs of patients and families, remembering that the nurse is a part of the health care delivery team.

PRETEST

1. What is the nurse's role in providing care for patients from a culture that is unfamiliar? (Select all that apply.)
   1. The nurse should provide for a way of communication with the patient and family.
   2. Appropriate resource people (such as interpreters) should be sought to participate in the care of the patient.
   3. A sincere attempt should be made by the nurse to gain knowledge related to the culture, thereby facilitating understanding.
   4. A collaborative approach should be taken when planning care.
2. How is cultural competence gained? By:
   1. Reading about a culture, a nurse will know how to care for anyone from that culture.

2. Remaining completely open-minded, letting go of personal beliefs and opinions.
3. Being sensitive to the needs of individual patients and their families and learning about the cultures with which there is frequent contact.
4. Watching a variety of documentaries about other countries.

3. Who is responsible to provide for spiritual care of the patient at the end of life? The:
   1. Patient's pastor and family
   2. Facility chaplain
   3. Nurse
   4. Health care team

4. What is the responsibility of the nurse when it comes to spiritual care of a patient at the end of life? To: (Select all that apply.)
   1. Identify spiritual needs through assessment.
   2. Provide appropriate nursing interventions to meet spiritual needs.
   3. Make appropriate referrals.
   4. Prioritize spiritual needs in the plan of care.

5. Why should the nurse have a self-awareness of spiritual beliefs and values? To:
   1. Be able to have the right things to say to a patient.
   2. Be sure that the patient's belief system is correct.
   3. Have a solid foundation from which to offer spiritual care to others.
   4. Be able to provide for spiritual needs without referring the patient to other professionals.

GLOSSARY

cultural competence   The knowledge and skills applicable to any patient or community cross-cultural encounter (Kemp, 2005, p. 44).

prayer   An intimate conversation between a person and God (Shelly & Fish, 1995).

religion   A system of beliefs, practices, and traditions that is based on spiritual values.

spirituality   That which allows a person to experience transcendent meaning in life (Puchalski & Romer, 2000, p. 129).

SECTION ONE: Culturally Competent Care at End of Life

Cultural competence has been widely discussed in recent years within nursing literature. As an integral part of the health care team, nursing professionals have taken a leading role in the promotion of culturally competent care. It must be conceded that perfection will never be achieved, so the pursuit of cultural competence is often viewed as a developmental journey (Garrett, Dickson, Lis-Young, Whelan, & Roberto-Forero, 2008). The primary prerequisite for making the journey successfully is the individual nurse's desire to become involved (Momeni, Jirwe, & Emami, 2008). Any progress toward the goal translates into significant strides toward improvement in patient care.

A crucial step in the development of cultural competence is self-assessment. A culturally competent person has a self-awareness of values, opinions, and beliefs that have developed from one's own culture (Crawley, Marshall, Lo, & Koenig, 2002). The culturally competent nurse must also be sensitive to the needs of individual patients and their families, maintain interest in and involvement with culturally diverse populations, learn about the cultures with which there is frequent contact, and be able to incorporate knowledge of various cultures into practice. In essence, the nurse must think globally in gaining understanding of various cultures, yet the nursing care provided must be offered according to individual patient perspectives.

Patients and families from diverse cultures may have very different views of dying, often resulting in being misunderstood by the health care team. Such misunderstanding increases the vulnerability of those who are experiencing the death of a loved one. A study by Murray, Grant, Grant, and Kendall (2003) described the dying experience of patients in developed and developing countries. They found that there were vast differences in the resources available, citing, for example, the fact that opioids for pain control are unavailable in many underdeveloped nations. Little or no morphine is used in one-half of the world's countries. People from diverse cultures have varying views about the death experience, and may also be hesitant about expressing needs, thus increasing the challenge of caregivers to meet family needs in a holistic way (Murray et al., 2003).

Sensitivity to Cultural Needs

Nurses have a wonderful opportunity to be involved with people from diverse cultures. Care must be exercised, however, when working with patients and families, to always be sensitive to the needs of the patient and family, and respectful of individual differences. The practice of patient-centered care goes hand in hand with cultural competence (Saha, Beach, & Cooper, 2008).

The nurse who is caring for a patient from an unfamiliar culture must practice discernment, looking at the situation through the viewpoint of the patient as well as the health care team. Since much of the health care system has been designed to meet the needs of the generic patient, those who are from other cultures may feel restricted in their abilities to pursue traditional customs surrounding times of illness and death (Mazanec & Tyler, 2003). For example, all of the extended family may wish to stay with the patient around-the-clock during the hospitalization. This may present a challenge when it comes to space for families in the patient's room or in the family lounges. In the alternative, tradition may dictate that substances be applied to the walls, or that incense be burned at particular times. Such situations may present challenges for the nurse who wishes to meet the needs of patient and family, while still following hospital regulations and respecting the rights of other patients and families.

If at all possible, the culturally competent nurse will provide an opportunity for the practice of traditional rituals. This may involve setting aside adequate space, providing necessary supplies, or assisting the family to locate an appropriate cultural or spiritual leader.

Allowing for privacy to practice rituals must be evaluated on a case-by-case basis. The patient and family may or may not want the nurse to be involved with traditional practices. If the practice conflicts with the belief system of the nurse, an appropriate representative should be involved in the place of the nurse such as a staff member from a similar cultural tradition or a chaplain or social worker. While provision of privacy is important, however, the nurse must be sure that attempts to provide privacy are not interpreted as attempts to isolate the patient or family.

The decision-making process related to end-of-life issues may also present a challenge for nurses. There are cultures in which tradition would dictate that decisions be made by a family leader, or by consensus, rather than by the patient alone. This may conflict with the traditional Western view of the patient's right to autonomy, right to privacy, or the pursuit of informed consent for procedures. This situation requires communication, collaboration between disciplines, and accurate documentation. If there is concern about protection of the patient's rights, or about possible violations related to policy, appropriate hospital personnel, including legal counsel, should be involved in the decision-making process. The nurse must not stand alone in such decisions, but rather should function as an integral part of the health care delivery team. If delivery of culturally competent care conflicts with the nurse's personal system of beliefs and values, it is reasonable to transfer the care of the patient to a provider who is more accepting of the belief system of the patient (Giger, Davidhizar, & Fordham, 2006).

When caring for the patient from a culture with which the nurse is unfamiliar, it is especially imperative that the nurse keep an open line of communication with the patient and the family leaders, maintaining an open mind and an attitude of respect for others (Kemp, 2005). Listening to the patient's story, which is discussed in greater detail in Chapter 8, is an important part of offering care to any patient, but is especially crucial when dealing with patients/families from diverse cultures. It is through listening that the feelings and experiences of the patient and family will be discovered (Donnelly, 2003).

Communication may be particularly challenging when patients or families do not wish to share much personal information due to culture, tradition, or individual preference. In these cases, it is the nurse's responsibility to seek to meet the needs of the patient and family, without trying to confer one's own belief system onto a family that is already hurting. Care and support must be offered within the context of the actual needs of patients and families, knowing that these needs will not be the same for everyone.

In summary, unless the nurse is able to maintain communication and sensitivity, the health care experience may become nontherapeutic for the patient and family, and often leads to mistrust, anger, and confrontation. The discerning nurse must be constantly aware of both verbal and nonverbal communication, addressing issues as they arise. There is generally a way to compromise in the interest of a satisfactory outcome. The nurse plays a key role as both advocate and facilitator in these situations, facilitating the provision of holistic care to patients and families from any culture, even those whose traditions are unfamiliar.

Becoming Familiar with Cultural Issues

Depending on the area where the nurse practices, there will often be one or more cultures that will be treated frequently within the health care system. Indeed, the demographics in the United States are rapidly changing. It is predicted that only about half of the population will be of European Caucasian descent by the year 2020 (Giger et al., 2006). It is therefore more and more common for nurses to be caring for people from various cultures wherever they practice.

As the number of multiple cultures continues to increase, it behooves the nurse to become as familiar as possible with the customs and traditions of various people groups. This is especially true for nurses who practice in settings where end-of-life care is provided. A nurse who is familiar with cultural rituals, beliefs, and traditions can serve as a source of great comfort to the family.

In some settings, certain nurses may be most familiar with particular cultures, while others would have increased familiarity with different cultures. These nurses could then be assigned to care for patients from the cultures with which they are most familiar, or they may serve as resources for other providers. Work groups may even be formulated by institutions or organizations to assist key nurses to become educated about diverse cultures. Those nurses could then be sent back to their work environment to teach others (Vergara, Lynch-Powers, Verhaeghe, & Hynes, 2006).

Developing familiarity with a culture is an ongoing responsibility for nurses. Some simple steps such as reading about the culture, attending festivals, and visiting with members of the population may prove invaluable in the nurse's practice. It is important that these steps be implemented prior to a crisis situation, when emotions may be hard to control and critical reasoning is hindered. A foundation of knowledge and understanding, therefore, will provide a solid base for nursing care during difficult times.

Even though a nurse may be very familiar with the traditions of a culture, it is always important to avoid stereotyping and assumptions. A person may be enmeshed in another culture through marriage, may have chosen not to participate in traditional practices, or may have developed variations of rituals and traditions. Although familiarity with a culture will still be helpful, the nurse must always assess cultural needs based on the individual patient and family. Asking about traditions and practices will provide a solid foundation on which to build a therapeutic plan of care. Assessment of cultural needs will most often be greatly appreciated by the patient and family, and will lead to more positive outcomes of care.

Incorporating Knowledge into Practice

Many communities are seeing an influx of immigrants or refugees from various areas who are seeking health care. This can present a unique challenge for health care providers. An immigrant or refugee has most probably faced many challenges to arrive at the current life situation. There may have been turmoil in the country of origin, loss of loved ones through death or separation, language barriers, and countless other struggles. Living in a new area will often leave such a person feeling isolated within a culture where everything seems new and strange. This feeling of isolation and loneliness may be exacerbated when facing one's own death or the death of a loved one (Kemp, 2005).

As a nurse, there are very practical things that may be done to help to alleviate the discomfort that is being experienced. Of prime importance is the ability to communicate with the patient and family. Patients and families who are unable to communicate in the language of their health care providers often experience additional stress, fear, or anxiety (Garrett et al., 2008). A nurse who is able to speak a few words of the patient's language is thus greatly appreciated. Even a rudimentary knowledge of the language conveys the message that the nurse values the people being served and wants to communicate with them. Unless one is fluent in the language, however, an expert interpreter should be sought. Most health care institutions have access to interpreters who speak the predominant languages of the area. If an interpreter is physically unavailable, a telephone interpretation service may be used. This may be less than ideal, as the nuances of the nonverbal communication may be missed, but should be considered if there are no other options available.

It should also be remembered that a patient or family member may nod and smile in response to a verbal message, but may not understand the message at all. Nodding may be done as a sign of respect or politeness, but may not indicate even partial understanding (Crawley et al., 2002).

Often a family member is selected to be the interpreter. This must be evaluated on a case-by-case basis. It must be verified that the family member is fluent in English and that the interpretation is not delivering a distorted message to the patient. Family members sometimes want to withhold negative findings in an attempt to protect the patient. It is therefore recommended to employ a professional interpreter for at least the first two or three visits to be sure that the family member is receiving valid information. It may also be unwise to have a young child as the interpreter. Frequently a child of 10 or 11 will be fluent in English due to school involvement. It may place an undue burden on the child, however, to be asked to interpret for a family member when the child may already be emotionally challenged related to the impending loss of a loved one.

Documentation related to communication and interpretation is especially important. The fact that the patient and family understand health care information, and that they are understood by health care personnel, must not be left in question. If a friend or family member is asked to interpret, there must also be adequate documentation that the patient has agreed to this arrangement. Such documentation alleviates any concerns about divulging confidential health information regarding the patient.

Another issue that may be a source of controversy is pain management. (Please refer to Chapter 4 for additional information about pain management at the end of life.) In some cultures, suffering pain may be viewed as a purifying process, a punishment for past sins, or a way of exhibiting strength within tribulation (Kemp, 2005). A nurse whose goal is to reduce pain may be conflicted about allowing a patient to suffer. In such a situation, communication with the patient and family is especially important. Patient involvement in development of the plan of care is also essential at such times, as the goals must be patient-centered rather than nurse-centered. Careful documentation related to pain management is equally essential.

Desired care of the body immediately after death is another area that varies from one culture to the next. Some families desire to be involved in washing the body, some want to place special articles or cloths on the body, and some request special positioning of the body. Some families may desire to sit with the body for an extended period of time, or they may want to bring the body home prior to the funeral ritual. Open communication with the family is of prime importance as the end of life approaches. There must be communication of family desires as well as discussion related to legal issues and institutional policies. A meeting of the minds prior to the time of death will often bring some degree of comfort immediately prior to and following the end of life.

SECTION ONE REVIEW

1. What is the nurse's role in providing care for patients from a culture that is unfamiliar? (Select all that apply.)
   1. The nurse should provide for a way of communication with the patient and family.
   2. Appropriate resource people (such as interpreters) should be sought to participate in the care of the patient.
   3. A sincere attempt should be made by the nurse to gain knowledge related to the culture, thereby facilitating understanding.
   4. The burden lies with the patient and family to thoroughly explain their cultural practices and preferences.

2. How is cultural competence gained?
   1. By reading about a culture, a nurse will know how to care for anyone from that culture.
   2. A nurse becomes culturally competent by remaining completely open-minded, letting go of personal beliefs and opinions.
   3. The culturally competent nurse is sensitive to the needs of individual clients and their families, is involved with culturally diverse populations, and attempts to learn about the cultures with which there is frequent contact.
   4. The best way to develop cultural competence is to watch a variety of documentaries about other countries.
3. How should a nurse be sure that the non-English-speaking patient has understood instructions related to medication?
   1. Explain the medication directions with pictures and hand gestures.
   2. Looking for affirmation from the patient such as nodding.
   3. Provide for an expert interpreter when explaining medications and receiving verbal feedback from the patient.
   4. Ask the patient's school-age child if the patient has any questions.

4. What is the nurse's role in providing culturally competent care? (Select all that apply.)
   1. Advocate
   2. Facilitator
   3. Resource person
   4. This is not within the nurse's scope
5. The family has requested to sit at the bedside of the hospitalized patient who has just passed away, as is their cultural tradition. They say that it will take two or three hours for the spirit to leave the room, and they wish to stay for that time. You have received a call saying that another patient is waiting to move into the not-yet-vacated bed. What should you do?
   1. Move the patient's body to a quiet area at the end of the hall, where the family can sit for as long as they like.
   2. Tell the family that they may stay for 30–40 minutes, but then you will have to ask them to leave.
   3. Explore other possibilities for finding a bed for the incoming patient.
   4. Explain that the patient won't know that they are there anyway, and it would be better for them to gather at home, where they can be more comfortable.

SECTION TWO: Spiritual Care at End of Life

Often going hand in hand with cultural issues, spiritual care is another important aspect of nursing care at the end of life. In order to address the needs of the patient and family, there are several issues that must be considered. First, a nurse must have self-awareness of personal values and beliefs. Second, the nurse must have a solid understanding of spirituality, and third, the nurse must be able to identify boundaries. It is not up to the nurse to be the sole provider of spiritual care, but rather to be a part of the team that provides for the needs of the patient and family.

Self-Awareness

Providing care for the whole person is an important aspect of nursing care, especially at the end of life. Meeting spiritual needs may be challenging, as spiritual issues often become more important as the end of life nears (Hermann, 2007). Since the nurse often spends more time with the patient than other members of the health care team do, there are prime opportunities to assess and address spiritual needs as they arise.

Identifying spiritual needs in others, however, may be difficult for nurses who do not have a clear picture of their own system of values, attitudes, and beliefs (Puchalski & Romer, 2000). The spiritual care provided to a patient will be affected by

lack of spiritual congruence within the nurse providing that care (Taylor, 1998). Nurses seeking to provide spiritual intervention for others should spend time defining their own spirituality. Becoming comfortable with one's own spirituality is the first step in increasing sensitivity to spirituality issues in others (Mitchell, Bennett, & Manfrin-Ledet, 2006).

Spirituality

Spirituality is defined as "that which allows a person to experience transcendent meaning in life" (Puchalski & Romer, 2000, p. 129). It may also be defined as an energy force within the human core that seeks to return to and commune with the God source from which it came (Neuman & Fawcett, 2002). Spirituality is often defined in broad terminology, since it can have a different meaning for each person. For example, one person's spirituality may center around a relationship with a supreme being, while another person may derive meaning in life from nature, family relationships, or any number of other life interests. Research related to people experiencing significant illness has shown that it is the patient's own spirituality that has proven to be the most powerful influence on coping ability (Narayanasamy, 2003).

Although there may be a relationship, it is important not to identify religiosity as spirituality. Religiosity, or religiousness, is typically related to the practice of traditions or beliefs, and it may flow from spirituality (Hodge, 2001). A person, however, may have a formal involvement with a specific **religion,** yet may not derive spiritual benefit from the traditions associated with it. It therefore becomes vital that nursing assessment include information that goes far beyond the question of religion or denominational involvement. Since health care professionals seek to build on the patient's strengths in order to enhance the helping process (Hodge, 2001), it is crucial to identify both positives and negatives in the spiritual realm. Baldree, Murphy, and Powers (1982) reported that, for patients who were facing a significant health crisis, formal religion, hope, prayer, and faith were important sources of strength and support.

There have been many instruments developed to assist nurses with spiritual assessment. Some are as simple as asking a few open-ended questions, while others involve more formal surveys and rating scales. It is believed that use of qualitative assessment methods, such as open-ended questions, contributes important information to the spiritual assessment (Hodge, 2001). Use of quantitative methods alone may allow vital information to be missed. The important thing is that each nurse finds a way of assessment that is easy to use and provides meaningful information. It is in learning about the patient's spiritual foundation that the nurse becomes able to identify and provide intervention for spiritual needs.

Two of the available assessment methods that have been found helpful in nursing assessment of spirituality are the SPIRIT model and the FICA model. The SPIRIT model (Maugans, 1996) prompts the nurse to investigate the areas related to spirituality depicted in Box 10–1.

The FICA Model (Puchalski & Romer, 2000) includes the areas depicted in Box 10–2.

Whatever method is used to assess spirituality, it is recommended that the nurse first do a self-assessment using the chosen

---

BOX 10–1   The SPIRIT Model

S – Spiritual belief system, including involvement in formal religious groups

P – Personal spirituality, including values and practices that are meaningful to the individual

I – Integration/Involvement with people who share common beliefs

R – Ritualized practices/restrictions (what the patient should or should not do)

I – Implications for health care (what may be encouraged or restricted)

T – Terminal events planning (what decisions have been made related to end of life, including existence of formal documents such as a living will)

Source: Maugans, 1996

BOX 10–2   The FICA Model

F – Faith/Beliefs (What does the patient consider to be meaningful?)

I – Importance/Influence (What personal significance does the patient's belief system have, how does it affect the patient in dealing with life circumstances?)

C – Community (What is the patient's support system, such as family, friends, worship community?)

A – Address (How can the health care team best address issues related to spirituality?)

Source: Puchalski & Romer, 2000

---

model. This helps to facilitate understanding of patients' responses. As the nurse becomes more comfortable doing spiritual assessments, the process often becomes less formalized and the nurse adapts and individualizes assessment techniques to meet the needs of the specific situation.

Identifying Boundaries

A nurse need not be solely responsible for meeting the needs of the patient and family at end of life. There will be many opportunities for identifying and meeting spiritual needs, but it should be anticipated that there will be occasions when it is necessary to provide referrals for spiritual assistance. For example, the patient may be a devoted follower of a religion that is unfamiliar to the nurse. Although there may be much spiritual strength that could be derived from practicing specific rituals, the nurse may not be able to provide what is needed for the patient in that situation. The nurse should take advantage of opportunities to involve, with the patient's permission, other resource people. There may be another member of the health care team who shares a similar belief system or a religious leader who may be consulted. It may be that the most therapeutic intervention would be to allow the family a time of privacy to practice sacred rituals.

Challenges and Opportunities in Spiritual Care

The more opportunities to practice spiritual assessment and care, the more comfortable the nurse will become. There are still students who graduate from nursing programs without having acquired basic knowledge related to providing nursing care at the end of life (Brajtman, Fothergill-Bourbonnais, Casey, Alain, & Fiset, 2007), yet building spiritual competence is an essential element in providing end-of-life nursing care (Mitchell et al., 2006). When starting out in a nursing position that involves end-of-life care, there will be much to learn, but spiritual care should be viewed as a priority no matter what the patient's situation may be.

A patient's spiritual assessment may reveal signs of negative religious coping, which may present greater challenges as the end of life approaches (Hills, Paice, Cameron, & Shott, 2005). For example, the patient may express a belief that illness is a punishment for misdeeds or that God no longer cares. A nurse should take advantage of opportunities to discuss the beliefs held by the patient, and should also explore positive experiences from the past. A nurse who is an active listener is greatly appreciated, but the services of the patient's spiritual leader or the facility chaplain may also be extremely valuable in such situations.

There may also be spiritual needs that need to be addressed in order to facilitate spiritual well-being. Forgiveness, for example, may be a need that arises. The patient may believe that forgiveness by God is necessary for entrance into heaven, or there may be a broken relationship for which the patient seeks forgiveness. Assisting the patient to explore the avenues to find reconciliation through forgiveness may be an important nursing intervention, helping the patient to find peace and restoration (Laukhuf & Werner, 1998).

Some patients may also deny that they have any spiritual interests. This may be challenging to the nurse who wishes to provide spiritual care. A brief spiritual assessment provides clues to the patient's spirituality. For example, asking questions related to how the patient finds meaning and purpose in life may help to grant insight into areas that the patient had not previously considered. A person who has not considered the meaning and significance of living may find it difficult to find meaning or purpose in dying (Mazanec & Tyler, 2003).

There may be times when the nurse struggles to find the right words to say. A nurse who has gained perspective related to the patient's spirituality develops a deeper relationship with the patient (Puchalski & Romer, 2000). Silence should not be uncomfortable when it is the nurse's presence that is providing strength for the spirit. A nurse's touch on the hand or a cool cloth on the brow may be as spiritually meaningful as a religious ritual.

Prayer and Religious Rituals

In conjunction with spirituality, religious rituals such as prayer have been widely studied. Defined as intimate conversation between a person and God (Shelly & Fish, 1995), **prayer** has proven to be a source of strength for patients and caregivers alike, particularly at the end of life. One study found that the results of private prayer during a time of health care crisis were long-lasting, and resulted in decreased incidence of depression even a year later (Ai, Dunkle, Peterson, & Bolling, 1998). Such long-term effects of prayer have great implications for those who are facing end-of-life issues.

Prayer has been identified as a nursing intervention that can provide a significant source of strength for patients, helping to provide them with both comfort and increased coping ability (Taylor, 2003; Taylor and Outlaw, 2002; Winslow & Winslow, 2003). Although prayer may add great depth to the nurse-patient relationship, however, it must be practiced with discretion, keeping in mind the needs of patient and nurse alike.

In addition to prayer, it is also appropriate for the nurse to offer the resources needed to assist patients to attend church services, spiritual support groups, or other resources that may contribute to strengthening of the spirit (Kantor & Houldin, 1999; Taylor, 2000). If unable to attend in person, patients and caregivers alike may be helped to cope by having opportunity to participate in watching religious services on television, reading or listening to Scripture, or practicing rituals such as communion (Theis, Diordi, Coeling, Nalepka, & Miller, 2003).

The importance of traditional religious rituals should not be downplayed. Practices such as prayer, anointing, and reading sacred literature may be a source of strength and encouragement to the patient. Even if a patient has not been involved in organized religion for many years, often religious traditions will be increasingly important as the time of death approaches (Mazanec & Tyler, 2003). To the greatest extent possible, opportunities should be allowed for the patient who desires to practice religious rituals.

Religious rituals may also be a key factor in assisting the family to cope at the time of death and immediately thereafter. In the case of an infant's death, for example, Christian baptism may be very important to the family. This may be performed by the pastor or chaplain, but often death will be approaching before there is time for the clergy to arrive. Christian baptism may be performed by any Christian in this situation, and it is often the nurse who will be asked by the family to perform the baptism. It is recommended that an outline of a baptism ceremony, along with a baptismal bowl, be kept available in areas such as neonatal intensive care units.

In summary, nursing has a tremendous opportunity to provide for the patient's spiritual needs at end of life. Spirituality, which can affect all other aspects of a patient's life (Hills et al., 2005), must remain a priority in planning end-of-life care. Unmet needs in this area may result in spiritual distress and negative outcomes, while building on identified strengths will promote spiritual well-being.

SECTION TWO REVIEW

1. A terminally ill patient is nearing death. Upon admission, the patient denied any spiritual or religious practices and stated that he did not believe in any "higher power." Today the patient is asking the nurse to send the chaplain to visit. The nurse understands that the reason for this request is likely which of the following?
   1. Spiritual issues become more important as the end of life nears.

2. The patient was not honest with his responses upon admission.
3. He believes that the chaplain may save his life.
4. The patient is not happy with the lack of spiritual care the nurse has provided.

2. A new nurse has started a position on an inpatient Hospice Unit. The precepting nurse realizes the best way to facilitate the new nurse's understanding of her own personal spiritual beliefs and values is to:
   1. Assign her to a patient with particularly challenging spiritual needs.
   2. Have her complete a spiritual assessment on her own beliefs.
   3. Arrange for her to present an in-service on spiritual care.
   4. Request that she visit various churches around the community.

3. What are rationales for a nurse supporting prayer practice with a patient at the end of life? Prayer: (Select all that apply.)
   1. Supports the holistic approach to patient care.
   2. Is a source of strength for patients.
   3. Is a means of coping for patients in stressful situations.
   4. Is a right of the patient.

4. A dying patient expresses the desire to speak with a religious leader in order to seek forgiveness for "something terrible" she did. What is the most appropriate response by the nurse?
   1. "Would you like for me to call the chaplain here at the hospital, or is there someone in the community you would like us to contact?"

2. "There is nothing so terrible that you could have done to wish to speak with the chaplain at this time in your life."
3. "Wouldn't you rather spend your time with your family and friends? I am sure that they forgive you."
4. "Our chaplain is very busy in the Emergency Room right now. Would you like to talk with me or the social worker?"

5. A terminally ill patient, likely experiencing her last days, tells the nurse that she usually attends a ladies prayer group from her church on Monday nights. She finds this to be a great source of comfort, spiritually uplifting, and social support. She says that the group was going to travel 50 miles to the hospital to visit her this Monday to hold the prayer group, but the weather has made travel that far prohibitive. She says that members of the group who are able to travel to the church were going to meet and that she wishes she could be there for what may be her last opportunity to do so. What is the nurse's best response?
   1. "Surely they will arrange to come here next week. In the meantime, I can ask our chaplain to stop by."
   2. "Would you like me to call and ask them to visit once the weather clears up?"
   3. "If they wanted to be here, they could make the trip. It is a shame they did not realize how much you enjoy the group."
   4. "This sounds very important to you. Let's see if we can arrange a conference call, so that you can participate in the prayer group."

Case Study 1

Gerald Crenshaw, 54 years old, is a man with developmental disabilities who was diagnosed with male breast cancer two years ago. An axillary lymph node dissection at the time of his mastectomy revealed that he had 12 positive nodes. Further testing identified metastasis to the liver. He lives alone with his elderly mother in a rural area. Earlier this evening, she found him unresponsive and she called an ambulance to bring him into the hospital. He has a do-not-resuscitate order. His vital signs are stable, and his mother decides to go home for the night, as she is very tired. Before she leaves, you notice that she is running her hands around the side rail of the bed. When you ask if you can help her, she states, "No, that's okay," and begins walking toward the door. You ask again if there is anything that she needs, to which she replies, "I was just going to kiss him good-night and say prayers like we do every night, but the bed is so high."

Question

What is the most practical way to provide spiritual care in this situation?

Suggested Response

As the nurse, you state that a good-night kiss and prayer are very meaningful to both of them and should not be overlooked. The bed is as low as it can go, but you lower the side rail, find a low footstool on which she can stand, and hold her arm as you assist her to reach her son's face. She kisses his cheek, says a prayer as she puts her hand on his forehead, and then you assist her back down from the stool. With tears in her eyes, she thanks you and leaves for home. When you come to check on Gerald during the night, you find that he has died. You feel pleased that the spiritual care you provided ensured that Gerald did not leave the world without one last good-night kiss and prayer from his mother.

CHAPTER SUMMARY

- As an integral part of the health care team, nursing professionals have taken a leading role in the promotion of culturally competent care, understanding that a critical step is self-assessment.
- A culturally competent person has a self-awareness of values, opinions, and beliefs that have developed from one's own culture.
- Patients and families from diverse cultures may have very different views of dying, resulting in the health care team misunderstanding the importance and relevance of aspects of the dying process.
- The decision-making process related to end-of-life issues may also present a challenge for nurses, as there are cultures in which tradition would dictate that decisions be made by a family leader, or by consensus, rather than by the patient alone.
- When caring for the patient from a culture with which the nurse is unfamiliar, it is especially imperative that the nurse keep an open line of communication with the patient and the family leaders, maintaining an open mind and an attitude of respect for others.

- A nurse who is familiar with cultural rituals, beliefs, and traditions will be a source of great comfort to the family.
- Though a patient or family member may nod and smile in response to a verbal message, nodding may be done as a sign of respect or politeness, but may not indicate even partial understanding.
- Providing care for the whole person includes meeting spiritual needs, as spiritual issues often become more important as the end of life nears.
- Although there may be a relationship, it is important not to identify religiosity as spirituality.
- Two assessment methods that assist nurses in the assessment of spirituality are the SPIRIT model and the FICA model.
- The more opportunities to practice spiritual assessment and care, the more comfortable the nurse will become.
- Religious rituals may also be a key factor in assisting the family to cope at the time of death and immediately thereafter.

CHAPTER REVIEW

Jennifer Vecci is a 31-year-old hospice patient who has a diagnosis of end-stage renal disease. She has decided to stop her treatments and "allow nature to take its course." She states that she just wants to die quietly at home, that she has made peace with God, and that she just wants to be "kept comfortable." She is not expected to live more than a few more days. She has no children and her husband was killed in an accident four years ago. She states that her mother-in-law is her only relative, but that she hesitates to have her visit, as she becomes very emotional and tries to convince Jennifer to participate in things that are of no interest to her. Her mother-in-law, an elderly Italian woman, contacts the nurse and insists that the priest be called, as she wants Jennifer to receive the Anointing of the Sick before she dies. She states that she wants to be with Jennifer and care for her.

Question

As a nurse, how can you address the cultural and spiritual issues that have arisen?

Suggested Response

Both Jennifer and her mother-in-law are alone. They would like to spend these last few days together, but Jennifer does not want to deal with the aggravation of her mother-in-law's demands. As a nurse, and with Jennifer's permission, you decide to have a family conference. Jennifer states that she would like to have her mother-in-law with her, but that she does not have the energy to argue with her. Jennifer's mother-in-law becomes tearful and states that she is worried about Jennifer's spiritual well-being, since she is not following the traditions with which she was raised. At the end of the conference, there is agreement that Jennifer's mother-in-law will be allowed to be with her, but that she will not make demands of her. Jennifer agrees that her mother-in-law will go to the church every day to pray for her, and agrees to having a rosary placed on her bedside table. Everyone seems pleased with the compromise that has been reached. Jennifer dies peacefully three days later as her mother-in-law sits at her bedside and holds her hand.

REFERENCES

Ai, A., Dunkle, R., Peterson, C., & Bolling, S. (1998). The role of private prayer in psychological recovery among midlife and aged patients following cardiac surgery. *The Gerontologist, 38*(5), 591–602.

Baldree, K., Murphy, S., & Powers, M. (1982). Stress identification and coping patterns in patients on hemodialysis. *Nursing Research, (31)*, 107–110.

Brajtman, S., Fothergill-Bourbonnais, F., Casey, A., Alain, D., & Fiset, V. (2007). Providing direction for change: Assessing Canadian nursing students' learning needs. *International Journal of Palliative Nursing, 13*(5), 213–221.

Crawley, L., Marshall, P., Lo, B., & Koenig, B. (2002). Strategies for culturally effective end-of-life care. *Annals of Internal Medicine, 136*(9), 673–679.

Donnelly, G. (2003). Integrate holistic care one patient at a time. *Holistic Nursing Practice, 17*(2), 117.

Garrett, P., Dickson, H., Lis-Young, M., Whelan, A., & Roberto-Forero, C. (2008). What do non-English speaking patients value in acute care: Cultural competency from the patient's perspective: A qualitative study. *Ethnicity and Health, 13*(5), 479–496.

Giger, J., Davidhizar, R., & Fordham, P. (2006). Multi-cultural and multi-ethnic considerations and advanced directives: Developing cultural competency. *Journal of Cultural Diversity, 13*(1), 3–9.

Hermann, C. (2007). The degree to which spiritual needs of patients near the end of life are met. *Oncology Nursing Forum, 34*(1), 70–78.

Hills, J., Paice, J., Cameron, J., & Shott, S. (2005). Spirituality and distress in palliative care consultation. *Journal of Palliative Medicine, 8*(4), 782–787.

Hodge, D. (2001). Spiritual assessment: A review of major qualitative methods and a new framework for assessing spirituality. *Social Work, 46*(3), 203–214.

Kantor, D., & Houldin, A. (1999). Breast cancer in older women: Treatment, psychosocial effects, interventions, and outcomes. *Journal of Gerontological Nursing, 25*(7), 19–28.

Kemp, C. (2005). Cultural issues in palliative care. *Seminars in Oncology Nursing, 21*(1), 44–52.

Laukhuf, G., & Werner, H. (1998). Spirituality: The missing link. *Journal of Neuroscience Nursing, 30*(1), 60–68.

Maugans, T. (1996). The SPIRITual history. *Archives of Family Medicine, 5*(1), 11–16.

Mazanec, P., & Tyler, M. (2003). Cultural considerations in end-of-life care. *American Journal of Nursing, 103*(3), 50–59.

Mitchell, D., Bennett, M., & Manfrin-Ledet, L. (2006). Spiritual development of nursing students: Developing competence to provide spiritual care to patients at the end of life. *Journal of Nursing Education, 45*(9), 365–370.

Momeni, P., Jirwe, M., & Emami, A. (2008). Enabling nursing students to become culturally competent—A documentary analysis of curricula in all Swedish nursing programs. *Scandinavian Journal of Caring Sciences, 22,* 499–506.

Murray, S., Grant, E., Grant, A., & Kendall, M. (2003). Dying from cancer in developed and developing countries: Lessons from two qualitative interview studies of patients and their careers. *British Medical Journal, 326*(7385), 368–378.

Narayanasamy, A. (2003). Spiritual coping mechanisms in chronically ill patients. *British Journal of Nursing, 11*(22), 1461–1470.

Neuman, B., & Fawcett, J. (2002). The Neuman systems model. Upper Saddle River, NJ: Prentice-Hall.

Puchalski, C., & Romer, A. (2000). Taking a spiritual history allows clinicians to understand patients more fully. *Journal of Palliative Medicine, 3*(1), 129–137.

Saha, S., Beach, M., & Cooper, L. (2008). Patient centeredness, cultural competence, and healthcare quality. *Journal of the National Medical Association, 100*(11), 1275–1285.

Shelly, J., & Fish, S. (1995). Praying with patients. *Journal of Christian Nursing, 12,* 9–13.

Taylor, E. (2003). Prayer's clinical issues and implications. *Holistic Nursing Practice, 17*(4), 179–189.

Taylor, E. (1998). Spirituality and the cancer experience. In R. Carroll-Johnson, L. Gorman, & N. Bush (Eds.) *Psychosocial nursing care: Along the cancer continuum.* Pittsburgh, PA: Oncology Nursing Press.

Taylor, E., & Outlaw, F. (2002). Use of prayer among persons with cancer. *Holistic Nursing Practice, 16*(3), 46–61.

Theis, S., Diordi, D., Coeling, H., Nalepka, C., & Miller, B. (2003). Spirituality in caregiving and care receiving. *Holistic Nursing Practice, 17*(1), 48–56.

Vergara, R., Lynch-Powers, B., Verhaeghe, L., & Hynes, P. (2006). End-of-life care in a multicultural society. *Dynamics of Critical Care 2006, 17*(2), 44–45.

Winslow, G., & Winslow, B. (2003). Examining the ethics of praying with patients. *Holistic Nursing Practice, 17*(4), 170–179.

Caring for the Caregiver

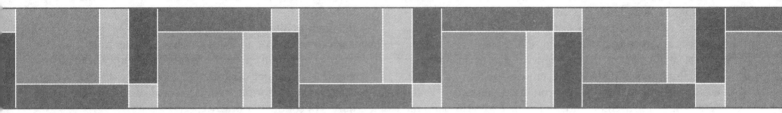

11.1. Differentiate between an informal and formal caregiver's needs.

11.2. Examine the economics of caregiving in America today.

11.3. Describe the impact of caregiving on the patient and caregiver.

11.4. Compare and contrast caregiver burnout with compassion fatigue.

This chapter introduces the roles of the informal and formal caregiver, differentiating the characteristics and needs for these caregivers as they assist persons at the end of life. The economic impact of caregiving in the United States is explored as is the impact of caregiving from both the patient's and caregiver's perspectives. The chapter concludes a discussion that compares and contrasts the concepts of caregiver burnout and compassion fatigue.

PRETEST

1. Most people with functional disabilities prefer to live as independently as possible with the care of:
   1. Nurses at home.
   2. Nurses in the hospital.
   3. Someone who knows them well.
   4. Their best friend.
2. More patients are being cared for in their homes and communities because:
   1. It is better financially for everyone.
   2. That is where they wish to continue to live.
   3. The desired and preferred caregiver is always a family member.
   4. Nursing homes are too crowded.
3. Being a nurse caregiver is a lifelong process. It involves integrating and balancing multiple dimensions of wellness, self-care, and:
   1. Professional growth.
   2. Confidentiality.
   3. Personal boundaries.
   4. Personal agenda.
4. The symptoms of caregiver burnout are similar to the symptoms of stress and:
   1. Agitation.
   2. Anxiety.
   3. Depression.
   4. Dementia.
5. Compassion fatigue may lead to work performance changes. There may be a: (Select all that apply.)
   1. Sense of hopelessness.
   2. Loss of purpose and anger toward God.
   3. Problem with sleep.
   4. Newly developed appreciation for the profession.

GLOSSARY

altruism   Selfless concern for the welfare of others.

caregiver   Person who attends to the holistic needs of a patient.

caregiver burnout   A psychological state of physical and emotional exhaustion thought to be a stress reaction to a reduced ability to meet the demands of one's occupation; symptoms include fatigue, insomnia, impaired work performance, and an increased susceptibility to physical illness and substance abuse.

care recipient   A person of any age who, due to an illness or disability, is unable to independently care for him- or herself.

compassion fatigue   Describes the condition that occurs as the stress of caring becomes more intensified over time and the caregiver becomes physically, mentally, and/or emotionally exhausted; sometimes called secondary traumatic stress disorder.

cumulative loss   The succession of individual deaths experienced by nurses with patients having life-threatening illnesses.

family caregiver   Any relative, partner, friend, or neighbor who has a significant personal relationship with the patient or family and provides a broad range of assistance.

formal caregiver   Encompasses the support and guidance provided by health and social service professionals, including physicians, nurses, social workers, and other members of the interdisciplinary health care team.

informal caregiver   An individual who provides care and/or support to a family member, friend, or neighbor, who has a physical or mental disability, is chronically ill or is frail; often having no formal training, they are not accountable to norms of conduct or practice.

sacred   Worthy of respect, highly valued and important, devoted exclusively to one service or use.

self-care   Care of self on all levels: physical, social, emotional, psychological, and spiritual.

SECTION ONE: Caregiving and the Informal Caregiver

Caregiving is the act of providing holistic assistance to someone who has an illness, including a terminal illness, or disability (cognitive, physical, or behavioral) and who is unable to adequately care for himself or herself. Most people who require caregiving assistance prefer to live as independently as possible while being provided this required assistance by someone who knows them well. Assistance that the **caregiver** provides may consist of supervision, direct provision of care, emotional support, maintenance of a safe environment, and/or coordination of care from the multiple caregivers who are needed for continuous care. The assistance may extend on a short- or long-term basis and can be provided by formal and/or informal caregivers.

Informal caregiving is an integral part of the United States health care system. The expectation that individuals care for each other has existed throughout much of history. In many cultures and societies, ill or disabled persons have been encouraged to care for themselves or designate a family member as custodian (Phillips & Crist, 2008). The vast majority of care is supplied by **informal caregivers,** who are family members or friends and who offer unpaid assistance for the physical and emotional needs of a loved one, ranging from partial assistance to 24-hour care. For example, high school–age students may be involved in driving grandparents to medical appointments or may assist a grandparent with shopping activities. Generally, these informal caregivers have had no formal training (American Nurses Association [ANA], 1995).

Informal caregivers often provide extraordinary, uncompensated care, primarily in the home setting, that may involve significant amounts of time and energy for months or even years. They are required to perform tasks that may be physically, emotionally, socially, or financially demanding (National Institute of Nursing Research [NINR], 2002). These individuals who care for family members fulfill an important role not only for the care recipient but for society as a whole.

There has been a societal shift away from institutional care, with increasingly more individuals receiving needed care in their homes and communities (End of Life Nursing Consortium [ELNEC], 2008). Family caregiving to an elderly parent when he or she is ill or disabled is expected in virtually all cultures of the world and is generally accepted as the norm in most developing countries. Usually this **family caregiver** is a spouse, adult child, or other relative of the care recipient such as sibling, niece, nephew, or grandchild. There is an increased demand for family caregiving with the increasing aging and frail population (NINR, 2002). Many Americans will be informal caregivers at some point during their lives and may provide informal care to more than one care recipient at various ages.

Caregivers play a critical role in keeping patients at home and out of institutions, both in acute care and long-term care (Roth, Haley, Wadley, Clay, & Howard, 2007). Frequently an adult child will balance work and family responsibilities while providing care of an aging parent, or a spouse will provide care for a loved one while struggling with his or her own chronic conditions. As the caregiving assistance increases, there is a progression from intermittent need or occasional chores to around-the-clock care. Eventually, demands on the caregiver become equivalent to having full-time employment. Thus, caregiving transitions to becoming an unpaid career with different stages, transitions, and stresses (Center on Aging, 2004).

Caregiving Population

Advances in medicine and nutrition have enabled individuals to live longer. However, living longer increases the risk of debilitating disease and the potential need for technical means to survive. The primary illnesses or conditions experienced by care recipients are usually described as age related, mobility problems, dementia, and various chronic diseases, including heart disease, cancer, stroke, arthritis, diabetes, and pulmonary disease. Functional disability also increases with age. Nearly three quarters of adults age 65 years and older have one or more chronic illnesses, and nearly half report two or more. Many chronic diseases are debilitating and may have a harmful effect on **self-care** functioning, requiring informal caregiving (National Family Caregivers Association [NFCA], 2004).

The greatest numbers of caregivers are estimated to be those caring for individuals with dementia and Alzheimer's disease (AD), which may or may not accompany concomitant diagnoses of end-of-life diseases and conditions. Approximately 5.2 million Americans are living with AD (Alzheimer's Association, 2008). The caregiving required for these individuals generally is intense, requiring assistance with activities of daily living (ADLS), incontinence, feeding, and transfer or use of a wheelchair or walker. The majority of AD caregivers are seniors. These caregivers are twice as likely to report physical strain and high levels of emotional distress from caregiving responsibilities. They are more likely to report family conflict, to spend less time with other family members, and to give up vacations, hobbies, and other personal activities. There is a high level of financial strain present for these caregivers as well (Vellone, Piras, Talucci, & Cohen, 2008).

Technological caregiving in the home is becoming more common. Examples of technology use for **care recipients** of all ages include kidney dialysis, intravenous lines, electronic monitoring, nutritional tube feedings, and ventilators. Care recipients who are technology-dependent may need continuous supervision, care, and monitoring. The success of informal technological caregiving is related to caregiver and care recipient abilities to share responsibilities, to understand tasks, and to coordinate efforts with multiple health care professionals. The use of technology in informal caregiving remains a major problem for caregivers and care recipients as technological advances become more common and more sophisticated (NINR, 2002).

More than 22.4 million informal and family caregivers provide care for a chronically ill, disabled, or aged family member or friend annually (Scott, 2006). People at all stages of life give and receive informal care. The majority of informal caregiving is provided by women, with current estimates that 61% of caregivers are women between the ages of 50 and 64 years of age. Additionally, the most common informal caregiving relationship is that of parent and child, with next category of caregiver relationship that of a spouse (Scott, 2006). Fortunately, trend data continues to show that most informal caregivers are not the sole caregiver (National Alliance for Caregiving and AARP, 2004; Takamura & Williams, 2000).

Though family and informal caregivers provide more than 80% of the long-term care required by elders (Bull & McShane, 2008), demographic trends have affected the availability of family caregivers. These demographic trends include higher divorce rates, lower birth rates, a highly mobile society, and an increased number of individuals living alone (Roth et al., 2007). These trends coincide with families who may desire to provide care for their loved one, but are unable to do so because of strained relationships, distance from the individual requiring care, or other responsibilities that prevent them from assuming this role. Despite problems associated with caregiving, the greatest gift that families report is being able to provide care to loved ones when they are terminally ill (Shugarman, Lorenz, Lynn, & Mularski, 2005).

Economics of Caregiving

Family caregivers comprise 13% of the workforce nationally. Over 50% of family caregivers who care for someone over the age of 18 either work or have been employed while providing care. Approximately 14.4 million employed caregivers balance outside work with caregiving. Cost of caregiving in lost productivity exceeds $11.4 billion (NAC and AARP, 2004).

While the majority of informal caregivers are employed, many of them have had to make significant adjustments to their work life, including reporting late to work or accepting part-time employment, at least temporarily. Some have been forced to resign from outside employment entirely. Informal caregiving cost estimates range from $117 to $292 billion a year for adults with a disability or chronic disease, with higher costs occurring in those caregivers assisting individuals with Alzheimer's disease. In 2000, the typical working family caregiver lost over $100 a day in wages and health benefits to provide full-time care for a loved one at home (Arno, 2006; Family Caregiver Alliance, 2006). This loss of revenue has a direct impact on the informal caregiver, as well as on the community as a whole. Lost revenue may be even further complicated if the caregiver has health problems of his or her own.

Informal caregivers have median incomes that are lower than non-caregivers. The value of the services family caregivers provide for "free" is estimated to be $306 billion a year, which is almost twice as much as is actually spent on homecare and nursing home services combined (Arno, 2006).

The fastest growing age group in America is people over 85, who are the most frail and potentially need the most health care assistance. Over half of people over 85 years of age need some help with personal care. By 2050, there will be only four potential caregivers for each person needing care, compared to eleven in 1990 (NFCA, 2004). These staggering statistics demonstrate the impact on both the caregiver and society. The need for care recipients by statistics may exceed the number of caregivers available.

Impact of Caregiving

Patients continue to be concerned about the possibility that they will become a burden to their families, both from the perspective of physical strain and financial hardship. Most caregivers report significant financial hardship as a result of being a caregiver, as well as physical strain and emotional stress (Akkerman & Ostwald, 2004; Majerovitz, 2007; Martin-Cook, Remakel-Davis, Svetlik, Hynan, & Weinger, 2003). Many caregivers admit to having some physical or emotional health problems directly related to caregiving; others have one or more preexisting health problems themselves (Pinquart & Sorenson, 2003; Schulz & Sherwood, 2008). More women than men caregivers report emotional stress and impaired physical health. Several issues affecting caregivers' well-being include depression, concern for future care, and caregiver burden. Burden was related, in various studies, to level of patient disability and psychological distress (NAC and AARP, 2004). Caregiver depression was related to the relationship with the patient, more concern for future care, fewer social contacts, more physical symptoms in the caregiver, and stroke patient symptoms. Caregiver fatigue and sleep difficulties were found to be significantly greater for spousal caregivers of individuals with AD, Parkinson's disease, or cancer (Schulz & Sherwood, 2008).

Dysfunctional family dynamics, including aggressive or abusive behaviors, inhibit healthy partnerships between informal caregivers and their care recipients, other family members, and formal health care providers, while placing further strain on the caregivers' own health. Ethical dilemmas faced by family-member caregivers and how the caregivers respond to these dilemmas influence the outcomes of caregiving for the caregivers and recipients. Alleviating dilemmas helps reduce the burden experienced by non-caregiving children or other family members and enhances their level of participation in caregiving (McCorkle & Pasacreta, 2001; NINR, 2002).

Family caregivers experiencing extreme stress have been shown to age prematurely. This level of stress can take as much as 10 years off a family caregiver's life (Arno, 2006). Family caregivers report having a chronic condition at more than twice the rate of non-caregivers. Seeing a beloved family member or friend through a terminal illness is always difficult and stressful, and is often seen as anticipatory loss.

Caregiver Self-Awareness and Unmet Needs

One of the greatest challenges family caregivers face is taking care of themselves while providing care to another (ANA, 2002).

This requires a level of understanding and self-awareness, which is often missing, as caregivers tend to neglect their own health needs as they care for their loved ones. Family caregivers often report the act of helping their loved one with personal care contributed to their self-identification as caregivers. Their loved one's diagnosis and their interaction with the health care system made them aware that they were family caregivers (NFCA, 2001). Many family caregivers become more proactive about seeking resources and skills they need to assist care recipients after they have self-identified their own needs. This self-identification as a caregiver often leads to acceptance and seeing services to help them be better and more effective caregivers (Coleman, 2003).

The most frequently reported unmet needs of caregivers included finding time for themselves, managing emotional and physical stress, and balancing work and family responsibilities. Caregivers note that they need help keeping the care recipient safe and finding activities that can be done with the care recipient. Many caregivers also report needing help talking with physicians and other health care professionals or making end-of-life decisions (NAC and AARP, 2004). Other areas for concern of caregiving families include finding services and resources, financial and legal assistance, when to seek medical care, transportation needs, home safety, social needs, and end-of-life issues (Duke, Hoover, & Kaplan, 2004). Respite and support services are often indicated and required.

Care for the Informal Caregiver

When the care of the person is transferred to a professional nurse, it is important and imperative that these nurses acknowledge what informal caregivers have done despite problems they may have incurred in delivering care to the ill or disabled person (Navaie-Waliser, Spriggs, Bonnell, & Peng, 2002). Issues that the caregivers may have faced include time constraints, ensuring the appropriate use of finances, and emotional and physical burdens. Family and informal caregivers should be included in discussions when these discussions concern the individual for whom they have cared. They need to be given choices and control in tasks yet to be done.

Often nurses forget to ask about the health and welfare of the caregiver. Because family caregivers are a core part of the health care team, it is important to recognize, respect, assess, and address their needs. Family caregivers desire and should be provided information about the patient, especially about those services that they may continue to provide. It is helpful to provide education about the disease process, risks, benefits, and anticipated outcomes (ELNEC, 2008).

It is important that professionals, including nurses and other members of the health care team, continue to recognize that involvement of family members in determining ongoing caregiving needs for the person. Ongoing and accurate assessment related to the care of the individual are of prime importance to family caregivers (ANA, 2002; Gill, Kaur, Rummans, Novotny, &

Sloan, 2003). There will frequently be a time when family members need to consider alternative choices regarding the individual's continuing care needs. Alternative yet realistic choices regarding continuing care may include discussing code levels and/or cardiopulmonary resuscitation, implementation of artificial hydration and nutrition, or the transition of the individual to a skilled nursing facility or other more appropriate health care setting. Primary comfort care measures and palliative care may not have been previously discussed and are now the more appropriate measures to address.

Finally, the issues surrounding withholding or withdrawing treatment after days, weeks, or months of caregiving can be devastating for the family caregiver. Choices regarding the dying process can be overwhelming and emotionally draining for family caregivers. Often the family caregivers will need adequate time to assimilate all of the options and to fully understand the ramifications of each of the options before they are able to make final decisions.

Nurses need to support and educate family caregivers as they assume more of the nursing role (ANA, 1995). Physical cares such as bathing, transferring, oral care, foot and nail care, along with turning and repositioning are taught, and demonstrated. Family members learn toileting or diapering, administering medications from drops in eyes and nose to rectal suppositories and opioid infusions on those who once took care of them and who have been independent and in control for so long. Technical skills with medical devices and equipment are taught and demonstrated. Family members do bolus tube feedings, catheter cares, oxygen therapy and treatments, suctioning, wound and dressing changes and injections. They learn to run infusion pumps. These can be daunting tasks to perform.

Along with daily routine physical cares, family caregivers must manage symptoms, such as fatigue, pain and comfort needs, nausea, vomiting, cough, congestion, constipation, and diarrhea. Many informal caregivers have never dealt with incontinence or breathlessness. It is difficult for caregivers to see their loved ones anxious and restless; at the same time they understand that the medications could provide some comfort, and relief for these symptoms may cause sedation and less awareness (Mittelman, 2005). Loss of appetite is often difficult for family caregivers to manage with the emotional distress of feeling they are starving their loved one.

Other symptoms families must manage include depression and hopelessness, drowsiness and lethargy, seizures, decreased activity and falls, bedsores, and pressure ulcers. These are not easy conditions or symptoms to manage. Staying awake with patients when they have insomnia can wear on the caregiver on a daily basis. Agitation, confusion, and any cognitive impairment adds more stress to the family caregiver. Some of the most distressing symptoms caregivers found most difficult to manage were constipation, confusion, and anorexia (Newton, Bell, Lambert, & Fearing, 2002).

It is imperative to help the family caregiver to take things one day at time. Families are facing continuous change. Their family relationships and roles are in flux. They are caring not only for their loved one's bodily needs, but must tend to his or her emotional, social, legal, and financial needs as well. There are decisions to make. The family must cope with the upheaval of the patient's health status as it waxes and wanes. Communication and support is vital (Scott, 2006). The overall goal is to maintain balance.

Nurses can improve the knowledge and abilities of caregivers for symptom management, caregiving procedures/activities with one-on-one instruction and support. Nurses work in conjunction with social services in providing information on appropriate health care/social services assistance and how to access them (Weman & Fagerberg, 2006). These include caregiver support and respite services as well as home health or hospice services. Symptom and medication management, prevention of complications, preventive care, changes in care needs when conditions improve or worsen, and troublesome behaviors are all issues family caregivers need to have knowledge about.

Listening to and learning from the family caregiver regarding the family's needs are the first steps in education. Allowing effective communication with clarification of information assists families to learn how to care for their loved ones both in hospital or long-term care settings and at home. Empathy and sympathy are necessary parts of care. Nurses should provide education according to the family's level of understanding. This process, and allowing choices, makes a patient-centered partnership and provides humanistic palliative care. There is always care that can be provided for them and their loved one.

Support is continuously required for the family caregiver so that he or she does not feel alone or abandoned. These individuals are often tired and fatigued. They may fear overdosing, giving the last dose, or killing their loved one. Anxiety and grief are high for them as their loved one is declining, with fears of the unknown. End-of-life caregivers commonly reported problems such as sleep disturbances, providing care when they themselves were ill, and worry over leaving their loved one alone (Gansler, 2007). Accepting that the loved one is no longer going to recover or get well may help the family caregiver with comfort care needs. Always ensure that other staff members also know of the caregiver's needs. Respond quickly and sympathetically to any crisis situation. Often therapeutic presence for the family caregiver is as important as for the patient.

Education is needed for the family and caregivers as the patient's end of life nears. The dying process can be openly or privately discussed. An excellent resource is Barbara Karnes's (2005) *Gone From My Sight: The Dying Experience*. This booklet helps patients and families understand what may be expected in the final months, weeks, days, and hours of life that helps alleviate the fear of the unknown. Awareness of nearing death is another subject that helps family caregivers understand the process. Family caregivers often have questions and will talk either privately or openly about what is happening to their loved one. Helping families cope with the imminent death is yet another role of the nurse.

After the loss, practical matters are handled with the family caregiver. Nurses can support other family members as well, including any children, grandchildren, and pets. It is important to recognize the end-of-life and dying process as a family affair. The final gifts that can be brought to the caregiver's attention include: love, support, presence, quality of life, dignity, honor, and respect. Those gifts constitute a legacy that will be remembered always.

SECTION ONE REVIEW

1. Many times an adult child will balance work and family responsibilities while providing care of an aging parent. This balancing affects: (Select all that apply.)
   1. Employment.
   2. Finances.
   3. Career opportunities.
   4. Personal well-being.
2. Informal caregivers are twice as likely to report physical strain and high levels of emotional distress from caregiving responsibilities when caring for patients who have:
   1. CVA or strokes.
   2. Alzheimer's disease.
   3. End-stage renal disease.
   4. Cancer.
3. Over 50% of family caregivers who care for someone over the age of 18 either work or have worked while providing care. The estimated economic value of this "free" care is:
   1. Over $250 billion annually.
   2. Approximately $1 million annually.
   3. Less than $1 million annually.
   4. Approximately $500,000 annually.
4. Caregivers admit to having physical or emotional health problems directly related to caregiving. Caregivers reporting emotional stress and impaired physical health are more likely to be:
   1. Spouses than children.
   2. Children than spouses.
   3. Women than men.
   4. Men than women.
5. The most frequently reported unmet needs of caregivers included managing emotional and physical stress, balancing work and family responsibilities, and:
   1. Finding resources for finances.
   2. Finding time for themselves.
   3. Obtaining legal support.
   4. Obtaining transportation.

SECTION TWO: Care for the Professional Caregiver

Formal caregiving is described as the support and guidance provided by health and social service professionals (Hudson, Aranda, & McMurray, 2002). These professions help facilitate assistance as care needs intensify, including assistance with transportation, home care, homemaking services, medical management, personal care, and financial care (Emanuel, Fairclough, Slutsman, & Emanuel, 2000). Nurses are essential members of the formal caregiver team, ensuring that personal and self-care needs of the individual are being met as effectively as possible. Nurses also concern themselves with the care of the caregiver, integrating and balancing the multiple dimensions of confronting the caregiver as he or she provides the assistance to an ill or disabled person.

For individuals who receive caregiving needs in a variety of health care settings, nurses are the main caregivers—thus nurses must be aware of their own self-care needs. Providing care for the nurse is a lifelong process of integrating and balancing wellness, self-care, and professional growth. Providing care for terminally ill patients and their families at the end of life may increase nurses' stress and have a negative effect on the nurses' state of health. However, this experience can also be viewed more positively as a journey with patients through the final phases of that person's life (Byock, 1996; Byock 1997). The journey involves not only the patient, but the family caregiver, other family members, and members of the health care team and may become a process of personal development and deepening of an individual's search for the meaning of life.

Setting goals is a healthy way to balance the multiple dimensions of work, home, and play. Nurses need to set aside specific time for themselves on a daily, weekly, and monthly basis. Self-awareness, self-reflection, and self-monitoring are keys to self-care (Meier & Beresford, 2006). Professional caregivers can create a personal checklist to include work/play balance, coping skills, hobbies and recreational interests, balance of family/friends with work, play dates, pets, and other passions, including civic and religious affiliations (Cramer, McCorkle, Cherlin, Johnson-Hurzeler, & Bradley, 2003).

Often **sacred** and spiritual self-care needs become neglected. It is important to honor what is sacred in life, such as the ideas, belief, concepts, and images that evoke praise and devotion that speak to one's heart or spiritual self of what is good. Silence, music, beauty, nature, arts, gardening, animals, God or a belief system, and loved ones can all become appropriate sacred self-care values for individual caregivers (Holland & Neimeyer, 2005). Such values are important to avoid the pitfalls of caregiver burnout or compassion fatigue, concepts that are described in a later section of this chapter.

Nurses' self-care can be at risk when varying aspects of nursing strain the caregiving role. Boundary issues can be one of the negative aspects of professional caregiving, such as knowing the limitations of relationships with patients and family members. It is important to maintain professionalism with personal care, treating all patients equally and with respect. Ultimately, providing comfort and support, developing meaningful relationships with patients and their family members, providing education, and receiving positive feedback from patients and their families are the aspects of caring for terminally ill patients that give greatest satisfaction to nurses. Additional sources of satisfaction include commitment to the organization, supportive supervision, job involvement, and feelings of effectiveness (Demmer, 2004).

Other barriers to nurses' professional self-care include multiple roles, **altruism,** setting a personal agenda or stage in work and life, time constraints, and overscheduling life in general. Cumulative loss can be a heavy burden on the professional caregiver. **Cumulative loss** is the succession of individual deaths experienced by nurses who work with patients who have life-threatening illnesses. Losses can accumulate on a daily basis. Nurses may experience anticipatory and normal grief before and after the death of a patient. Loss is inevitable and often painful. Many times nurses do not have time to resolve the grief issues. Then there is symbolic loss, a feeling that security has been violated. Often the feeling of loss diminishes trust, as well as liberty and pursuing happiness and well-being. It is vital to manage these barriers to regain balance.

Several factors influence the adaptation of nurses in their professional role as a caregiver. Professional education and training is the first factor in this process. Nurses who work with patients at the end of their lives also have their own personal history with death. Life changes and the aging process put nurses at different levels of adaptation. And support systems, both formal and informal, will influence nurses' ability to adjust and adapt to the stages of health, dying, and death (Laird & Massey, 2006).

Balancing day-to-day care of patients is essential so that compassionate, quality care can be given to patients at the end of their lives with personal satisfaction to nurses working as professionals (Laird & Massey, 2006). Nurses can seek support systems within their work environment, formal and informal. Informal support is often given by the team members and staff within a short period of time after delivery of care. Formal support is usually found in set aside, preplanned gatherings, debriefings, or ceremonies. Having input and support from instructors and mentors is also very helpful for professional care. Nurses can also benefit professionally and personally from ongoing education in end-of-life care. Seeking support from spiritual counselors, chaplains, and pastors may be overlooked, but is advised. At times, it may be necessary to gain individual, facilitated support through professional counseling. Employers may have employee assistance programs that assist nurses with this needed counseling.

SECTION TWO REVIEW

1. Providing care for patients and their families in terminal conditions and at the end of their lives may increase the burden of nursing well-being; experiences during the final phases of a person's life may be called a:
   1. Dilemma.
   2. Trial.
   3. Journey.
   4. Rollercoaster.
2. Nurses need to set aside time for themselves on a daily, weekly, and monthly basis. One's own life plan should reflect aspects of physical, psychological, emotional, social/relationships, cultural, and:
   1. Medical well-being.
   2. Recreational well-being.
   3. Community well-being.
   4. Spiritual well-being.
3. Barriers to professional self-care include multiple roles, altruism, setting a personal agenda, stage in work and life, time constraints, and:
   1. Overscheduling life in general.
   2. Spending too much time with the patient's family discussing the patient.
   3. Working a second job.
   4. Reading journal articles on a patient's disease.
4. There are several factors that influence the adaptation of nurses in their professional role as a caregiver. The first factor in this process is:
   1. Being a team player.
   2. Professional education and training.
   3. Working the night shift alone.
   4. Caring for a dying patient.
5. Nurses can seek support within their work environment, including formal and informal support. Formal support includes:
   1. Team members.
   2. Other staff members.
   3. A friend outside the hospital.
   4. Debriefings and ceremonies.

SECTION THREE: Caregiver Burnout

Caregiver burnout is a state of physical, emotional, and mental exhaustion that is generally accompanied by a change in a positive and caring attitude to one that is more negative and unconcerned (Keidel, 2002). Burnout can occur when caregivers do not receive needed assistance or if requested to exceed their capabilities and qualifications. Caregiver burnout is work related and encompasses emotional and physical fatigue caused by constant levels of high stress resulting from feelings of being overworked, underappreciated, and/or confused about job expectations. Caregiver burnout is especially common in individuals who serve as caregivers to persons at the end of life, especially if the care is prolonged over an extended period of time (Fayed, 2008). The underlying work environment, demanding workload and stress related to the dying process are considered to be the contributing factors causing burnout (deValk & Oostrom, 2007). Burnout may also be related to changes in the work situation and feelings of lack of control over work.

Burnout may be assumed to be the inevitable outcome of care and is sometimes referred to as a fatal disease of caring. Although caregiving has natural ebbs and flow, burnout describes an end stage of a much more complex issue. Symptoms of caregiver burnout include physical and emotional exhaustion, lack of motivation, poor patient/customer service, increased conflict with coworkers, and chronic worry about work. The symptoms of caregiver burnout are similar to the symptoms of stress and depression and are outlined in Box 11–1.

Caregivers often become so busy caring for others that they tend to neglect their own emotional, physical, and spiritual health. The demands on a caregiver's body, mind, and emotions can easily seem overwhelming, leading to fatigue and hopelessness, and ultimately to burnout. Other factors that can lead to caregiver burnout include unrealistic expectations, lack of control, and unreasonable demands or work expectations (Neufold, 2002).

BOX 11–1   Symptoms of Emotional and Physical Exhaustion

- Loss of interest in job and activities previously enjoyed
- Withdrawal from coworkers, friends, family, and other loved ones
- Feeling depressed, irritable, hopeless, and/or helpless
- Changes in appetite, weight, or both
- Changes in sleep patterns
- Increasing illness
- Irritability

Source: Sherman, 2004

With caregiver burnout it is important to find someone to trust, such as a friend, coworker, or neighbor to talk to about feelings and frustrations. The nurse should set realistic goals and accept that a team approach is needed and that caregiving is a shared responsibility. The professional caregiver should be realistic about the level of care an individual can provide, knowing that education is critical in preventing burnout. The more knowledge one has about an illness, the more effective one can become in caring for the person with the illness. Additionally, taking care of the caregiver through proper diet, exercise, and sleep and knowing when to set limits also assist in preventing caregiver burnout.

Finally, evaluating the level of work stress is critical. Questions that elicit greater understanding regarding the work environment, a realistic picture of the emotional needs that a dying person may have, and potential changes in a specific job and/or how employing additional help might assist the caregiver begin to play major roles in the prevention of caregiver burnout.

SECTION THREE REVIEW

1. Caregiver burnout is work-related emotional and physical fatigue caused by constant levels of high stress. Contributing factors include demanding workload and: (Select all that apply.)
   1. Attitude.
   2. Personal strength.
   3. Hours of work.
   4. Personality.
2. Which of these is not a manifestation of caregiver burnout?
   1. Emotional and physical exhaustion
   2. Increased hours of work
   3. Changes in appetite, weight, or both
   4. Poor patient/customer service

3. Caregivers often are so busy caring for others that they tend to neglect their own emotional, physical, and:
   1. Spiritual health.
   2. Social health.
   3. Cultural health.
   4. Biological health.
4. The professional caregiver should be realistic about the level of care the nurse can provide, based on the patient's needs. The key is:
   1. Proficiency.
   2. Education.
   3. Teamwork.
   4. Disease.

5. A psychological state of physical and emotional exhaustion thought to be a stress reaction to a reduced ability to meet the demands of one's occupation; symptoms include fatigue, insomnia, impaired work performance, and an increased susceptibility to physical illness and substance abuse defines:

1. Caregiving.
2. Compassion fatigue.
3. Informal caregiver.
4. Caregiver burnout.

SECTION FOUR: Compassion Fatigue

Compassion fatigue is a gradual lessening of the ability to feel compassion over time (Joinson, 1992). As the stress of caring becomes more intensified and the caregiver becomes physically, mentally, and/or emotionally exhausted, the caregiver begins to experience what has come to be known as compassion fatigue or secondary traumatic stress disorder, generally first recognized as the individual begins losing patience more easily and becoming much more cynical. First recognized in the early 1990s, compassion fatigue can have detrimental effects on an individual, both personally and professionally (Flemister, 2006).

Compassion fatigue is frequently seen in the health care profession, especially with those professionals who work with vulnerable populations. Nurses who provide assistance and support to those with pain, suffering, and other symptom management issues at the end of life are at high risk for compassion fatigue. The risks for developing compassion fatigue are increased by one's high expectations concerning making a difference in someone's life, lack of self-care behaviors, and/or insufficient education in working with patients and families at the end of life (Figley, 2004).

Symptoms of compassion fatigue are very similar to classic stress symptoms and include intense somatic illnesses, sleeplessness, helplessness, re-experiencing negative aspects of a patient's care, depression, and workaholism (Flemister, 2006). Nurses may become detached and avoid situations that cause emotional stress or avoid specific persons altogether. There may be increased irritability or anger along with physical and emotional exhaustion. The inability to maintain a balance of empathy and objectivity occurs. The caregiver feels hopelessness and has less ability to feel joy (Pfifferling & Gilley, 2000).

Compassion fatigue is increased by lack of time for self-care, lack of qualified and sufficient support, the inability to balance empathy and objectivity, and a lack of hopefulness. In compassion fatigue, there is decreased concentration and self-esteem. There may be increasing confusion and forgetfulness. Images of the stressors such as agony, pain, and death reappear (Figley, 2004). For self-preservation, the caregiver becomes apathetic, can feel anxious, guilty, numb, or fearful. Depression and feelings of being overwhelmed occur.

A caregiver with compassion fatigue may experience sleep disturbances or nightmares, become increasingly impatient and/or irritable, and start using negative coping methods such as smoking, alcohol, and other substance use. Other physical symptoms may include shock, tachycardia, diaphoresis, dizziness, and other somatic changes. Spiritually, a caregiver with compassion fatigue may question the meaning of life, with loss of purpose and anger toward God or belief system, which may further question the meaning of faith and spirit.

Compassion fatigue generally leads to changes in work performance. There may be a decreased sense of morale, avoidance of responsibilities, increased negativity and absenteeism, poor performance, and an increase in conflict among staff members. Though similar to caregiver burnout, compassion fatigue is thought to have a faster rate of onset and be more attributable to emotional and cognitive strain and stress rather than true physical fatigue (Keidel, 2002). Additionally, compassion fatigue has been historically ascribed as unique to people in the caregiving professions (Joinson, 1992).

Treatment for compassion fatigue includes having someone to talk to and processing the emotions and feelings that the individual is experiencing. It is important to understand that the pain felt with compassion fatigue is normal. Self-care, as mentioned earlier, with physical exercise and proper diet is essential. Caregivers need to obtain additional amounts of restful

---

BOX 11-2   Positively Coping with Compassionate Fatigue and Caregiver Burnout

- Avoid the tendency to become over involved, asking whose needs are being met, the patient's or your needs.
- See things from the family's perspectives rather than feeling your emotions and reacting to those emotions.
- Set attainable goals for yourself and give yourself rewards when the goals are attained.
- Learn to say no and ask for what you need.
- Share distress and get support from friends and family members, remembering not to discuss work issues with everyone.
- Discuss concerns with supportive coworkers and members of the interdisciplinary health team.
- Combat stress by eating healthy foods, exercising, and getting adequate amount of sleep.
- Above all, strive for balance in your personal and professional life.

Source: Adapted from Keidel, 2002

sleep when compassion fatigue is experienced. At times, the caregiver may need to take some time away from his or her caregiving responsibilities and develop interests outside of health care (Huggard, 2003). Box 11–2 lists some ways of positively coping with compassion fatigue and caregiver burnout in end-of-life situations.

SECTION FOUR REVIEW

1. Nurses who provide assistance and support to those with pain, suffering, and other symptom management issues at the end of life are at high risk for compassion fatigue. Also at risk are personality traits of high:
   1. Anxiety and agitation.
   2. Depression and fatigue.
   3. Empathy and compassion.
   4. Energy and stress.
2. Often nurses may become detached and avoid situations or certain patients and families. A caregiver with compassion fatigue may feel:
   1. Joyful.
   2. Hopeless.
   3. Respectful.
   4. Sympathetic.
3. A caregiver with compassion fatigue may experience sleep disturbances, nightmares, become increasingly impatient and/or irritable, and start using: (Select all that apply.)

1. Alcohol.
2. Cigarettes.
3. Illicit drugs.
4. More sick leave or vacation time.
4. Compassion fatigue differs from caregiver burnout because it has:
   1. Different onset and recovery.
   2. Different physical characteristics.
   3. Mental exhaustion.
   4. Coworker issues.
5. It is important to understand that the pain felt with compassion fatigue is normal. Self-care, including physical exercise and proper diet is essential, along with:
   1. Medications.
   2. Restful sleep.
   3. Leave of absence.
   4. Change of job.

CHAPTER SUMMARY

- Caregiving is the act of providing holistic assistance to someone with an illness, including a terminal illness, or disability who is unable to care for himself or herself.
- Informal caregiving describes care provided by family and friends of the ill or disabled person.
- The economic impact of informal caregiving is staggering, with cost estimates ranging from $117 to $292 billion a year.
- One of the greatest challenges for family caregivers is taking care of themselves while providing care to another person.

- Formal caregiving is described as the support and guidance provided by health and social service professionals, with nurses being an essential component of the interdisciplinary health care team.
- Caregiver burnout is a state of physical, emotional, and mental exhaustion that is generally accompanied by a change in a positive and caring attitude to one that is more negative and unconcerned.
- Compassion fatigue is a gradual lessening of the ability to feel compassion over time.

CHAPTER REVIEW

Douglas Smith is an 84-year-old widowed gentleman with end-stage renal disease, who is receiving peritoneal dialysis and supplemental oxygen. He had been living alone on his farm until this admission. He is being discharged to his daughter Julie's home after having a new Tenckhoff dialysis line placed. Julie is married, with four school-aged children and her husband works independently as a truck driver. She works as a teacher in their school. She has taken family leave to bring her father home. The nurse who is assisting them has worked several days in a row, but has not been taking care of Douglas.

Questions

1. What may the nurse's reaction be to this patient and his discharge needs?
2. Which disciplines need to be involved in this discharge planning?
3. What are basic but specific things that need to be considered before discharge?

4. How will Douglas's move into Julie's home affect Douglas and Julie's family?

5. What may Julie be thinking or planning for the future?

Suggested Responses

1. The nurse may experience caregiver burnout, compassion fatigue, normal processing, basic overload, helpful or helpless feelings, and may need other's assistance.

2. Other disciplines that should be involved in this patient's discharge planning include, but are not limited to, social work/case management, renal dialysis, clinical nurse specialists, respiratory therapists, pharmacists, home health nurses, home health care aides, physical therapists, occupational therapists, and respite care or caregiver support groups.

3. Specific teaching needs include care and use of Tenckhoff catheter, care and storage of supplies, oxygen use, and information about any equipment and supplies that are unfamiliar to the patient and his daughter.

4. There are multiple ways in which this move may affect the family. Julie's leave may or may not cause financial hardship. Physical and emotional strain are possible for Julie as her Dad's primary caregiver. Questions that should be answered before deciding the effects on the family include: What was the relationship of Julie and her family with her father before this admission? Was the family close and did the grandchildren have a good relationship with their grandfather? Will Douglas have his own room? Who will be doing the dialysis procedure, Douglas or Julie? What is Douglas's level of activity? What is the house arrangement? Will Julie's husband be home to assist Julie in caring for her father or to assist her in caring for their children? Once these questions are answered, the nurse can begin to work with all concerned parties in ensuring that the transition of Douglas to his daughter's home is positive.

5. Julie may be thinking in terms of days, weeks, months, or years. Is she aware of her father's prognosis and his ability or inability to return to his own home? Will he be strong enough to return to his farm and live independently? Is dying and death in the foreseeable future? At this stage, there are too many unknowns to fully answer this question, but there are several possibilities that the nurse should consider.

REFERENCES

Akkerman, R. L., & Ostwald, S. K. (2004). Reducing anxiety in Alzheimer's disease family caregivers: The effectiveness of a nine-week cognitive behavioral program. *American Journal of Alzheimer's Disease and Other Dementias, 19*(2), 117–123.

Alzheimer's Association. (2008). *2008 Alzheimer's Disease facts and figures.* Chicago: Author.

American Association of Retired Persons Public Policy Institute. (2005). Caregiving in the United States fact sheet. Retrieved from http://assets.aarp.org/rgcenter/il/fs111_caregiving.pdf

American Nurses Association. (1995). Position statement: Informal caregiving. Retrieved from http://www.nursingworld.org/MainMenuCategories/HealthcareandPolicyIssues/ANAPositionStatements/social/sccare14501.aspx

American Nurses Association. (2002). Helping nurses help caregivers. Retrieved from http://www.nursingworld.org/TAN/mayjun02/helping.htm

Arno, P. (2006). *Economic value of informal caregiving.* Presented at the Care Coordination and the Caregiving Forum, Department of Veterans Affairs, Bethesda, MD: January 25–27, 2006.

Bull, M. J., & McShane, R. E. (2008). Seeking what's best during transition to adult day health services. *Qualitative Health Research, 18*(5), 597–605.

Byock, I. (1996). The nature of suffering and the nature of opportunity at the end of life. *Clinics in Geriatric Medicine, 12*(2): 237–251.

Byock, I. (1997). *Dying well: The prospect for growth at the end of life.* New York: Riverhead Books.

Center on Aging. (2004). Informal caregiving. Donald A. Reynolds Institute on Aging. Retrieved from http://centeronaging.uams.edu/patients/informal_caregiving.asp

Coleman, E. (2003). Falling through the cracks: Challenges and opportunities for improving transitional care for persons with continuous complex care needs. *Journal of the American Geriatrics Society, 51*, 549–555.

Cramer, L., McCorkle, R., Cherlin, E., Johnson-Hurzeler, R., & Bradley, E. (2003). Nurses' attitudes and practice related to hospice care. *Journal of Nursing Scholarship, 35*, 249–255.

Demmer, C. (2004). Burnout: The health care worker as survivor. *AIDS Leader, 14*(10), 522–537.

deValk, M., & Oostrom, C. (2007). Burnout in the medical profession: Causes, consequences and solutions. Retrieved from http://www.intermedic.nl/Proof.pdf

Duke, B., Hoover, S., & Kaplan, M. (2004). Family caregivers: Outreach and assistance in our communities. Retrieved from http://caregiverpa.psu.edu/info/3Facilitator%20Guidebook.doc

Emanuel, E. J., Fairclough, D. L., Slutsman, J., & Emanuel, L. L. (2000). Understanding economic and other burdens of terminal illness: The experience of patients and their caregivers. *Annuals of Internal Medicine, 132*, 451–459.

End of Life Nursing Consortium. (2008). *Advanced end of life nursing care: ELNEC supercore training program 2008.* Washington, DC: American Association of Colleges of Nursing.

Family Caregiver Alliance. (2006). *Caregiver assessment: Principles, guidelines and strategies for change. Report from a national consensus development conference.* Volume I. San Francisco: Family Caregiver Alliance; Retrieved from http://www.caregiver.org/caregiver/jsp/content/pdfs/v1_consensus.pdf

Fayed, L. (2008). *Cancer caregiver burnout: How to recognize it, and how to prevent it.* Retrieved from http://cancer.about.com/od/howtocope/a/burnout.htm

Figley, C. (2004). *Compassion fatigue: An introduction.* Retrieved from http://www.traumatologyacademy.org/Training/2004/Blackmountain/CFT-Workbook_v2.pdf

Flemister, B. (2006). Be aware of compassion fatigue. *Journal of Wound Ostomy and Continence Nursing, 33*(5), 465–466.

Gansler, T. (2007). End-of-life caregiving often like a full time job. *A Cancer Journal for Clinicians, 57*, 128–129.

Gill, P., Kaur, J., Rummans, T., Novotny, P., & Sloan, J. (2003). The hospice patient's primary caregiver. What is their quality of life? *Journal of Psychosomatic Research, 55*, 445–451.

Holland, J., & Neimeyer, R. (2005). Reducing the risk of burnout in end-of-life care settings: The role of daily spiritual experiences and training. *Palliative and Supportive Care, 3*, 173–181.

Hudson, P., Aranda, S., & McMurray, N. (2002). Intervention development for enhanced lay palliative caregiver support: The use of focus groups. *European Journal of Cancer Care, 11*, 262–270.

Huggard, P. (2003). Compassion fatigue: How much can I give? *Medical Education, 37*(2), 163–164.

Joinson, C. (1992). Coping with compassion fatigue. *Nursing 1992, 22*(4), 116–121.

Karnes, B. (2005). *Gone from my sight: The dying experience.* Vancouver, WA: Barbara Karnes Books.

Keidel, G. C. (2002). Burnout and compassion fatigue among hospice caregivers. *American Journal of Hospice and Palliative Care, 19*(3), 200–205.

Laird, J., & Massey, S. (2006). Survival guide for palliative care RNs. Retrieved from http://www.medicalnewstoday.com/articles/38233.php

Majerovitz, S. D. (2007). Predictors of burden and depression among nursing home family caregivers. *Aging and Mental Health, 11*(3), 323–329.

Martin-Cook, D., Remakel-Davis, B., Svetlik, D., Hynan, L., & Weinger, M. F. (2003). Caregiver attrition and resentment in dementia care. *American Journal of the Alzheimer's Disease and Other Dementias, 18*(6), 366–374.

McCorkle, R., & Pasacreta, J. (2001). Enhancing caregiver outcomes in palliative care. *Cancer Control, 8*(1), 36–45.

Meier, D., & Beresford, L. (2006). Preventing burnout. *Journal of Palliative Medicine, 9*(5), 1045–1048.

Mittelman, M. (2005). Taking care of the caregivers. *Current Opinion of Psychiatry, 18*(6), 633–639.

National Alliance for Caregiving and AARP. (2004). *Caregiving in the U.S.* [Ebook]. Retrieved from http://www.caregiving.org/data/04finalreport.pdf

National Family Caregivers Association. (2004). Caregiving statistics: Family caregivers and family caregiving. Retrieved from http://www.nfcacares.org/who_are_family_caregivers/care_giving_stat.stics.cfm

National Family Caregivers Association & Family Caregivers Alliance. Estimated prevalence and economic value of family caregiving, (2004). Retrieved from http://www.thefamilycaregiver.org/pdfs/State_Caregiving_Databystate2006.pdf

National Institute of Nursing Research, the National Institute of Child Health and Human Development, and the National Institute of Mental Health. (2002). Informal caregiving research for chronic conditions. Retrieved from http://grants.nih.gov/grants/guide/pa-files/PA-02-155.html

Navaie-Waliser, M., Spriggs, A., Bonnell, C., & Peng, T. (2002). Informal and formal home health caregivers: The disconnect between providers in patient care systems. *Abstracts of the Academy of Health Service Research and Health Policy Meeting, 19*, 19.

Neufold, S. (2002). Coping with Caregiver Burnout. Retrieved from http://www.healthology.com/caregiving/article336.htm

Newton, M., Bell, D., Lambert, S., & Fearing, A. (2002). Concerns of hospice patient caregivers. *ABNF J, 13*, 140–144.

Pfifferling, J.-H., & Gilley, K. (2000). Overcoming compassion fatigue. *Family Medical Practitioner. 7*(4), 39–42.

Phillips, L. R., & Crist, J. (2008). Social relationships among family caregivers: A cross-cultural comparison between Mexican Americans and non-Hispanic White caregivers. *Journal of Transcultural Nursing, 19*(4), 326–337.

Pinquart, M., & Sorenson, S. (2003). Differences between caregivers and noncaregivers in psychological health and physical health: A meta-analysis. *Psychology of Aging, 18*(2), 250–267.

Roth, D. L., Haley, W. E., Wadley, V. G., Clay, O. J., & Howard, G. (2007). Race and gender differences in perceived caregiver availability for community-dwelling middle-aged and older adults. *The Gerontologist, 47*(6), 721–729.

Schulz, R., & Sherwood, P. (2008). Physical and mental health effects of family caregiving. *American Journal of Nursing, 108*(9), 23–27.

Scott, J. A. (2006). *Informal caregiving.* Prepared for the Blaine House Conference on Aging, September 2006. Orono, ME: University of Maine Center on Aging.

Sherman, D. (2004). Nurses' stress & burnout: How to care for yourself when caring for patients and their families experiencing life-threatening illness. *American Journal of Nursing, 104*(5), 48–56.

Shugarman, L., Lorenz, K., Lynn, J., & Mularski, R. A. (2005). Patient and caregiver satisfaction with care at her end of life: A review of the evidence. *Abstracts of the Academy of Health Meeting, 22* (#3910).

Takamura, J., & Williams, B. (2000). *Informal caregiving: Compassion in action.* Washington, DC: U.S. Department of Health and Human Services (DHHS).

Vellone, E., Piras, G., Talucci, C., & Cohen, M. Z. (2008). Quality of life for caregivers of people with Alzheimer's disease. *Journal of Advanced Nursing, 61*(2), 222–231.

Weman, K., & Fagerberg, I. (2006) Registered nurses working together with family members of older people. *Journal of Clinical Nursing, 15*(3), 281.

Review Question Answers
and Rationales

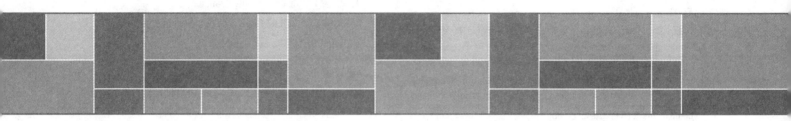

CHAPTER 1

Pretest

1. **ANSWER:** 3

   RATIONALE: Palliative care involves aggressively treating symptoms of the illness and ensuring the patient's comfort. Palliative care does not treat or focus on recovery from a disease. It is also important for more than just terminally ill patients.

   NURSING PROCESS STEP: Implementation

   CATEGORY OF CLIENT NEED: Physiological Integrity

   KNOWLEDGE LEVEL: Comprehension

2. **ANSWER:** 4

   RATIONALE: Those working in health care now recognize and value the quality of life more so than the quantity of life, and futile measures are avoided. Quality care is still difficult to provide at the end of life, and unfortunately pain is still ignored and/or overlooked.

   NURSING PROCESS STEP: Evaluation

   CATEGORY OF CLIENT NEED: Physiological Integrity

   KNOWLEDGE LEVEL: Comprehension

3. **ANSWER:** 1

   RATIONALE: Those caring for elderly patients must take special needs such as safety into account when providing care. The elderly frequently find it difficult to express their needs, are frequently dependent on others, and usually exhibit more impairments than other adults.

   NURSING PROCESS STEP: Evaluation

   CATEGORY OF CLIENT NEED: Physiological Integrity

   KNOWLEDGE LEVEL: Comprehension

4. **ANSWER:** 4

   RATIONALE: Hospice started as a means to assist patients and their families living with life-threatening and life-limiting illnesses. It has existed for several decades, has consistent qualification guidelines, and is not the same as palliative care.

NURSING PROCESS STEP: Evaluation

CATEGORY OF CLIENT NEED: Physiological Integrity

KNOWLEDGE LEVEL: Comprehension

5. **ANSWER:** 3

   RATIONALE: Palliative care differs from hospice care, as the goal of palliative care is to maintain the highest quality of life with rigorous treatment. It can address multiple patient health issues, decreases burden and stressors, and is provided in multiple settings.

   NURSING PROCESS STEP: Implementation

   CATEGORY OF CLIENT NEED: Physiological Integrity

   KNOWLEDGE LEVEL: Comprehension

Section One Review

1. **ANSWER:** 2

   RATIONALE: Nurses can provide palliative care in any setting or unit because it focuses on maximizing quality of life and minimizing suffering. It does not focus on patients with terminal illnesses, is individualized based on client needs, and is provided by a multidisciplinary team.

   NURSING PROCESS STEP: Evaluation

   CATEGORY OF CLIENT NEED: Physiological Integrity

   KNOWLEDGE LEVEL: Application

2. **ANSWER:** 2, 3, and 4

   RATIONALE: Palliative care includes the physical, psychosocial, cultural, spiritual, and emotional needs of the client and family.

   NURSING PROCESS STEP: Implementation

   CATEGORY OF CLIENT NEED: Physiological Integrity

   KNOWLEDGE LEVEL: Application

3. **ANSWER:** 1

   RATIONALE: Palliative care as defined by the World Health Organization does not include speeding up or delaying death. It does include providing relief from distressing symptoms and integrating physiological and spiritual aspects of care.

NURSING PROCESS STEP: Evaluation

CATEGORY OF CLIENT NEED: Physiological Integrity

KNOWLEDGE LEVEL: Analysis

4. **ANSWER:** 1, 2, 3, 4

   RATIONALE: Palliative care is useful in assisting patients in all areas. Physical disabilities may include weakness, fatigue, cachexia; changes in sensorium include alterations in touch, sight, hearing, taste, or smell; psychological responses include anxiety, depression, delirium, and coping responses; emotional distress includes joy, sadness, anger, and/or denial.

   NURSING PROCESS STEP: Assessment

   CATEGORY OF CLIENT NEED: Physiological Integrity

   KNOWLEDGE LEVEL: Application

5. **ANSWER:** 3

   RATIONALE: Palliative care includes an interdisciplinary approach to patient and family needs. This is both difficult to define and describe, as it varies for each patient. It is not separate from medical treatment but parallel, and all aspects of care are included.

   NURSING PROCESS STEP: Assessment

   CATEGORY OF CLIENT NEED: Physiological Integrity

   KNOWLEDGE LEVEL: Comprehension

6. **ANSWER:** 4

   RATIONALE: Palliative care focuses on individual aspects of care, not the community aspects of care. The structure and process of palliative care are included in this practice as well as the psychosocial, psychiatric, spiritual, religious, and existential needs of the patient and family.

   NURSING PROCESS STEP: Evaluation

   CATEGORY OF CLIENT NEED: Physiological Integrity

   KNOWLEDGE LEVEL: Analysis

Section Two Review

1. **ANSWER:** 1

   RATIONALE: During the 1900s, advances in health care extended life by approximately 30 years because the focus of medical care shifted from alleviating suffering to curing disease. Dying in a hospital became the preferred situation and dying was viewed as a failure in health care technology. The individual patient became more important as the overall welfare of the community was minimized or ignored.

   NURSING PROCESS STEP: Evaluation

   CATEGORY OF CLIENT NEED: Physiological Integrity

   KNOWLEDGE LEVEL: Comprehension

2. **ANSWER:** 2, 3, 5

   RATIONALE: Palliative care teams work with families and patients to ensure understanding of medical futility, the right to undergo or refuse procedures and/or therapies, and discussing advances in technology and medicine available in the specific situation. Decision-making difficulties for the team members, family, and patient do not stem from questions about inheritances. The only correct decision is the one the patient, family, and team members work through and arrive at together.

   NURSING PROCESS STEP: Evaluation

   CATEGORY OF CLIENT NEED: Physiological Integrity

   KNOWLEDGE LEVEL: Application

3. **ANSWER:** 3

   RATIONALE: The existence of a comorbid condition in a dying patient means the nurse must also take that condition into consideration when working through planning and implementing the patient's care, just as with any other patient. Abandonment and suffering are never an alternative, regardless of the existence of comorbid conditions. All options should be made available to the patient to ensure the appropriate decision is made for the particular patient's situation.

   NURSING PROCESS STEP: Implementation

   CATEGORY OF CLIENT NEED: Physiological Integrity

   KNOWLEDGE LEVEL: Analysis

4. **ANSWER:** 2

   RATIONALE: In those with life-threatening or terminal illnesses, much of the fear experienced is related to the uncertainty of how the illness might change appearances or body smells. Fear is not tangible and can also be related to pain.

   NURSING PROCESS STEP: Assessment

   CATEGORY OF CLIENT NEED: Physiological Integrity

   KNOWLEDGE LEVEL: Application

5. **ANSWER:** 3

   RATIONALE: The aging population will consume an increased proportion of health care services and funding as health care costs will continue to rise. Due to the increase in technology, more people will live with chronic illnesses as they grow older. The aging will outnumber the young as the aging will live longer than ever before.

   NURSING PROCESS STEP: Evaluation

   CATEGORY OF CLIENT NEED: Physiological Integrity

   KNOWLEDGE LEVEL: Analysis

Section Three Review

1. **ANSWER:** 3

   RATIONALE: Research and medical treatments are aimed at more positive outcomes for patients with life-threatening and life-altering illnesses. Unfortunately, it is becoming more difficult for nurses to provide quality care since more nurses are needed than are available. Pain and suffering are not overlooked in health care, but sometimes patient desires and treatments given are not always in agreement.

NURSING PROCESS STEP: Assessment

CATEGORY OF CLIENT NEED: Physiological Integrity

KNOWLEDGE LEVEL: Application

2. **ANSWER:** 1, 2, 3

RATIONALE: Nurses working in palliative care must be familiar with the signs and symptoms of the dying process to give anticipatory guidance to patients and family members. Treatment options must also be discussed in detail and can be done so in an interdisciplinary manner so that the patient, family, and team members are aware of topics that have been discussed. Any nurse is capable of working in palliative care regardless of experience with dying patients, and does not work alone but with many other team members.

NURSING PROCESS STEP: Implementation

CATEGORY OF CLIENT NEED: Physiological Integrity

KNOWLEDGE LEVEL: Application

3. **ANSWER:** 1

RATIONALE: The palliative care nurse is always wholly honest with the patient about the current state of the disease, including anticipatory guidance as applicable. It is up to the patient to decide when and if the family is made fully aware of the situation.

NURSING PROCESS STEP: Implementation

CATEGORY OF CLIENT NEED: Physiological Integrity

KNOWLEDGE LEVEL: Analysis

4. **ANSWER:** 2

RATIONALE: As a patient undergoes palliative care, he or she may exhibit a decreased functional capacity to continue the things that are meaningful and valuable, thus leading the patient to feel a loss of control over his or her life. Quality of life varies on a daily basis and over time, independence suffers. The family role will also change as the patient may become less able to function in the same capacity as before the illness.

NURSING PROCESS STEP: Evaluation

CATEGORY OF CLIENT NEED: Physiological Integrity

KNOWLEDGE LEVEL: Analysis

Section Four Review

1. **ANSWER:** 4

RATIONALE: The citizens of the United States are overall more likely to attempt to defy death by using every technological advance available to them through medical interventions. Deficiencies are present in the systems of care for those at the end of life, in part because of social and economic forces.

NURSING PROCESS STEP: Assessment

CATEGORY OF CLIENT NEED: Physiological Integrity

KNOWLEDGE LEVEL: Application

2. **ANSWER:** 2

RATIONALE: Since interventions in palliative care are aimed at keeping the patient comfortable, the focus is not on treatments but simply doing as requested and needed as well as spending time with the patient. Stabilizing all conditions is not possible and, thus the goals of care may change over the course of the illness.

NURSING PROCESS STEP: Planning

CATEGORY OF CLIENT NEED: Physiological Integrity

KNOWLEDGE LEVEL: Application

3. **ANSWER:** 1, 4

RATIONALE: According to the theoretical basis for palliation, interdisciplinary care is given to the patient and the family. Thus, care does not cease when the patient dies; it continues until after the family is also ready to end the relationship.

NURSING PROCESS STEP: Implementation

CATEGORY OF CLIENT NEED: Safe, Effective Care Environment

KNOWLEDGE LEVEL: Analysis

4. **ANSWER:** 3

RATIONALE: Patients fear a prolonged death during which suffering occurs with little intervention. People also fear dying alone in the hospital.

NURSING PROCESS STEP: Planning

CATEGORY OF CLIENT NEED: Psychosocial Integrity

KNOWLEDGE LEVEL: Knowledge

5. **ANSWER:** 2, 3, 4

RATIONALE: The goals of palliative care include ensuring both patient and family understand the disease prognosis, and to ensure the overall goals of care are understood. Palliative care does not include making it easier for caregivers to avoid the situation.

NURSING PROCESS STEP: Planning

CATEGORY OF CLIENT NEED: Physiological Integrity

KNOWLEDGE LEVEL: Analysis

Section Five Review

1. **ANSWER:** 3

RATIONALE: As the United States health care system currently focuses on disease and curing, end-of-life care is not well covered in medical school and nursing school. Thus, the benefits of palliative care and hospice care are not well known.

NURSING PROCESS STEP: Implementation

CATEGORY OF CLIENT NEED: Safe, Effective Care Environment

KNOWLEDGE LEVEL: Comprehension

2. **ANSWER:** 1

RATIONALE: Both hospice and palliative care allow the patient to remain in the home and out of the hospital with fewer procedures.

NURSING PROCESS STEP: Implementation

CATEGORY OF CLIENT NEED: Physiological Integrity

KNOWLEDGE LEVEL: Knowledge

3. **ANSWER:** 4

RATIONALE: Palliative care allows the focus to remain on comfort care while still treating the illness or disease. Palliative care can occur for longer than six months, does not have to be used only in terminal illness, and can be given in any department within the hospital.

NURSING PROCESS STEP: Implementation

CATEGORY OF CLIENT NEED: Safe, Effective Care Environment

KNOWLEDGE LEVEL: Application

4. **ANSWER:** 2

RATIONALE: Hospice ensures each patient's needs are met by an individualized plan for pain management and symptom control. Hospice uses a family-centered approach and focuses on not only the patient's needs, but also on the family's needs.

NURSING PROCESS STEP: Implementation

CATEGORY OF CLIENT NEED: Physiological Integrity

KNOWLEDGE LEVEL: Application

5. **ANSWER:** 1, 3, 5

RATIONALE: There are only four levels of hospice care according to Box 1-8; Outpatient Respite and General Outpatient Care are not included in the levels.

NURSING PROCESS STEP: Implementation

CATEGORY OF CLIENT NEED: Safe, Effective Care Environment

KNOWLEDGE LEVEL: Application

Section Six Review

1. **ANSWER:** 3

RATIONALE: Measurement of quality of life includes the physical, psychological, social, and spiritual dimensions. The emotional, human, and secular dimensions are not part of quality-of-life measurement.

NURSING PROCESS STEP: Assessment

CATEGORY OF CLIENT NEED: Health Promotion and Maintenance

KNOWLEDGE LEVEL: Knowledge

2. **ANSWER:** 2

RATIONALE: Since the dimensions of quality of life are interrelated, any change in any dimension affects the overall quality of life. Thus, when an illness is diagnosed and/or there is a worsening of a condition, all aspects of quality of life must be considered at every stage of the process.

NURSING PROCESS STEP: Planning

CATEGORY OF CLIENT NEED: Safe, Effective Care Environment

KNOWLEDGE LEVEL: Application

3. **ANSWER:** 1

RATIONALE: When a patient experiences support from and good communication with health care providers and family members, this enhances psychological well-being, which in turn can affect physical well-being. The other options include all negative or mind-altering components, which do not affect psychological well-being as readily as positive communication and support.

NURSING PROCESS STEP: Implementation

CATEGORY OF CLIENT NEED: Psychosocial Integrity

KNOWLEDGE LEVEL: Application

4. **ANSWER:** 4

RATIONALE: Family structures may be endangered by disruptions in relationships and roles, which may cause turmoil and dysfunction. Family structures are always related to the patient and his or her prognosis and overall status.

NURSING PROCESS STEP: Assessment

CATEGORY OF CLIENT NEED: Psychosocial Integrity

KNOWLEDGE LEVEL: Comprehension

5. **ANSWER:** 3

RATIONALE: It is not uncommon for health care providers to overlook spiritual care as it lacks importance compared to physical and psychological components of care. Spiritual care does not necessarily mean religious practices.

NURSING PROCESS STEP: Assessment

CATEGORY OF CLIENT NEED: Psychosocial Integrity

KNOWLEDGE LEVEL: Comprehension

Section Seven Review

1. **ANSWER:** 1

RATIONALE: The first step of the nursing process is assessment, and the nurse needs to initiate discussion before asking questions, alleviating fears, or taking notes.

NURSING PROCESS STEP: Implementation

CATEGORY OF CLIENT NEED: Psychosocial Integrity

KNOWLEDGE LEVEL: Application

2. **ANSWER:** 4

RATIONALE: Completing life is a very individual experience but progresses through inner and outer perspectives. The outer perspective includes those affairs outside the person and outside the immediate circle of family and friends.

NURSING PROCESS STEP: Evaluation

CATEGORY OF CLIENT NEED: Psychosocial Integrity

KNOWLEDGE LEVEL: Analysis

3. **ANSWER:** 2

RATIONALE: Early signs of the dying process include changes in outward behavior. The remaining options are physical changes, which occur later in the process.

NURSING PROCESS STEP: Assessment

CATEGORY OF CLIENT NEED: Psychosocial Integrity

KNOWLEDGE LEVEL: Knowledge

4. **ANSWER:** 3

RATIONALE: It is not unusual for the dying patient to hallucinate as the process of dying continues. Periods of apnea, unresponsiveness, and an energy surge occur as death is imminent.

NURSING PROCESS STEP: Assessment

CATEGORY OF CLIENT NEED: Psychosocial Integrity

KNOWLEDGE LEVEL: Knowledge

5. **ANSWER:** 1

RATIONALE: As death approaches, the patient's eyes may remain open but are unseeing. Talking usually ceases, breathing becomes erratic (usually in a Cheyne-Stokes pattern), and the skin becomes mottled as blood circulation slows.

NURSING PROCESS STEP: Implementation

CATEGORY OF CLIENT NEED: Physiological Integrity

KNOWLEDGE LEVEL: Analysis

Section Eight Review

1. **ANSWER:** 2

RATIONALE: A good death is personal but usually occurs when positive thoughts and events emerge from the dying process. Thus, denying the death process is a part of life, not reviewing life, and not becoming more aware of spiritual aspects of self may discourage the perception of a good death.

NURSING PROCESS STEP: Implementation

CATEGORY OF CLIENT NEED: Psychosocial Integrity

KNOWLEDGE LEVEL: Comprehension

2. **ANSWER:** 1

RATIONALE: Hope should never be lost. The nurse can encourage the continuance of hope but discuss switching from the hope for a cure to the hope for a quality death. The focus should remain on the life lived and the important contributions made.

NURSING PROCESS STEP: Assessment

CATEGORY OF CLIENT NEED: Physiological Integrity

KNOWLEDGE LEVEL: Comprehension

3. **ANSWER:** 3

RATIONALE: Family members must be aware that the care they provide shows love. While care can instill hope and provide nutrients, it is more important that the family is aware it shows love.

NURSING PROCESS STEP: Implementation

CATEGORY OF CLIENT NEED: Psychosocial Integrity

KNOWLEDGE LEVEL: Application

4. **ANSWER:** 4

RATIONALE: The nurse who accepts death as a natural event is able to focus on the patient, not on personal fears.

NURSING PROCESS STEP: Implementation

CATEGORY OF CLIENT NEED: Psychosocial Integrity

KNOWLEDGE LEVEL: Application

5. **ANSWER:** 2, 4, 5

RATIONALE: Patients with cancer, chronic obstructive pulmonary disease, and Alzheimer's disease are more likely to have time to work through the dying process than are those who die from a traumatic or sudden event or illness.

NURSING PROCESS STEP: Assessment

CATEGORY OF CLIENT NEED: Psychosocial Integrity

KNOWLEDGE LEVEL: Analysis

Section Nine Review

1. **ANSWER:** 2

RATIONALE: Primary prevention is the nurse's first responsibility in any area of nursing or medical care. Primary prevention involves education for patients and families.

NURSING PROCESS STEP: Implementation

CATEGORY OF CLIENT NEED: Physiological Integrity

KNOWLEDGE LEVEL: Application

2. **ANSWER:** 1

RATIONALE: Rest periods for family members are imperative to assist them to relieve stress and distress. They should assist in care, have conversations as needed with the patient, and should get assistance from others as necessary.

NURSING PROCESS STEP: Implementation

CATEGORY OF CLIENT NEED: Physiological Integrity

KNOWLEDGE LEVEL: Comprehension

3. **ANSWER:** 1, 2, 3, 4

RATIONALE: Nurses should function as advocates, consultants, educators, social support, and cheerleaders for patients and families. In most circumstances, nurses do not do errands.

NURSING PROCESS STEP: Implementation

CATEGORY OF CLIENT NEED: Safe, Effective Care Environment

KNOWLEDGE LEVEL: Analysis

4. **ANSWER:** 3

RATIONALE: Palliative care nursing coordinates and communicates care for patients and their families. Palliative care nursing does not limit treatment, focus only on long-term needs, or function independently.

NURSING PROCESS STEP: Implementation

CATEGORY OF CLIENT NEED: Physiological Integrity

KNOWLEDGE LEVEL: Application

5. **ANSWER:** 3, 4

RATIONALE: It is difficult to maintain continuity of care in palliative care because health care providers have differing views about its necessity and the best way to provide care. In addition, staffing in palliative care is frequently understaffed and thus, less time is available per patient. Patients do not frequently refuse palliative care and multiple family members are encouraged to ask questions.

NURSING PROCESS STEP: Implementation

CATEGORY OF CLIENT NEED: Physiological Integrity

KNOWLEDGE LEVEL: Analysis

CHAPTER 2

Pretest

1. **ANSWER:** 2

RATIONALE: Ethics determines the reasons behind individual actions, not those of society as a whole. Laws are enforced through statutes and the judiciary.

NURSING PROCESS STEP: Implementation

CATEGORY OF CLIENT NEED: Safe, Effective Care Environment

KNOWLEDGE LEVEL: Comprehension

2. **ANSWER:** 2

RATIONALE: Deontology is the classification of ethics derived from one person's duties. Situation ethics is a subset of deontology and takes the particular situation into account when focusing on one's duty to act. Teleological theories (or utilitarianism) of ethics focus on outcomes. This means the end outcome of the situation justifies the means used to get there.

NURSING PROCESS STEP: Assessment

CATEGORY OF CLIENT NEED: Safe, Effective Care Environment

KNOWLEDGE LEVEL: Comprehension

3. **ANSWER:** 2

RATIONALE: The patient benefit model facilitates decision making for the incompetent patient and attempts to decide an issue how a patient would.

NURSING PROCESS STEP: Implementation

CATEGORY OF CLIENT NEED: Safe, Effective Care Environment

KNOWLEDGE LEVEL: Knowledge

4. **ANSWER:** 1

RATIONALE: Therapeutic jurisprudence considers the patient's well-being when faced with legal and ethical issues.

NURSING PROCESS STEP: Implementation

CATEGORY OF CLIENT NEED: Safe, Effective Care Environment

KNOWLEDGE LEVEL: Comprehension

5. **ANSWER:** 2

RATIONALE: When advocating for a patient, the advocator considers the patient and/or family values when making decisions. Thus, there is information sharing to empower the individual.

NURSING PROCESS STEP: Implementation

CATEGORY OF CLIENT NEED: Safe, Effective Care Environment

KNOWLEDGE LEVEL: Comprehension

Section One Review

1. **ANSWER:** Ethics

RATIONALE: Ethics is the science related to moral actions and values. It is these values and attitudes which determine decisions about whether one action or another should be undertaken.

NURSING PROCESS STEP: Implementation

CATEGORY OF CLIENT NEED: Safe, Effective Care Environment

KNOWLEDGE LEVEL: Application

2. **ANSWER:** 1

RATIONALE: Laws are created by people and are to protect people from actions by others. Keeping the patient away from others and making sure the others take their own medications allows the offending patient to walk away without penalty for wrongdoing. The ethics committee has no power in this situation as it is a legal issue.

NURSING PROCESS STEP: Implementation

CATEGORY OF CLIENT NEED: Safe, Effective Care Environment

KNOWLEDGE LEVEL: Application

3. **ANSWER:** 1, 2, 5

RATIONALE: Values are personal beliefs about behaviors appropriate in society. Thus, being honest, kind, and doing unto others as they do unto you are all examples of values. Justice is an ethical term meaning all people should be treated fairly, and the term maleficence should be nonmaleficence meaning the duty to do no harm.

NURSING PROCESS STEP: Implementation

CATEGORY OF CLIENT NEED: Safe, Effective Care Environment

KNOWLEDGE LEVEL: Comprehension

4. **ANSWER:** 3

RATIONALE: While values are individualistic and vary because of many aspects of a person's life and upbringing, race does not necessarily affect a person's values. Religion, family orientation, and a person's age may all account for differences in values.

NURSING PROCESS STEP: Evaluation

CATEGORY OF CLIENT NEED: Safe, Effective Care Environment

KNOWLEDGE LEVEL: Analysis

Section Two Review

1. **ANSWER:** 1

   RATIONALE: Normative ethics describes the standards of behavior applying to the actions of everyday life. Personal beliefs describe values, ethics about conflicts in clinical setting is called principalism, and substituted judgment describes making decisions for those unable to make decisions for themselves.

   NURSING PROCESS STEP: Implementation

   CATEGORY OF CLIENT NEED: Safe, Effective Care Environment

   KNOWLEDGE LEVEL: Comprehension

2. **ANSWER:** 2

   RATIONALE: The deontological theories of ethics state the deciding factor in choosing between two actions is the duties human beings owe one another by virtue of commitments made and roles assumed. Deontology looks at what is meant by the action and not the end result. Teleological theories believe actions are chosen based on the end result obtained by a particular action. If the result is desirable, then the action is ethical. Utilitarian ethics decides an action based on the greatest good for the greatest number, and non-normative ethics is not applicable to clinical situations as it looks at meanings behind moral statements.

   NURSING PROCESS STEP: Implementation

   CATEGORY OF CLIENT NEED: Safe, Effective Care Environment

   KNOWLEDGE LEVEL: Application

3. **ANSWER:** 4

   RATIONALE: Act utilitarianism believes the most ethical action is the one that causes the least harm or suffering, if the greatest happiness to one individual is not possible. Thus, allowing the physician to discontinue the ventilator allows the family member to die quietly and when the time is right.

   NURSING PROCESS STEP: Implementation

   CATEGORY OF CLIENT NEED: Safe, Effective Care Environment

   KNOWLEDGE LEVEL: Application

4. **ANSWER:** deontology or situation ethics

   RATIONALE: The deontological theories of ethics state the deciding factor in choosing between two actions is the duties human beings owe one another by virtue of commitments made and roles assumed. The decision maker takes into account the unique characteristics of each individual, the caring relationship between the person and the caregiver, and the most humanistic course of action given the circumstances.

   NURSING PROCESS STEP: Assessment

   CATEGORY OF CLIENT NEED: Safe, Effective Care Environment

   KNOWLEDGE LEVEL: Comprehension

Section Three Review

1. **ANSWER:** 1, 3, 4, 5

   RATIONALE: Veracity is truthfulness during the discussion to give the whole truth and answer questions honestly; Nonmaleficence is "doing no harm"; Beneficence involves always doing good for the patient and family, which in end of life care may be just listening and supporting decisions; Fidelity involves keeping promises and commitments to the patient and family members. Paternalism should not apply, as it is making decisions for another without their consent or input.

   NURSING PROCESS STEP: Planning

   CATEGORY OF CLIENT NEED: Safe, Effective Care Environment

   KNOWLEDGE LEVEL: Application

2. **ANSWER:** 2

   RATIONALE: Double effect occurs when the nurse decides upon an action that is at least "morally neutral" with only good intentions, knowing an undesirable and unintended effect will also occur. The desirable effects must also outweigh the undesirable. The other options do not describe a double effect.

   NURSING PROCESS STEP: Implementation

   CATEGORY OF CLIENT NEED: Physiological Integrity

   KNOWLEDGE LEVEL: Application

3. **ANSWER:** 4

   RATIONALE: Autonomy is most likely to be in conflict for this nurse as the patient moves in and out of lucidity. If a patient is incompetent part of the time, it is difficult for the nurse to determine the patient's wishes. Veracity is truthfulness in caring for the patient. Nonmaleficence is "doing no harm"; Beneficence involves always doing good for the patient, which in end of life care may be just listening and supporting decisions.

   NURSING PROCESS STEP: Implementation

   CATEGORY OF CLIENT NEED: Safe, Effective Care Environment

   KNOWLEDGE LEVEL: Application

4. **ANSWER:** 2, 3, 5

   RATIONALE: The nurse would consider all the options, who should be involved, and the consequences of each option. In addition, the applicable rules and/or guidelines should be a consideration, as well as the desired outcomes for all parties involved. The nurse would not want to make the decision independently or decide when the decision would have to be made.

   NURSING PROCESS STEP: Planning

   CATEGORY OF CLIENT NEED: Safe, Effective Care Environment

   KNOWLEDGE LEVEL: Application

Section Four Review

1. **ANSWER:** 2, 4

   RATIONALE: The respect for persons model, also called the patient advocate model, specifically requires the nurse to value the patient as a person. In doing this, the nurse must act in whatever manner will protect the rights of the patient.

   NURSING PROCESS STEP: Assessment

   CATEGORY OF CLIENT NEED: Safe, Effective Care Environment

   KNOWLEDGE LEVEL: Comprehension

2. ANSWER: 3

RATIONALE: The values-based model specifically requires the nurse to discuss the patient's values and assist in making the decision most consistent with those values.

NURSING PROCESS STEP: Assessment

CATEGORY OF CLIENT NEED: Safe, Effective Care Environment

KNOWLEDGE LEVEL: Comprehension

3. ANSWER: 2, 3, 4

RATIONALE: The patient advocacy models rely on beneficence, as the nurse must do "good" as perceived by the patient, justice in treating all patients fairly and equally, and veracity, requiring the nurse to always be honest. The nurse cannot be a true advocate for patients if these principles are not followed. Respect for others is the other principle that applies to patient advocacy.

NURSING PROCESS STEP: Implementation

CATEGORY OF CLIENT NEED: Safe, Effective Care Environment

KNOWLEDGE LEVEL: Application

Section Five Review

1. ANSWER: 4

RATIONALE: When an ethics committee makes decisions for an incompetent patient based on the beliefs of that patient, this is called the patient benefit model of committee structure. Social justice models discuss the issue based on the effect on the health care institution.

NURSING PROCESS STEP: Implementation

CATEGORY OF CLIENT NEED: Safe, Effective Care Environment

KNOWLEDGE LEVEL: Analysis

2. ANSWER: 4

RATIONALE: Ethical rounds in health care arenas assist those working in the clinical area with the ethical principles within which decisions can be made. It is through these rounds that staff begin to understand considerations necessary when confronted with ethical dilemmas.

NURSING PROCESS STEP: Implementation

CATEGORY OF CLIENT NEED: Safe, Effective Care Environment

KNOWLEDGE LEVEL: Comprehension

3. ANSWER: 3

RATIONALE: Ethics committees meet to discuss and decide ethical dilemmas with and for the patient with only the concerns and best interest of the patient in mind. These committees do provide structure and guidelines, but function on more than an "as needed" basis.

NURSING PROCESS STEP: Evaluation

CATEGORY OF CLIENT NEED: Safe, Effective Care Environment

KNOWLEDGE LEVEL: Application

Section Six Review

1. ANSWER: 4

RATIONALE: The dying process is an individual experience differing widely from one person to another. Trying to understand the perceptions of each patient assists the health care professional to better serve the patient's and family's specific needs.

NURSING PROCESS STEP: Evaluation

CATEGORY OF CLIENT NEED: Psychosocial Integrity

KNOWLEDGE LEVEL: Application

2. ANSWER: 1

RATIONALE: Open communication is the foundation for the Respectful Death Model as all parties must be willing to discuss the positive and negative aspects of the process. The other options are correct but are secondary to open communication in this model of end-of-life care.

NURSING PROCESS STEP: Implementation

CATEGORY OF CLIENT NEED: Psychosocial Integrity

KNOWLEDGE LEVEL: Analysis

3. ANSWER: 3

RATIONALE: It is imperative for the nurse to spend time reflecting upon and clarifying his or her own values and beliefs about death and dying, as it is these topics that are discussed with the family and patient in the Respectful Death Model. The nurse's feelings about the dying process are discussed with both family and patient and the nurse does not have to have the same religious background as the patient. Opening communication in all aspects forms the foundation of the model, but the nurse must be aware of, and be able to discuss his or her own feelings.

NURSING PROCESS STEP: Planning

CATEGORY OF CLIENT NEED: Psychosocial Integrity

KNOWLEDGE LEVEL: Comprehension

CHAPTER 3

Pretest

1. ANSWER: 3

RATIONALE: As technology in the mid-1970s made it possible to be resuscitated and placed on life support, individuals questioned whether or not they would have the right to refuse such treatment. Courts began hearing cases of individuals and/or families requesting the right to refuse.

NURSING PROCESS STEP: Implementation

CATEGORY OF CLIENT NEED: Safe, Effective Care Environment

KNOWLEDGE LEVEL: Comprehension

2. ANSWER: 1, 2

RATIONALE: A durable power of attorney for health care allows an individual to choose a person to make health care decisions for the patient, should the patient become incompetent to make his or her own decisions and the natural death act also has provisions for the selection of a surrogate decision maker. The Death with Dignity Act is the law in Oregon and Washington State allowing physician-assisted suicide and the Physician Orders for Life-Sustaining Treatment form is most frequently used by emergency medical personnel in the determination of treatments or procedures to be done/not done when the patient is transported from home.

NURSING PROCESS STEP: Implementation

CATEGORY OF CLIENT NEED: Safe, Effective Care Environment

KNOWLEDGE LEVEL: Comprehension

3. **ANSWER:** 1, 3

RATIONALE: Oregon was the first state to allow physician-assisted suicide (PAS), doing so in 1994. In November 2008, Washington State also legalized PAS. The measure did not pass in California.

NURSING PROCESS STEP: Implementation

CATEGORY OF CLIENT NEED: Safe, Effective Care Environment

KNOWLEDGE LEVEL: Knowledge

4. **ANSWER:** 1

RATIONALE: Even after consent has been given, it can be revoked any time prior to the beginning of the treatment or procedure, regardless of whether it was originally written or verbal.

NURSING PROCESS STEP: Implementation

CATEGORY OF CLIENT NEED: Safe, Effective Care Environment

KNOWLEDGE LEVEL: Application

5. **ANSWER:** 4

RATIONALE: When a valid natural death act is in place, it allows the dying person to determine which treatments and/or procedures will be or will not be done at the time of arrest. It also protects the health care worker who follows the natural death act provisions from being found guilty of a criminal or civil crime.

NURSING PROCESS STEP: Implementation

CATEGORY OF CLIENT NEED: Safe, Effective Care Environment

KNOWLEDGE LEVEL: Application

Section One Review

1. **ANSWER:** 1

RATIONALE: The parents of Karen Quinlan were the first to ask the courts' permission allowing their daughter to die. Nancy Cruzan was next, and finally Terri Schiavo. Jack Kevorkian is a physician who helped numerous patients die and was sent to prison after multiple lawsuits were filed.

NURSING PROCESS STEP: Implementation

CATEGORY OF CLIENT NEED: Safe, Effective Care Environment

KNOWLEDGE LEVEL: Knowledge

2. **ANSWER:** 2

RATIONALE: The doctrine of substituted judgment is a subjective determination of how persons, were they capable of making their opinions and wishes known, would have chosen to exercise their right to accept or refuse therapy.

NURSING PROCESS STEP: Implementation

CATEGORY OF CLIENT NEED: Safe, Effective Care Environment

KNOWLEDGE LEVEL: Comprehension

3. **ANSWER:** 4

RATIONALE: Courts must clarify ambiguous statements to assist families, patients, and health care professionals in making decisions and to help protect themselves from lawsuits such as those involving Terri Schiavo, Karen Quinlan, and Nancy Cruzan.

NURSING PROCESS STEP: Planning

CATEGORY OF CLIENT NEED: Safe, Effective Care Environment

KNOWLEDGE LEVEL: Application

Section Two Review

1. **ANSWER:** 2

RATIONALE: The Durable Power of Attorney for Health Care supersedes all other directives, first because it is a Federal law, and second because the person who signs the power of attorney names someone who can make decisions for the patient. It can be relied upon in most circumstances.

NURSING PROCESS STEP: Planning

CATEGORY OF CLIENT NEED: Safe, Effective Care Environment

KNOWLEDGE LEVEL: Knowledge

2. **ANSWER:** 4

RATIONALE: After a person has signed and executed a natural death act, those health care personnel abiding by it cannot be penalized legally.

NURSING PROCESS STEP: Implementation

CATEGORY OF CLIENT NEED: Safe, Effective Care Environment

KNOWLEDGE LEVEL: Application

3. **ANSWER:** 4

RATIONALE: The reason advance directives became more popular was not due to the final requests of competent patients being ignored. It was more to ensure final wishes were known by both family members and health care professionals, and to ensure the legal safety of health care professionals if they follow the final requests.

NURSING PROCESS STEP: Planning

CATEGORY OF CLIENT NEED: Safe, Effective Care Environment

KNOWLEDGE LEVEL: Application

4. **ANSWER:** 1, 2

RATIONALE: The reason durable power of attorney for health care documents are preferred is to provide a better understanding of the patient's wishes. They are state specific.

NURSING PROCESS STEP: Planning

CATEGORY OF CLIENT NEED: Safe, Effective Care Environment

KNOWLEDGE LEVEL: Application

Section Three Review

1. **ANSWER:** 1, 3

   RATIONALE: Respecting Choices and Physician Orders for Life-Sustaining Treatment are both programs in several states in the United States. The other options do not exist.

   NURSING PROCESS STEP: Implementation

   CATEGORY OF CLIENT NEED: Safe, Effective Care Environment

   KNOWLEDGE LEVEL: Knowledge

2. **ANSWER:** 2

   RATIONALE: The Respecting Choices program is an education and role-defining program designed to make health care personnel, family members, and patients more aware of the legal implications of end-of-life decisions. The POLST involves information for not only emergency services personnel, but also other health care settings, making each aware of procedures or life-saving measures accepted or refused by the patient for whom they are transporting or providing care. Both are less complex and easier to implement than advance directive documents.

   NURSING PROCESS STEP: Implementation

   CATEGORY OF CLIENT NEED: Safe, Effective Care Environment

   KNOWLEDGE LEVEL: Analysis

3. **ANSWER:** 4

   RATIONALE: Advance care planning does not constitute advance directives, but is used in many health care settings, including prehospital, to make others aware of preferences for future care. Nurses have a role in assisting patients prepare these documents, as nurses work in all environments. Finally, patients are urged to have both advance care planning and advance directives in place to ensure their wishes are well known, regardless of location in the health care system.

   NURSING PROCESS STEP: Implementation

   CATEGORY OF CLIENT NEED: Safe, Effective Care Environment

   KNOWLEDGE LEVEL: Analysis

Section Four Review

1. **ANSWER:** 2

   RATIONALE: The main reason for obtaining informed consent is to protect patients' rights to choose what is or is not done to or for them. There is no assurance that health care deliverers will not be sued, even if consent is obtained or there is no adverse outcome. Patients are made aware of the Bill of Rights regardless of whether they request or not.

   NURSING PROCESS STEP: Evaluation

   CATEGORY OF CLIENT NEED: Safe, Effective Care Environment

   KNOWLEDGE LEVEL: Application

2. **ANSWER:** 3

   RATIONALE: The goal when making decisions for incompetent patients is an attempt to make decisions as the patient would have wanted. Family members, health care professionals, and any other surrogate decision makers must work together to decide what that decision should be.

   NURSING PROCESS STEP: Planning

   CATEGORY OF CLIENT NEED: Safe, Effective Care Environment

   KNOWLEDGE LEVEL: Application

3. **ANSWER:** 1

   RATIONALE: The standard becoming more accepted when deciding decisional capacity is that each decision must be decided separately. The other options are already standards in use when deciding decisional capacity for patients.

   NURSING PROCESS STEP: Implementation

   CATEGORY OF CLIENT NEED: Safe, Effective Care Environment

   KNOWLEDGE LEVEL: Comprehension

4. **ANSWER:** 2

   RATIONALE: Surrogate decision makers can be appointed by the court, chosen and named by the patient in advance directives, clinically designated family members (spouses first, then adult children), and those family members designated by statute.

   NURSING PROCESS STEP: Implementation

   CATEGORY OF CLIENT NEED: Safe, Effective Care Environment

   KNOWLEDGE LEVEL: Comprehension

5. **ANSWER:** 2, 3, 5

   RATIONALE: The explanation of the procedure or therapy must be complete, including the name and qualifications of those involved, that the patient can refuse it once it is initiated, and palliative care will continue if desired.

   NURSING PROCESS STEP: Implementation

   CATEGORY OF CLIENT NEED: Safe, Effective Care Environment

   KNOWLEDGE LEVEL: Application

Section Five Review

1. **ANSWER:** 3

   RATIONALE: The American Nurses Association believes assisted suicide is unethical, as nurses cannot and should not make life and death decisions. Nurses are patient advocates and cannot assist in causing another's life to end.

   NURSING PROCESS STEP: Implementation

   CATEGORY OF CLIENT NEED: Safe, Effective Care Environment

   KNOWLEDGE LEVEL: Comprehension

2. **ANSWER:** 1

   RATIONALE: They describe the role of nurses in ensuring that all people experience a peaceful death.

NURSING PROCESS STEP: Implementation

CATEGORY OF CLIENT NEED: Physiological Integrity

KNOWLEDGE LEVEL: Comprehension

3. **ANSWER:** 3

   RATIONALE: The Death with Dignity Act in Oregon requires that the patient must know that he or she can change her mind at any moment in the process of the suicide. The patient does not have to be within 6 months of death, but must be a resident of Oregon at the time the request is made.

   NURSING PROCESS STEP: Implementation

   CATEGORY OF CLIENT NEED: Physiological Integrity

   KNOWLEDGE LEVEL: Comprehension

4. **ANSWER:** 1, 2, 3, 6

   RATIONALE: The ethical principles applying to the patient are autonomy and paternalism, as the patient feels he or she has lost autonomy and is being treated paternalistically. The ethical principles applying to the physician, which are in direct conflict, are nonmaleficence and beneficence, as the physician has to decide whether "doing good" means assisting this patient, or "doing no harm" means assisting this patient.

   NURSING PROCESS STEP: Evaluation

   CATEGORY OF CLIENT NEED: Safe, Effective Care Environment

   KNOWLEDGE LEVEL: Analysis

5. **ANSWER:** 4

   RATIONALE: There are four safeguards in place to ensure patients are requesting assistance of their own free will. These are 1) that they are competent to understand their situation completely, including their medical condition and prognosis; 2) that he or she makes the request freely at least twice; 3) that he or she is fully informed of the process; and 4) that he or she acknowledges the right to change his or her mind at any time.

   NURSING PROCESS STEP: Implementation

   CATEGORY OF CLIENT NEED: Safe, Effective Care Environment

   KNOWLEDGE LEVEL: Comprehension

CHAPTER 4

Pretest

1. **ANSWER:** 3

   RATIONALE: When a patient is dying, pain requires comprehensive assessment and interventions. Pain and comfort care become the focus of care at the end of life.

   NURSING PROCESS STEP: Planning

   CATEGORY OF CLIENT NEED: Physiological Integrity

   KNOWLEDGE LEVEL: Application

2. **ANSWER:** 2

   RATIONALE: Vital signs in chronic or end of life pain change and vary in each individual. It is considered a fifth vital sign, but isn't measurable. It doesn't always match the patient's intensity level of pain.

NURSING PROCESS STEP: Assessment

CATEGORY OF CLIENT NEED: Physiological Integrity

KNOWLEDGE LEVEL: Application

3. **ANSWER:** 1, 3, 4

   RATIONALE: Pain at the end of life includes many aspects such as spiritual and psychological care, family's perception and barriers to pain, as well as financial needs should they arise. These aspects can lower pain tolerance. A patient's emotional reactions may also cause stress, which can increase all aspects of pain. Likewise, pain intensity can lead to or exacerbate other conditions. Environmental conditions do not necessarily correlate with pain.

   NURSING PROCESS STEP: Assessment

   CATEGORY OF CLIENT NEED: Physiological Integrity

   KNOWLEDGE LEVEL: Application

4. **ANSWER:** 1

   RATIONALE: Cancer or the underlying disease usually increases the pain experienced at the end of life. Family's presence often will help decrease pain intensity. The inability to swallow and implementing a bowel program do not apply to this question.

   NURSING PROCESS STEP: Assessment

   CATEGORY OF CLIENT NEED: Physiological Integrity

   KNOWLEDGE LEVEL: Application

5. **ANSWER:** 3

   RATIONALE: Finances, age, and culture are some of the barriers to pain control, which may create difficulty in management of pain at the end of life. Treatment modalities, pain scale usage, and medications are not barriers to pain control but are often used to help manage pain.

   NURSING PROCESS STEP: Planning

   CATEGORY OF CLIENT NEED: Physiological Integrity

   KNOWLEDGE LEVEL: Analysis

Section One Review

1. **ANSWER:** 3

   RATIONALE: Pain is a complex phenomenon requiring a comprehensive assessment. Pain is more common as the individual ages; not as common in younger people. Each individual experiences pain differently, thus making assessment of pain more challenging.

   NURSING PROCESS STEP: Assessment

   CATEGORY OF CLIENT NEED: Physiological Integrity

   KNOWLEDGE LEVEL: Application

2. **ANSWER:** 1, 2, 3, 4

   RATIONALE: The nurse must assess the patient at regular time intervals to include a subjective report of pain from the patient, how the patient is eating and sleeping, and what pain goals the patient hopes to achieve. The nurse will also want to assess objective data such as facial expressions, physical movements such as swaying or rocking motions, and nonverbal vocalizations such as grunting or groaning that might also be clues to the presence of pain.

NURSING PROCESS STEP: Assessment

CATEGORY OF CLIENT NEED: Physiological Integrity

KNOWLEDGE LEVEL: Application

3. **ANSWER:** 1, 2, 3

RATIONALE: A patient's pain intensity can be linked to his or her current and past medical history. Comorbidities should be assessed to be certain that the current pain is not related to a treatable comorbidity, to understand if the current pain is different than previous pain, and to manage the current pain appropriately. Helping find a cure for the illness is not related to assessing comorbidities and is not a realistic goal.

NURSING PROCESS STEP: Assessment

CATEGORY OF CLIENT NEED: Physiological Integrity

KNOWLEDGE LEVEL: Synthesis

4. **ANSWER:** 2, 4

RATIONALE: A comprehensive pain scale includes several additional factors beyond the location and intensity of the pain. It includes a physical exam, psychological factors, and duration, aggravating and relieving factors, as well as treatments that may or may not have been effective. Family history and how many times pain is resolved are not factors that play a role in a comprehensive pain assessment.

NURSING PROCESS STEP: Assessment

CATEGORY OF CLIENT NEED: Physiological Integrity

KNOWLEDGE LEVEL: Application

5. **ANSWER:** 1, 3, 4

RATIONALE: A nurse's own comfort level may impact the nurse's assessment of the patient's spiritual, emotional, and psychological aspects due to the nurse's belief system, his or her own fears and anxiety, and prior personal loss.

NURSING PROCESS STEP: Assessment

CATEGORY OF CLIENT NEED: Physiological Integrity

KNOWLEDGE LEVEL: Synthesis

Section Two Review

1. **ANSWER:** 1

RATIONALE: The older adult may have difficulty verbalizing pain. Thus the nurse will base interventions on assessment data such as alteration in mental status. While the nurse will utilize facial expressions and body language to assess for pain, the nurse should not assign a numeric rating to such observations. The nurse also knows that pain is common in the older adult, not uncommon. Pain medication may eventually reach the dosages used for younger adults, but should be started with lower dosages initially, given slowly, and titrated aggressively as needed.

NURSING PROCESS STEP: Implementation

CATEGORY OF CLIENT NEED: Physiological Integrity

KNOWLEDGE LEVEL: Analysis

2. **ANSWER:** 1

RATIONALE: Stoicism is common in some cultures and must be considered as the nurse plans for the patient's care. Not all patients, based upon their cultural practices, will discuss pain. In some cultures, medication is not considered an option for treatment. Language is a barrier when rating or treating pain in patients.

NURSING PROCESS STEP: Planning

CATEGORY OF CLIENT NEED: Health Promotion and Maintenance

KNOWLEDGE LEVEL: Application

3. **ANSWER:** 2

RATIONALE: Since finances and health care costs can be significant barriers to some patients' treatment plans for pain management, one option is to contact pharmaceutical companies that provide for patient assistance programs.

NURSING PROCESS STEP: Implementation

CATEGORY OF CLIENT NEED: Safe, Effective Care Environment

KNOWLEDGE LEVEL: Application

4. **ANSWER:** 1, 2, 3

RATIONALE: Realistic goals for the patient with a history of addiction include setting limits and being consistent. Treating the underlying issues may reduce the chances of a relapse and make pain control more effective. Medications may still be utilized, but limitations and other practices may need to be put into place.

NURSING PROCESS STEP: Planning

CATEGORY OF CLIENT NEED: Psychosocial Integrity

KNOWLEDGE LEVEL: Application

5. **ANSWER:** 3

RATIONALE: As the nurse plans care for the dying child, it is important for the nurse to understand that pain tolerance increases with age, so younger children may experience higher levels of pain. Parent's fear of opioid addiction for the child may need to be addressed. Parents should be consulted regarding the child's pain since the goal of treatment is to treat pain as early as possible. The younger child has the developed systems necessary to experience pain.

NURSING PROCESS STEP: Planning

CATEGORY OF CLIENT NEED: Physiological Integrity

KNOWLEDGE LEVEL: Application

Section Three Review

1. **ANSWER:** 2

RATIONALE: A goal of pain management should be to allow the patient the quality of life and ability to function that the patient desires. The patient should be able to have pain under control without heavy sedation. While family plays a vital role in the care of the patient, it should be the patient who primarily directs the goal of pain management.

NURSING PROCESS STEP: Planning

CATEGORY OF CLIENT NEED: Physiological Integrity

KNOWLEDGE LEVEL: Analysis

2. **ANSWER:** 4

RATIONALE: The patient must understand that continuous pain control medications will be given, with breakthrough pain medications available when needed. Health care professionals should be available whenever the patient has questions, not just during normal working hours. The best pain control comes with managing pain before it becomes unbearable. Pain medications should be available 24/7.

NURSING PROCESS STEP: Implementation

CATEGORY OF CLIENT NEED: Physiological Integrity

KNOWLEDGE LEVEL: Synthesis

3. **ANSWER:** 2, 3, 4

RATIONALE: Chronic, persistent pain creates a management challenge for the terminally ill patient's pain control. However, frequent assessments, frequent interventions—usually medication related, and a systematic, written structured treatment plan will assist in the goal of effective pain management.

NURSING PROCESS STEP: Implementation

CATEGORY OF CLIENT NEED: Physiological Integrity

KNOWLEDGE LEVEL: Synthesis

Section Four Review

1. **ANSWER:** 3

RATIONALE: The WHO Cancer pain relief ladder combines non-opioids, opioids, and adjuvants for pharmacotherapy. The pain relief ladder demonstrates a model for decision making based upon the intensity of pain reported by the patient. It is effective for all types of pain.

NURSING PROCESS STEP: Planning

CATEGORY OF CLIENT NEED: Safe, Effective Care Environment

KNOWLEDGE LEVEL: Analysis

2. **ANSWER:** 1

RATIONALE: To enhance pain management in patients at the end of life, nurses should give appropriate doses in a timely manner. Timed release medications may be used for chronic, as well as ongoing acute pain. Constipation should be anticipated and managed before it becomes an issue. Fentanyl patches are best used for chronic pain management.

NURSING PROCESS STEP: Implementation

CATEGORY OF CLIENT NEED: Physiological Integrity

KNOWLEDGE LEVEL: Analysis

3. **ANSWER:** 2

RATIONALE: Non-opioids can be used for minor pain and often are used effectively in combination with opioids to manage pain. Rebound pain can occur with over-the-counter non-opioids when taking them on a routine basis and then stopping the medication.

NURSING PROCESS STEP: Implementation

CATEGORY OF CLIENT NEED: Physiological Integrity

KNOWLEDGE LEVEL: Application

4. **ANSWER:** 4

RATIONALE: When the nurse is preparing for patient teaching, it is important for the nurse to understand the following: that opioids are the same as narcotics, that all opioids have some risk of addiction, that few people actually have a true allergy to opioids, and while methadone is best known for addiction withdrawal, it is also useful in the management of chronic cancer and neuropathic pain.

NURSING PROCESS STEP: Implementation

CATEGORY OF CLIENT NEED: Physiological Integrity

KNOWLEDGE LEVEL: Analysis

5. **ANSWER:** 3

RATIONALE: Adjuvants are effective when combined with pain medications to treat chronic pain. Adjuvants have been shown to enhance the effects of pain medications and can be prescribed with or without the patient having the condition for which the drug is primarily used.

NURSING PROCESS STEP: Implementation

CATEGORY OF CLIENT NEED: Physiological Integrity

KNOWLEDGE LEVEL: Analysis

6. **ANSWER:** 2

RATIONALE: Propoxyphene and meperidine are considered poor choices for persistent and end-of-life pain due to the buildup of toxic metabolites when used long term.

NURSING PROCESS STEP: Implementation

CATEGORY OF CLIENT NEED: Physiological Integrity

KNOWLEDGE LEVEL: Application

Section Five Review

1. **ANSWER:** 1, 2, 3, 4

RATIONALE: Adjuvant therapies that may be used include pharmacological based, relaxation techniques, rehabilitative approach, and prayer, as well as a host of other options. Adjuvant therapies enhance other pain control measures.

NURSING PROCESS STEP: Implementation

CATEGORY OF CLIENT NEED: Physiological Integrity

KNOWLEDGE LEVEL: Analysis

2. ANSWER: 1

RATIONALE: Before deciding if the adjuvant therapy massage has been effective, the nurse should review the documentation of the patient's response to treatment, as well as utilizing other communication with the patient and health care workers. The intake and output, the family's cultural background, and the patient's medical history play no role in whether massage is an effective adjuvant therapy.

NURSING PROCESS STEP: Evaluation

CATEGORY OF CLIENT NEED: Physiological Integrity

KNOWLEDGE LEVEL: Analysis

3. ANSWER: 1, 3, 4

RATIONALE: Nonpharmacological interventions that might be employed in an effort to relieve pain include surgical intervention, diversion therapy, and deep breathing. Medications are a pharmacological intervention.

NURSING PROCESS STEP: Implementation

CATEGORY OF CLIENT NEED: Physiological Integrity

KNOWLEDGE LEVEL: Analysis

Section Six Review

1. ANSWER: 1

RATIONALE: Poor or inadequate pain control can result in the reduction of the patient's quality of life that impacts them physically, mentally, socially, and spiritually.

NURSING PROCESS STEP: Implementation

CATEGORY OF CLIENT NEED: Physiological Integrity

KNOWLEDGE LEVEL: Application

2. ANSWER: 3

RATIONALE: Pain can have harmful effects on humans that include decreased gastric motility as well as increased anxiety, decreased pulmonary function, and decreased output.

NURSING PROCESS STEP: Planning

CATEGORY OF CLIENT NEED: Physiological Integrity

KNOWLEDGE LEVEL: Application

3. ANSWER: 2

RATIONALE: When providing palliative care, health care professionals should be aware that the intent to relieve pain that might also unintentionally hasten death versus providing medication to deliberately cause death is called double effect.

NURSING PROCESS STEP: Implementation

CATEGORY OF CLIENT NEED: Physiological Integrity

KNOWLEDGE LEVEL: Application

CHAPTER 5

Pretest

1. ANSWER: 3

RATIONALE: Fatigue is reported by more than 90% of patients at the end of life. In cancer-related cases, many patients experience pain (70–90%) at the end of life; however, fatigue is still more common (80–90%). Pain or the underlying disease can cause anorexia and constipation.

NURSING PROCESS STEP: Assessment

CATEGORY OF CLIENT NEED: Psychosocial Integrity

KNOWLEDGE LEVEL: Analysis

2. ANSWER: 2

RATIONALE: Depression, delirium, and anxiety are most often confused. Delirium is an acute confused state in which the incidence increases with age. Sadness, decreased self-worth, and discouragement characterize depression. Anxiety is a feeling of fear and apprehension with or without respiratory distress.

NURSING PROCESS STEP: Planning

CATEGORY OF CLIENT NEED: Psychological Integrity

KNOWLEDGE LEVEL: Analysis

3. ANSWER: 1, 2, 4

RATIONALE: Manifestations of delirium include poor concentration, misinterpretations, rambling incoherent speech, impaired level of consciousness, and impaired short-term memory.

NURSING PROCESS STEP: Diagnosis

CATEGORY OF CLIENT NEED: Psychological Integrity

KNOWLEDGE LEVEL: Application

4. ANSWER: 1

RATIONALE: Nonpharmacological interventions for dyspnea include a fan, cool environment, and diversion. A cool breeze may trigger receptors of the trigeminal nerve that reduce the perception of dyspnea. The fan helps with the perception of air movement and temperature control.

NURSING PROCESS STEP: Implementation

CATEGORY OF CLIENT NEED: Physiological Integrity

KNOWLEDGE LEVEL: Application

5. ANSWER: 1, 2, 3, 4

RATIONALE: The symptoms from renal disease cross into multiple body systems and include hiccups, muscle cramps, infections, and metallic taste in the mouth. Symptoms increase as the disease progresses.

NURSING PROCESS STEP: Assessment

CATEGORY OF CLIENT NEED: Physiological Integrity

KNOWLEDGE LEVEL: Application

Section One Review

1. **ANSWER:** 3

   RATIONALE: Basic nursing care for dyspnea may include elevating the head of the bed or having the patient sit forward in an upright position. Breathing techniques, a fan, raising the head of the bed, relaxation techniques, and medication may also be utilized to treat dyspnea.

   NURSING PROCESS STEP: Implementation

   CATEGORY OF CLIENT NEED: Physiological Integrity

   KNOWLEDGE LEVEL: Application

2. **ANSWER:** 2

   RATIONALE: Comfort alteration is the best choice for this patient with metastatic lung cancer. There is no evidence to support airway clearance impairment or knowledge deficit of his disease process. Alteration in body elimination might also be appropriate due to the constipation. However, increased shortness of air, anorexia, fatigue, insomnia, and constipation would cause alteration in this patient's comfort.

   NURSING PROCESS STEP: Diagnosis

   CATEGORY OF CLIENT NEED: Physiological Integrity

   KNOWLEDGE LEVEL: Synthesis

3. **ANSWER:** 4

   RATIONALE: Offering the patient lukewarm, bland food is a nursing intervention that is more comforting than cold, hot, or textured foods. Water only will not supply enough nutrients.

   NURSING PROCESS STEP: Implementation

   CATEGORY OF CLIENT NEED: Physiological Integrity

   KNOWLEDGE LEVEL: Synthesis

4. **ANSWER:** 1, 2, 3

   RATIONALE: Relief of distressing symptoms, such as pain and odor, wound healing, and prevention of further skin breakdown may all be appropriate goals for this patient depending upon the patient's condition, disease status, and wishes. It is not practical to think you might be able to eliminate the disease process.

   NURSING PROCESS STEP: Planning

   CATEGORY OF CLIENT NEED: Physiological Integrity

   KNOWLEDGE LEVEL: Analysis

Section Two Review

1. **ANSWER:** 1, 2, 4

   RATIONALE: Interventions for end-stage renal disease may include treating the itching, Haldol (haloperidol) for nausea or delirium, and a fan to assist with the dyspnea. Morphine should be avoided in ESRD.

   NURSING PROCESS STEP: Implementation

   CATEGORY OF CLIENT NEED: Physiological Integrity

   KNOWLEDGE LEVEL: Application

2. **ANSWER:** 1

   RATIONALE: Treating the distressing symptoms, for most terminal diseases, yields the greatest benefit for the patient, thereby creating a better quality of life. Distressing symptoms for the patient may include pain, itching, cough, constipation, depression, dry mouth, fatigue, breathlessness, and so on.

   NURSING PROCESS STEP: Implementation

   CATEGORY OF CLIENT NEED: Physiological Integrity

   KNOWLEDGE LEVEL: Analysis

3. **ANSWER:** 1, 3, 4

   RATIONALE: The nurse plays a vital role in patient advocacy, frequent patient assessments, and communication with other health care providers to ensure optimum patient care. While the nurse will assist with activity of daily living tasks for the patient, these tasks may also be assigned to unlicensed personnel or the family and are not vital to optimum patient care.

   NURSING PROCESS STEP: Assessment

   CATEGORY OF CLIENT NEED: Safe, Effective Care Environment

   KNOWLEDGE LEVEL: Application

CHAPTER 6

Pretest

1. **ANSWER:** 3

   RATIONALE: The health care delivery team must work together with the patient and family by presenting impartial and unbiased information (the benefits, risks, and expected outcomes), thereby allowing the patient and family to participate and make decisions in the treatment plan. Even the language used when discussing the benefits and risks can distort a patient's decision. While discussing the treatment options with other health care providers, understanding the basic concepts and options for the patient and discussing the differences between nutrition and hydration options are useful, but alone, these will not allow for working with the client and family.

   NURSING PROCESS STEP: Planning

   CATEGORY OF CLIENT NEED: Safe, Effective Care Environment

   KNOWLEDGE LEVEL: Application

2. **ANSWER:** 1, 2, 3

   RATIONALE: The nurse should support a patient's decision. The nurse may support the decision by reinforcing the risks, benefits, and potential outcomes of their decision, and by advocating for the patient by keeping the physician and other health care providers informed.

   NURSING PROCESS STEP: Planning

   CATEGORY OF CLIENT NEED: Safe, Effective Care Environment

   KNOWLEDGE LEVEL: Analysis

3. **ANSWER:** 1

   RATIONALE: As advances in technology have allowed artificial nutrition and hydration to become a common health care practice, it has also created a dilemma regarding potential benefits versus harm.

   NURSING PROCESS STEP: Planning

   CATEGORY OF CLIENT NEED: Psychosocial Integrity

   KNOWLEDGE LEVEL: Analysis

4. **ANSWER:** 2

   RATIONALE: Artificial hydration and nutrition may become an issue for discussion when treatments are first started to assist with recovery but when the patient's condition changes. It isn't always easy for health care providers or families to recognize when to stop treatment.

   NURSING PROCESS STEP: Planning

   CATEGORY OF CLIENT NEED: Psychosocial Integrity

   KNOWLEDGE LEVEL: Application

5. **ANSWER:** 1

   RATIONALE: Because many societies intertwine food with cultural rituals, health care providers, particularly nurses, may have difficulty separating the concept of nurturing from the idea of providing nutrition. Nurses relate feeding as part of basic nursing care.

   NURSING PROCESS STEP: Assessment

   CATEGORY OF CLIENT NEED: Safe, Effective Care Environment

   KNOWLEDGE LEVEL: Synthesis

Section One Review

1. **ANSWER:** 3

   RATIONALE: The goals for intake and socialization may be separate. Socialization often includes settings where food is the central theme. Intake involves the goal of nourishment. Many times individuals overlook that separate goals exist—eating and drinking for nourishment versus eating and drinking for socialization.

   NURSING PROCESS STEP: Assessment

   CATEGORY OF CLIENT NEED: Psychosocial Integrity

   KNOWLEDGE LEVEL: Synthesis

2. **ANSWER:** 1

   RATIONALE: Advances in technology have allowed artificial nutrition and hydration to become a common health care practice, while also creating difficult and, at times, uncomfortable choices for patients and families.

   NURSING PROCESS STEP: Planning

   CATEGORY OF CLIENT NEED: Safe, Effective Care Environment

   KNOWLEDGE LEVEL: Application

3. **ANSWER:** 4

   RATIONALE: The current aging population has more chronic health problems that will likely increase the frequency with which artificial hydration or nutrition is offered. Patients should be part of any discussion regarding their health care, especially the risks, benefits, and expected outcomes of artificial hydration and nutrition.

   NURSING PROCESS STEP: Assessment

   CATEGORY OF CLIENT NEED: Safe

   KNOWLEDGE LEVEL: Knowledge

4. **ANSWER:** 3

   RATIONALE: When a person's health is failing, natural anorexia and loss of appetite are common. The loss of appetite is frequently distressing for families. As organs decrease or cease their normal functioning, a patient's physical needs become less and natural dehydration may be more comfortable for the patient.

   NURSING PROCESS STEP: Planning

   CATEGORY OF CLIENT NEED: Psychosocial Integrity

   KNOWLEDGE LEVEL: Synthesis

5. **ANSWER:** 2

   RATIONALE: A swallow study is commonly used to evaluate dysphagia. It is often hard for the family to accept dysphagia. Survival and outcomes with long-term use of feeding tubes, according to data, is generally pretty poor.

   NURSING PROCESS STEP: Assessment

   CATEGORY OF CLIENT NEED: Psychosocial Integrity

   KNOWLEDGE LEVEL: Synthesis

Section Two Review

1. **ANSWER:** 2

   RATIONALE: Treatment options such as artificial hydration and nutrition can be viewed as medical procedures since patients do not chew, swallow, or taste with artificial nutrition and hydration. Therefore, the natural intake of nutrition and hydration allows patients control over the consumption of their intake.

   NURSING PROCESS STEP: Assessment

   CATEGORY OF CLIENT NEED: Psychosocial Integrity

   KNOWLEDGE LEVEL: Analysis

2. **ANSWER:** 1

   RATIONALE: A patient's refusal of food and drink is a sign of the last phase of a terminal condition. The decrease of appetite and intake decreases nausea and vomiting for many patients, as well as fewer complaints of hunger. There is no evidence to support that a diminishing appetite and decreased thirst increases pain or a painful death.

   NURSING PROCESS STEP: Evaluation

   CATEGORY OF CLIENT NEED: Psychosocial Integrity

   KNOWLEDGE LEVEL: Evaluation

3. **ANSWER:** 2

   RATIONALE: Other symptoms, such as headache, nausea and vomiting, abdominal cramps, and delirium, do not usually accompany end-stage dehydration as they do with dehydration from other causes. Dehydration of any type can often be improved with IV fluids, even if it is short term. Xerostomia may have several other causes besides dehydration.

   NURSING PROCESS STEP: Evaluation

   CATEGORY OF CLIENT NEED: Physiological Integrity

   KNOWLEDGE LEVEL: Analysis

4. **ANSWER:** 4

   RATIONALE: The patient who would benefit the most from artificial nutrition and hydration is the patient with a short-term condition who has the ability to recover from the disease process. The patient with tongue cancer can continue with natural nutrition and hydration once the tongue is healed from the surgery. The stroke patient, end-stage renal patient, and the stomach cancer patient all have illnesses that may benefit from artificial nutrition and hydration but are not short-term conditions.

   NURSING PROCESS STEP: Evaluation

   CATEGORY OF CLIENT NEED: Physiological Integrity

   KNOWLEDGE LEVEL: Analysis

5. **ANSWER:** Xerostomia

   RATIONALE: Xerostomia, dry mouth, can be treated with offering the patient popsicles, ice chips, mouth swabs, lemon or peppermint drops, and sports gum.

   NURSING PROCESS STEP: Implementation

   CATEGORY OF CLIENT NEED: Physiological Integrity

   KNOWLEDGE LEVEL: Application

Section Three Review

1. **ANSWER:** 3

   RATIONALE: A time-limited trial of artificial nutrition or hydration is ethical and legal and may have different results for different individual patients. While there may be a designated end point for reassessment and evaluation, it is not required. There are no set protocols that are followed for each eligible patient since this is a very individualized matter.

   NURSING PROCESS STEP: Implementation

   CATEGORY OF CLIENT NEED: Physiological Integrity

   KNOWLEDGE LEVEL: Application

2. **ANSWER:** Goals

   RATIONALE: Health care providers need to be informed regarding the patient's health care goals so that treatment options can be tailored to meet those goals. The provider should discuss with the patient and family how artificial nutrition and hydration would support or hinder the patient's goals.

   NURSING PROCESS STEP: Planning

   CATEGORY OF CLIENT NEED: Safe, Effective Care Environment

   KNOWLEDGE LEVEL: Application

3. **ANSWER:** 1, 2

   RATIONALE: If the patient makes the decision to refuse nutrition and hydration, health care providers should ensure that the patient is not suffering from depression or inadequate pain control. If these conditions are absent or managed effectively, the health care providers need to support the patient's decision by discussing the patient's decision with the family and providing them with support. Asking for a different nursing assignment is not an appropriate option in most cases. The family does not necessarily need to leave the patient alone to rest based upon the patient's decision to stop nutrition and hydration.

   NURSING PROCESS STEP: Implementation

   CATEGORY OF CLIENT NEED: Safe, Effective Care Environment

   KNOWLEDGE LEVEL: Analysis

4. **ANSWER:** 1

   RATIONALE: When determining if artificial nutrition and hydration are appropriate for the patient, the patient's underlying belief system should be taken into consideration. The patient's education and family history play no role in whether artificial nutrition and hydration would be an appropriate choice for the patient. Withdrawing treatment is appropriate in most instances when there is no reason to continue it.

   NURSING PROCESS STEP: Planning

   CATEGORY OF CLIENT NEED: Physiological Integrity

   KNOWLEDGE LEVEL: Application

CHAPTER 7

Pretest

1. **ANSWER:** 2

   RATIONALE: Open communication, listening to the expressions of grieving, and assistance with the grieving process by health care workers are among the greatest benefits for the grieving family.

   NURSING PROCESS STEP: Planning

   CATEGORY OF CLIENT NEED: Psychosocial Integrity

   KNOWLEDGE LEVEL: Application

2. **ANSWER:** 3

   RATIONALE: Patients in the last hours of their lives require more skilled nursing care in settings that respect the privacy needs of the person. These settings may include acute care facilities or the home. While it is important to consider the ease of care for the caregivers, the patient's needs will take a higher priority.

   NURSING PROCESS STEP: Planning

   CATEGORY OF CLIENT NEED: Safe, Effective Care Environment

   KNOWLEDGE LEVEL: Application

3. **ANSWER:** 3

   RATIONALE: The best interest standard of decision making should be the standard for making decisions for neonates. This model requires acting for another's good, irrespective of the parents' wishes or desires. Putting the parents' needs first, or what they see as best for the child, is the paternalistic model for decision making.

NURSING PROCESS STEP: Planning

CATEGORY OF CLIENT NEED: Psychosocial Integrity

KNOWLEDGE LEVEL: Application

4. **ANSWER:** 1, 2, 3

RATIONALE: Parents who have a dying child need someone to listen to their thoughts and concerns, information about the child's illness, prognosis, and treatment plans, and outside help when they are not available. They do not need assistance with making decisions, but rather require adequate information from health care workers to make their own informed decisions.

NURSING PROCESS STEP: Implementation

CATEGORY OF CLIENT NEED: Safe, Effective Care Environment

KNOWLEDGE LEVEL: Analysis

5. **ANSWER:** 3

RATIONALE: Denial often lasts longer in the terminally ill young adult because the adult does not anticipate death and therefore is left unprepared to handle the subsequent processes.

NURSING PROCESS STEP: Assessment

CATEGORY OF CLIENT NEED: Psychosocial Integrity

KNOWLEDGE LEVEL: Application

Section One Review

1. **ANSWER:** 1

RATIONALE: Over the last century, health care has shifted from Americans dying at ages of less than 50 years old due to acute illnesses to Americans dying at ages greater than 77 years old from slower, more lingering chronic illnesses. The health care provided has gone from families providing care at home to, currently, providing care in an acute care setting with paid caregivers.

NURSING PROCESS STEP: Assessment

CATEGORY OF CLIENT NEED: Safe, Effective Care Environment

KNOWLEDGE LEVEL: Analysis

2. **ANSWER:** 2

RATIONALE: Although the definition of family has changed over the last century, the importance of the family in the patient's care has not changed. The loss of a family member continues to be a very personal and traumatic event and needs to be a consideration for the nursing care. While the family member may assist with care when the nurse is unavailable, this potentially could be true of friends as well. The other options are not pertinent to the question.

NURSING PROCESS STEP: Assessment

CATEGORY OF CLIENT NEED: Safe, Effective Care Environment

KNOWLEDGE LEVEL: Analysis

3. **ANSWER:** 4

RATIONALE: When the nurse is assessing the family dynamics, respect for each other, honesty in discussing difficult topics, and setting mutual goals are characteristics of healthy communication patterns among family members that might be observed. All family members present and discussing the patient's care, with one person talking at a time would demonstrate respect for what each has to say, as well as attempting to understand other's points of view. Everyone talking at once, talking negatively about other family members, and arguing about care with the patient do not demonstrate respect or honesty.

NURSING PROCESS STEP: Assessment

CATEGORY OF CLIENT NEED: Safe, Effective Care Environment

KNOWLEDGE LEVEL: Application

Section Two Review

1. **ANSWER:** 2

RATIONALE: Adolescence is the stage of identity versus role confusion. The person begins to develop self-esteem during this developmental period. Should the adolescent be unable to fully complete this stage of role development and self-identity, there is a potential for role confusion later in life.

NURSING PROCESS STEP: Assessment

CATEGORY OF CLIENT NEED: Health Promotion and Maintenance

KNOWLEDGE LEVEL: Synthesis

2. **ANSWER:** 1

RATIONALE: Trust develops in infancy as the parent or caregiver provides close contact and care for the infant. This stage in infancy is called trust versus mistrust according to Erickson.

NURSING PROCESS STEP: Assessment

CATEGORY OF CLIENT NEED: Health Promotion and Maintenance

KNOWLEDGE LEVEL: Application

3. **ANSWER:** 4

RATIONALE: The school-age child develops more social skills and begins to rely more on friends than on close family ties. This is the developmental stage (according to Erickson) of industry versus inferiority, and unsuccessful completion of this stage could result in feelings of incompetence and low self-esteem later in life.

NURSING PROCESS STEP: Assessment

CATEGORY OF CLIENT NEED: Health Promotion and Maintenance

KNOWLEDGE LEVEL: Application

4. **ANSWER:** 1, 2, 4

RATIONALE: An understanding of the developmental stages of the person assists the nurse in having a fuller appreciation for the emotions that the person and family may be experiencing, as well as assist the nurse in planning nursing interventions. An understanding of developmental stages is important among all health care providers, but doesn't, in itself, create better communication between health care providers.

NURSING PROCESS STEP: Implementation

CATEGORY OF CLIENT NEED: Psychosocial Integrity

KNOWLEDGE LEVEL: Application

Section Three Review

1. **ANSWER:** 4

   RATIONALE: The nurse will want to educate the family of a 2-year-old child, who is in the early childhood stage of development, on continuing familiar routines and utilizing simple explanations. The 2-year-old child is developing a sense of autonomy and is very dependent upon the family. A 2-year-old is likely to have occasional temper tantrums as part of normal development and not related to the grieving process. An earlier bedtime will be of no help, and may serve to accentuate issues for the child, particularly for the mid-childhood and school-age child, since they are more likely to grieve when they are alone. The 2-year-old child will not utilize peers as part of his or her developmental process.

   NURSING PROCESS STEP: Implementation

   CATEGORY OF CLIENT NEED: Psychosocial Integrity

   KNOWLEDGE LEVEL: Synthesis

2. **ANSWER:** 2

   RATIONALE: The mid-childhood–stage children are most likely to exhibit fears and regression in normal development, especially when losing a parent to violence. Family members need to be reassured that this is common during this developmental stage as a product of grief.

   NURSING PROCESS STEP: Assessment

   CATEGORY OF CLIENT NEED: Psychosocial Integrity

   KNOWLEDGE LEVEL: Analysis

3. **ANFSWER:** 1, 2, 3, 4

   RATIONALE: Palliative care includes comfort care, end of life decision making, and bereavement support. Pain control, emotional support, reassurance to the family regarding withdrawal of life support measures, and follow-up care for families are all considered palliative care.

   NURSING PROCESS STEP: Implementation

   CATEGORY OF CLIENT NEED: Psychosocial Integrity

   KNOWLEDGE LEVEL: Analysis

4. **ANSWER:** 2

   RATIONALE: A possible nursing diagnosis for this situation might be compromised family coping since the otherwise supportive family has just been told about the terminal stage for the young patient. Failure to thrive, disturbed thought process, and knowledge deficit do not apply to this situation since the issues are about coping with the grieving process. Besides the care for the patient, support for the family must be included.

   NURSING PROCESS STEP: Diagnosis

   CATEGORY OF CLIENT NEED: Health Promotion and Maintenance

   KNOWLEDGE LEVEL: Analysis

Section Four Review

1. **ANSWER:** 1

   RATIONALE: The nurse can anticipate the need to assist the family with acceptance and closure of the young adult's death since these deaths are usually sudden and unanticipated and often extend the grieving process. Frequently there is a desire to blame someone for the death. It is not helpful to the family or health care provider to encourage discussions on who is to blame. Encouraging health promotion is often not necessary in this age group, as the young adult is frequently very active. Rarely has the family already come to terms with the death, thus requiring, not forgoing, bereavement measures.

   NURSING PROCESS STEP: Implementation

   CATEGORY OF CLIENT NEED: Psychosocial Integrity

   KNOWLEDGE LEVEL: Application

2. **ANSWER:** 3

   RATIONALE: The death of a young adult is often difficult for health care providers to overcome because young people are not supposed to die. Health care providers can see themselves in similar situations as a family member.

   NURSING PROCESS STEP: Assessment

   CATEGORY OF CLIENT NEED: Psychosocial Integrity

   KNOWLEDGE LEVEL: Application

3. **ANSWER:** 2

   RATIONALE: One's peer group may avoid contact with the dying younger adult because they are closest in age to the dying younger adult and feel threatened by this person's death as their own mortality comes into question. They may not know how to express sympathy, may have busy lives, and may fail to appreciate the severity of the diagnosis, but none of those options is the primary reason for avoiding contact.

   NURSING PROCESS STEP: Assessment

   CATEGORY OF CLIENT NEED: Psychosocial Integrity

   KNOWLEDGE LEVEL: Application

4. **ANSWER:** 1

   RATIONALE: Bereavement measures may be the most important aspect of palliative care with a young adult because these deaths may be sudden, and frequently family members are first approached after the person has died.

   NURSING PROCESS STEP: Implementation

   CATEGORY OF CLIENT NEED: Psychosocial Integrity

   KNOWLEDGE LEVEL: Application

Section Five Review

1. **ANSWER:** 1, 3, 4

   RATIONALE: During the initial assessment, the nurse will want to assess for the presence of other chronic illnesses/comorbidities, the presence of potential family caregivers, and any financial concerns the mid-adulthood and late adulthood terminally ill patient might have. The developmental stage, not particularly the exact age, of the patient is relevant to the nursing history. The patient's age can be obtained in other ways.

NURSING PROCESS STEP: Assessment

CATEGORY OF CLIENT NEED: Physiological Integrity

KNOWLEDGE LEVEL: Analysis

2. **ANSWER:** 3

RATIONALE: The mid-adulthood and late adulthood terminally ill patient and family will need to be able to recognize symptoms that are related to chronic illnesses, and thus treatable, versus expected symptoms that are related to the terminal illness.

NURSING PROCESS STEP: Implementation

CATEGORY OF CLIENT NEED: Physiological Integrity

KNOWLEDGE LEVEL: Analysis

3. **ANSWER:** 1, 3

RATIONALE: Barriers to planning care for the mid-adulthood, terminally ill patient include the potential for no family being available to assist with care since this age group often has children who have other obligations, parents who are elderly with their own health problems, and spouses who are still employed in demanding careers. The family also desires the patient to be hospitalized, while the terminally ill patient prefers to be at home for care. The patient's desire for realistic information regarding his or her disease and request for financial support are not barriers to care, but rather information that can be utilized as part of the plan of care.

NURSING PROCESS STEP: Planning

CATEGORY OF CLIENT NEED: Psychological Integrity

KNOWLEDGE LEVEL: Synthesis

4. **ANSWER:** 3

RATIONALE: Because of the patient in the late adulthood developmental stage reflecting upon life accomplishments and declining peer group, this patient is at higher risk for depression if the patient has a sense of failure. Suicide is more common in the young adult developmental stage. Cancer and skin disorders, while more prevalent in the older adult, can happen at any point and are not related to the associated developmental tasks.

NURSING PROCESS STEP: Assessment

CATEGORY OF CLIENT NEED: Health Promotion and Maintenance

KNOWLEDGE LEVEL: Application

Section Six Review

1. **ANSWER:** 1

RATIONALE: According to recent research, patients are increasingly asking questions about the progression of their illness and what they might expect. These questions are more holistic in nature and not focused on themselves directly, but on the impact their lives have had overall.

NURSING PROCESS STEP: Implementation

CATEGORY OF CLIENT NEED: Health Promotion and Maintenance

KNOWLEDGE LEVEL: Analysis

2. **ANSWER:** 3

RATIONALE: Recent research indicates terminally ill patients want to leave lasting memories with their families upon their death. While family discussions and a family portrait have some meaning, a videotape provides the impression of a face-to-face conversation for those left after the patient's death. A will is impersonal and only distributes keepsakes to family members.

NURSING PROCESS STEP: Implementation

CATEGORY OF CLIENT NEED: Health Promotion and Maintenance

KNOWLEDGE LEVEL: Application

CHAPTER 8

Pretest

1. **ANSWER:** 1

RATIONALE: Loss of a patient, particularly one that a nurse has developed a close relationship with, should be considered a significant loss and the nurse will likely experience the grieving process. Avoiding contact with the family, trying not to think about the death, and crying only when alone do not foster a healthy approach for dealing with loss.

NURSING PROCESS STEP: Planning

CATEGORY OF CLIENT NEED: Psychosocial Integrity

KNOWLEDGE LEVEL: Application

2. **ANSWER:** 3

RATIONALE: Communication regarding end-of-life issues is best supported by a trusting relationship with ample opportunity for assessment of needs and time for open communication. Nurses do not necessarily receive the best communication training of all health disciplines, nurses are not required to be the sole source of end-of-life information, and this is not advocated by nurse practice acts.

NURSING PROCESS STEP: Implementation

CATEGORY OF CLIENT NEED: Psychosocial Integrity

KNOWLEDGE LEVEL: Application

3. **ANSWER:** 1, 3, 4

RATIONALE: Examining coping abilities, evaluating the support system, and seeking professional help are all appropriate actions for burn out. Discussing burnout with patients and families is inappropriate and unprofessional.

NURSING PROCESS STEP: Evaluation

CATEGORY OF CLIENT NEED: Psychosocial Integrity

KNOWLEDGE LEVEL: Application

4. **ANSWER:** 2, 3, 4

   RATIONALE: Informed decision making, economic benefits, and decreased anxiety for patients and families are all benefits of open communication with the health care team. Open communication does not increase staff independence in decision making, but facilitates collaboration.

   NURSING PROCESS STEP: Implementation

   CATEGORY OF CLIENT NEED: Psychosocial Integrity

   KNOWLEDGE LEVEL: Application

Section One Review

1. **ANSWER:** 4

   RATIONALE: Identifying the need, desiring improvement, and taking action are the first steps in fulfilling a learning need and improving practice. Referring communication issues to others and scripting will not give the nurse the opportunity to improve practice. Asking patients and families for tips will only provide opinions specific to their need, not a general framework for therapeutic communication.

   NURSING PROCESS STEP: Planning

   CATEGORY OF CLIENT NEED: Psychosocial Integrity

   KNOWLEDGE LEVEL: Application

2. **ANSWER:** 1

   RATIONALE: If nurses demonstrate distancing from patients and families experiencing loss, it may be a reflection of their own unmet needs regarding mortality or support. The nurse's concern may initiate self-reflection about her beliefs and needs. Facilitating more interactions, transferring the nurse, or taking a class may be next steps, after further assessment of the underlying issue.

   NURSING PROCESS STEP: Evaluation

   CATEGORY OF CLIENT NEED: Psychosocial Integrity

   KNOWLEDGE LEVEL: Analysis

3. **ANSWER:** 3

   RATIONALE: It is of utmost importance that the nurse providing end-of-life care also receives the support needed to deal with the emotional impact of loss and grief. Changing exercise and eating habits, meeting with the supervisor, and taking a leave of absence may be necessary at some point.

   NURSING PROCESS STEP: Evaluation

   CATEGORY OF CLIENT NEED: Psychosocial Integrity

   KNOWLEDGE LEVEL: Analysis

Section Two Review

1. **ANSWER:** 1, 2, 3

   RATIONALE: Meetings, active listening, and assessing level of understanding all promote open, supportive exchange of information. Referring the family to the nurse manager inhibits open and supportive communication with the nurses and may further isolate and frustrate the family.

   NURSING PROCESS STEP: Planning

   CATEGORY OF CLIENT NEED: Psychosocial Integrity

   KNOWLEDGE LEVEL: Analysis

2. **ANSWER:** 3

   RATIONALE: Open communication will promote better overall planning and care. Patients may want to change advance directives at any time. The other options do not support open communication throughout the period of care.

   NURSING PROCESS STEP: Planning

   CATEGORY OF CLIENT NEED: Psychosocial Integrity

   KNOWLEDGE LEVEL: Application

3. **ANSWER:** 1, 2, 4

   RATIONALE: Actively listening, asking open-ended questions, assessing knowledge level, and offering a family conference demonstrate support and allow for informed decision making. Lack of support from the family does not permit the nurse to alter from the patient's wishes.

   NURSING PROCESS STEP: Implementation

   CATEGORY OF CLIENT NEED: Psychosocial Integrity

   KNOWLEDGE LEVEL: Analysis

4. **ANSWER:** 1, 2, 3, 4

   RATIONALE: Communication is a priority in end-of-life care. Therapeutic communication includes active listening and supportive body language. Nurses also should know that patients may change the plan of care at any point.

   NURSING PROCESS STEP: Evaluation

   CATEGORY OF CLIENT NEED: Psychosocial Integrity

   KNOWLEDGE LEVEL: Analysis

Section Three Review

1. **ANSWER:** 1, 2, 3

   RATIONALE: Storytelling helps keep the memory of the patient alive, allows the family to share the patient's story, and helps build respect and trust. Storytelling does not isolate the family.

   NURSING PROCESS STEP: Planning

   CATEGORY OF CLIENT NEED: Psychosocial Integrity

   KNOWLEDGE LEVEL: Application

2. **ANSWER:** 3

   RATIONALE: Storytelling serves as a distraction for some patients. It would be presumptuous to assume that the patient is taking more medication than needed or that the nurses are not meeting pain control needs, or that there is inaccurate documentation, if the patient's pain assessments are accurate.

NURSING PROCESS STEP: Evaluation

CATEGORY OF CLIENT NEED: Psychosocial Integrity

KNOWLEDGE LEVEL: Analysis

3. **ANSWER:** 2

   RATIONALE: This is honest and open communication, and lets the family and patient hear that the nurse has a genuine interest in the patient, but must also prioritize care. Saying that the story can be told another time, advising the family to talk about the trip without the nurse, and saying there are more important things to discuss do not foster therapeutic communication or value storytelling.

   NURSING PROCESS STEP: Implementation

   CATEGORY OF CLIENT NEED: Psychosocial Integrity

   KNOWLEDGE LEVEL: Application

4. **ANSWER:** 4

   RATIONALE: This response is supportive and provides factual information about storytelling. The other statements do not facilitate therapeutic communication and are not the best response to support storytelling.

   NURSING PROCESS STEP: Implementation

   CATEGORY OF CLIENT NEED: Psychosocial Integrity

   KNOWLEDGE LEVEL: Analysis

CHAPTER 9

Pretest

1. **ANSWER:** 1, 2, 3

   RATIONALE: The nurse should clean and position the body, remove medical equipment from the room, and provide a quiet environment to view the body. Lines and tubes should not be removed in cases for which an autopsy will be performed.

   NURSING PROCESS STEP: Implementation

   CATEGORY OF CLIENT NEED: Psychosocial Integrity

   KNOWLEDGE LEVEL: Application

2. **ANSWER:** 3

   RATIONALE: Positive coping minimizes additional stressors for the patient and the family, but it will not eliminate stressors, anger, or psychosocial issues.

   NURSING PROCESS STEP: Evaluation

   CATEGORY OF CLIENT NEED: Psychosocial Integrity

   KNOWLEDGE LEVEL: Application

3. **ANSWER:** 4

   RATIONALE: Nurses have varying levels of expertise and should counsel within their professional ability, recognizing that there are situations that are better addressed by other professionals.

NURSING PROCESS STEP: Implementation

CATEGORY OF CLIENT NEED: Psychosocial Integrity

KNOWLEDGE LEVEL: Application

Section One Review

1. **ANSWER:** 4

   RATIONALE: The changes that the death of a loved one brings to a family will create a new sense of normalcy.

   NURSING PROCESS STEP: Assessment

   CATEGORY OF CLIENT NEED: Psychosocial

   KNOWLEDGE LEVEL: Knowledge

2. **ANSWER:** 3

   RATIONALE: The patient's safety is the nurse's priority. Addressing the negative coping mechanism in a therapeutic manner may assist getting the son the help he needs to better cope with his mother's death and promote the maintenance of that relationship.

   NURSING PROCESS STEP: Implementation

   CATEGORY OF CLIENT NEED: Psychosocial Integrity

   KNOWLEDGE LEVEL: Application

3. **ANSWER:** 3

   RATIONALE: Expressing sympathy and inquiring about the family's well-being allows for open discussion and an opportunity to assist if needed. Explaining that the parent is young enough to have another child, stating that a support group will know how she feels, or avoiding the discussion do not facilitate therapeutic communication or demonstrate empathy.

   NURSING PROCESS STEP: Implementation

   CATEGORY OF CLIENT NEED: Psychosocial Integrity

   KNOWLEDGE LEVEL: Application

Section Two Review

1. **ANSWER:** 1

   RATIONALE: The issue at hand is that the caregiver may be consumed with the needs of his wife and neglecting himself. Assessing the situation and making appropriate referrals is indicated. Assuming that the wife needs to be admitted to a facility, sending the husband home, and calling the adult children do not directly address the issue.

   NURSING PROCESS STEP: Implementation

   CATEGORY OF CLIENT NEED: Psychosocial

   KNOWLEDGE LEVEL: Analysis

2. **ANSWER:** 2

   RATIONALE: Talking directly to the nurse and pointing out the observed change in behaviors deals directly with the issue and may assist the nurse in realizing the change in her behaviors. Reporting it to the manager, asking the chaplain to talk with the nurse, and avoiding terminal patients may be steps to take in the future if the nurse is aware of the behavior and is unable to change the behavior.

NURSING PROCESS STEP: Implementation

CATEGORY OF CLIENT NEED: Psychosocial

KNOWLEDGE LEVEL: Application

3. **ANSWER:** 1, 2, 4

    RATIONALE: Children may feel guilty and believe that illness is a punishment for something they have done, may fear the separation from their parents, and may have siblings who feel isolated and unimportant. The nurse should explore these possibilities with the child. The nurse should try to build a therapeutic relationship with the child, and not assume he will only talk to his parents.

    NURSING PROCESS STEP: Evaluation

    CATEGORY OF CLIENT NEED: Psychosocial

    KNOWLEDGE LEVEL: Application

4. **ANSWER:** 4

    RATIONALE: The primary focus of care is the patient's best interests. The life partner should be involved as the patient desires, and treated as an equal significant other.

    NURSING PROCESS STEP: Implementation

    CATEGORY OF CLIENT NEED: Psychosocial Integrity

    KNOWLEDGE LEVEL: Application

CHAPTER 10

Pretest

1. **ANSWER:** 1, 2, 3, 4

    RATIONALE: Communication, resources, knowledge about culture, and collaborating for care planning are all part of providing care for a patient with an unfamiliar culture.

    NURSING PROCESS STEP: Planning

    CATEGORY OF CLIENT NEED: Psychosocial Integrity

    KNOWLEDGE LEVEL: Application

2. **ANSWER:** 3

    RATIONALE: Reading about culture, letting go of personal beliefs and opinions, and watching documentaries do not ensure that a nurse is culturally competent. Providing culturally sensitive care and learning about cultures with which the nurse has frequent contact, is the best way to become competent.

    NURSING PROCESS STEP: Planning

    CATEGORY OF CLIENT NEED: Psychosocial Integrity

    KNOWLEDGE LEVEL: Application

3. **ANSWER:** 4

    RATIONALE: The entire health care team is responsible for providing spiritual care at the end of life. No one is solely responsible—not the patient's pastor and family, not the chaplain, and not the nurse.

    NURSING PROCESS STEP: Planning

    CATEGORY OF CLIENT NEED: Psychosocial Integrity

    KNOWLEDGE LEVEL: Application

4. **ANSWER:** 1, 2, 3, 4

    RATIONALE: It is the nurse's responsibility to identify spiritual needs through assessment, provide appropriate interventions, make referrals, and prioritize spiritual needs at the end of life.

    NURSING PROCESS STEP: Planning

    CATEGORY OF CLIENT NEED: Psychosocial Integrity

    KNOWLEDGE LEVEL: Application

5. **ANSWER:** 3

    RATIONALE: Self-awareness of spiritual beliefs provides a solid foundation from which to offer spiritual care to others; it does not provide the ability to say the right things to a patient, ensure that the patient's belief system is correct, or prevent referrals.

    NURSING PROCESS STEP: Planning

    CATEGORY OF CLIENT NEED: Psychosocial Integrity

    KNOWLEDGE LEVEL: Application

Section One Review

1. **ANSWER:** 1, 2, 3

    RATIONALE: The nurse should provide communication means, an interpreter or other resources, and should attempt to learn about a culture; the nurse should not expect the patient and family to thoroughly explain cultural practices and preferences without assessment.

    NURSING PROCESS STEP: Implementation

    CATEGORY OF CLIENT NEED: Psychosocial Integrity

    KNOWLEDGE LEVEL: Application

2. **ANSWER:** 3

    RATIONALE: Reading about culture, letting go of personal beliefs and opinions, and watching documentaries do not ensure that a nurse is culturally competent. Providing culturally sensitive care and learning about cultures with which the nurse has frequent contact is the best way to become competent.

    NURSING PROCESS STEP: Planning

    CATEGORY OF CLIENT NEED: Psychosocial Integrity

    KNOWLEDGE LEVEL: Application

3. **ANSWER:** 3

    RATIONALE: Explaining the medication with pictures and hand gestures does not ensure the patient understands the content. Nodding may be a cultural means of showing respect and may not indicate understanding. The patient's school-age child is not the best means to provide information, in case there is a misunderstanding of content. An expert interpreter is the most reliable means to provide education and evaluate understanding.

NURSING PROCESS STEP: Planning

CATEGORY OF CLIENT NEED: Safe, Effective Care Environment

KNOWLEDGE LEVEL: Application

4. **ANSWER:** 1, 2, 3

   RATIONALE: Culturally competent care is within the nurse's scope and the nurse should serve as advocate, facilitator, and as a resource person.

   NURSING PROCESS STEP: Implementation

   CATEGORY OF CLIENT NEED: Psychosocial Integrity

   KNOWLEDGE LEVEL: Application

5. **ANSWER:** 3

   RATIONALE: Exploring other possibilities for a bed for the incoming patient allows the family to practice important cultural practices. Moving the patient's body to the end of the hall does not allow for privacy. Limiting the time with the patient does not allow for the cultural practice to be done in its entirety. Encouraging the family to go home is not a culturally sensitive response by the nurse.

   NURSING PROCESS STEP: Implementation

   CATEGORY OF CLIENT NEED: Psychosocial Integrity

   KNOWLEDGE LEVEL: Analysis

Section Two Review

1. **ANSWER:** 1

   RATIONALE: Spiritual issues do become more important as the end of life nears. One should not assume that the patient was not honest upon admission, that he believes the chaplain can save his life, or that he is unhappy with the care the nurse has provided.

   NURSING PROCESS STEP: Implementation

   CATEGORY OF CLIENT NEED: Psychosocial Integrity

   KNOWLEDGE LEVEL: Analysis

2. **ANSWER:** 2

   RATIONALE: Completing a spiritual self-assessment is the best way to explore one's own spiritual beliefs. Assigning a particularly challenging patient, arranging for an in-service presentation, and visiting churches in the community are not the best ways to explore personal spiritual beliefs and values, compared to answering the questions on a spiritual assessment, which are designed to do so.

   NURSING PROCESS STEP: Assessment

   CATEGORY OF CLIENT NEED: Psychosocial Integrity

   KNOWLEDGE LEVEL: Application

3. **ANSWER:** 1, 2, 3, 4

   RATIONALE: Prayer supports the holistic approach to patient care, is a patient right, and can be a source of strength and coping for the patient.

   NURSING PROCESS STEP: Implementation

   CATEGORY OF CLIENT NEED: Psychosocial Integrity

   KNOWLEDGE LEVEL: Application

4. **ANSWER:** 1

   RATIONALE: Asking specifically with whom the patient would like to talk validates her wishes and facilitates meeting her spiritual needs with the appropriate referral. Reassuring the patient that nothing she could have done is terrible enough to seek consultation belittles the patient's experience, is nonsupportive, and not therapeutic. Encouraging the patient to spend time with family and friends, or offering for the patient to speak with the nurse or social worker does not address her expressed concerns and wishes.

   NURSING PROCESS STEP: Implementation

   CATEGORY OF CLIENT NEED: Psychosocial Integrity

   KNOWLEDGE LEVEL: Analysis

5. **ANSWER:** 4

   RATIONALE: Validating the patient's value of the prayer group and making arrangements for her to participate that evening is the most appropriate response by the nurse. Postponing the experience does not address the patient's immediate needs or her priority spiritual need. Criticizing the group, which the patient finds to be very supportive, is not therapeutic and does not address the issue at hand.

   NURSING PROCESS STEP: Planning

   CATEGORY OF CLIENT NEED: Psychosocial Integrity

   KNOWLEDGE LEVEL: Analysis

CHAPTER 11

Pretest

1. **ANSWER:** 3

   RATIONALE: Most people prefer someone they know well to provide care rather than a nurse at home or at the hospital; it does not have to be their best friend.

   NURSING PROCESS STEP: Planning

   CATEGORY OF CLIENT NEED: Psychosocial Integrity

   KNOWLEDGE LEVEL: Knowledge

2. **ANSWER:** 2

   RATIONALE: Patients are being cared for in their homes and communities because that is where they wish to live; it is not necessarily due to finances, caregivers are not always family members, and nursing homes are not too crowded.

   NURSING PROCESS STEP: Planning

   CATEGORY OF CLIENT NEED: Psychosocial Integrity

   KNOWLEDGE LEVEL: Knowledge

3. ANSWER: 1

RATIONALE: The nurse cares for himself or herself to prolong professional survival by balancing wellness, self-care, and professional growth; confidentiality, personal boundaries, and personal agenda are aspects of nursing professional experience, but are not key factors to professional survival.

NURSING PROCESS STEP: Planning

CATEGORY OF CLIENT NEED: Psychosocial Integrity

KNOWLEDGE LEVEL: Knowledge

4. ANSWER: 3

RATIONALE: Symptoms of stress and depression are similar to caregiver burnout; not symptoms of agitation, anxiety, or dementia.

NURSING PROCESS STEP: Evaluation

CATEGORY OF CLIENT NEED: Psychosocial

KNOWLEDGE LEVEL: Application

5. ANSWER: 1, 2, 3

RATIONALE: Caregiver fatigue may cause a sense of hopelessness, loss of purpose and anger toward God, and problems with sleep; it will not improve the appreciation for the profession.

NURSING PROCESS STEP: Evaluation

CATEGORY OF CLIENT NEED: Psychosocial

KNOWLEDGE LEVEL: Knowledge

Section One Review

1. ANSWER: 1, 2, 3, 4

RATIONALE: An adult child caring for an aging parent while working and addressing family responsibilities will impact employment, finances, career opportunities, and personal well-being.

NURSING PROCESS STEP: Evaluation

CATEGORY OF CLIENT NEED: Psychosocial Integrity

KNOWLEDGE LEVEL: Knowledge

2. ANSWER: 2

RATIONALE: Alzheimer's disease and the related symptomology correlate with higher levels of emotional distress from caregivers, over CVA, ESRD, and Cancer.

NURSING PROCESS STEP: Planning

CATEGORY OF CLIENT NEED: Psychosocial Integrity

KNOWLEDGE LEVEL: Knowledge

3. ANSWER: 1

RATIONALE: This is a statistical fact.

NURSING PROCESS STEP: Planning

CATEGORY OF CLIENT NEED: Safe, Effective Care Environment

KNOWLEDGE LEVEL: Knowledge

4. ANSWER: 3

RATIONALE: This is a statistical fact; female caregivers are more likely than spouses, children, and men to report emotional stress and impaired physical health.

NURSING PROCESS STEP: Evaluation

CATEGORY OF CLIENT NEED: Psychosocial Integrity

KNOWLEDGE LEVEL: Knowledge

5. ANSWER: 2

RATIONALE: Caregivers rank finding time for themselves a higher unmet need, over finding resources for finances, obtaining legal support, and obtaining transportation.

NURSING PROCESS STEP: Planning

CATEGORY OF CLIENT NEED: Psychosocial Integrity

KNOWLEDGE LEVEL: Knowledge

Section Two Review

1. ANSWER: 3

RATIONALE: Viewing the final phases of a person's life as a journey does not carry the negative connotation of dilemma, trial, or rollercoaster and may assist with more positive coping mechanisms.

NURSING PROCESS STEP: Planning

CATEGORY OF CLIENT NEED: Psychosocial Integrity

KNOWLEDGE LEVEL: Application

2. ANSWER: 4

RATIONALE: Physical, psychological, emotional, social relationships, cultural and spiritual well-being encompass the holistic health approach. Medical, recreational, and community well-being are encompassed by these aspects.

NURSING PROCESS STEP: Planning

CATEGORY OF CLIENT NEED: Psychosocial

KNOWLEDGE LEVEL: Knowledge

3. ANSWER: 1

RATIONALE: Over-scheduling life is a barrier to professional self care. Spending time with the patient's family and reading journal articles on the patient's disease promote professional self care. Working a second job is encompassed by the "multiple role" in the stem of the question.

NURSING PROCESS STEP: Planning

CATEGORY OF CLIENT NEED: Psychosocial

KNOWLEDGE LEVEL: Knowledge

4. ANSWER: 2

RATIONALE: Professional education and training is the first factor in adaptation of nurses in their professional role as caregiver. Being a team player, caring for a dying patient, and working the night shift alone are all factors that come after education and training.

NURSING PROCESS STEP: Planning

CATEGORY OF CLIENT NEED: Safe, Effective Care Environment

KNOWLEDGE LEVEL: Knowledge

5. **ANSWER:** 4

    RATIONALE: Team members, other staff members, and friends outside of the work place are examples of informal support. Debriefings and ceremonies are formal support.

    NURSING PROCESS STEP: Planning

    CATEGORY OF CLIENT NEED: Psychosocial Integrity

    KNOWLEDGE LEVEL: Knowledge

Section Three Review

1. **ANSWER:** 1, 2, 3, 4

    RATIONALE: Attitude, personal strength, hours of work, and personality may all contribute to caregiver burnout.

    NURSING PROCESS STEP: Planning and Evaluation

    CATEGORY OF CLIENT NEED: Psychosocial Integrity

    KNOWLEDGE LEVEL: Knowledge

2. **ANSWER:** 2

    RATIONALE: Emotional exhaustion, changes in appetite and weight, and poor patient service are all manifestations of caregiver burnout. Increasing hours of work is not.

    NURSING PROCESS STEP: Assessment

    CATEGORY OF CLIENT NEED: Psychosocial Integrity

    KNOWLEDGE LEVEL: Knowledge

3. **ANSWER:** 1

    RATIONALE: Social, cultural, and biological health are secondary to emotional, physical, and spiritual health.

    NURSING PROCESS STEP: Planning

    CATEGORY OF CLIENT NEED: Psychosocial Integrity

    KNOWLEDGE LEVEL: Knowledge

4. **ANSWER:** 2

    RATIONALE: Education is the foundation of the level of care that the nurse can provide. Proficiency, teamwork, and disease are secondary to education.

    NURSING PROCESS STEP: Planning

    CATEGORY OF CLIENT NEED: Safe, Effective Care Environment

    KNOWLEDGE LEVEL: Knowledge

5. **ANSWER:** 4

    RATIONALE: This is the definition of caregiver burnout.

    NURSING PROCESS STEP: Evaluation

    CATEGORY OF CLIENT NEED: Psychosocial Integrity

    KNOWLEDGE LEVEL: Knowledge

Section Four Review

1. **ANSWER:** 3

    RATIONALE: Personality traits of high empathy and compassion are at high risk for compassion fatigue, over anxiety and depression, depression and fatigue, and energy and stress.

    NURSING PROCESS STEP: Evaluation

    CATEGORY OF CLIENT NEED: Psychosocial Integrity

    KNOWLEDGE LEVEL: Knowledge

2. **ANSWER:** 2

    RATIONALE: Hopelessness, not joy, respect, or sympathy, is associated with compassion.

    NURSING PROCESS STEP: Evaluation

    CATEGORY OF CLIENT NEED: Psychosocial Integrity

    KNOWLEDGE LEVEL: Knowledge

3. **ANSWER:** 1, 2, 3, 4

    RATIONALE: Taking time off of work, using alcohol, cigarettes, and/or illicit drugs are negative coping mechanisms associated with compassion fatigue.

    NURSING PROCESS STEP: Evaluation

    CATEGORY OF CLIENT NEED: Psychosocial Integrity

    KNOWLEDGE LEVEL: Knowledge

4. **ANSWER:** 1

    RATIONALE: Both compassion fatigue and caregiver burnout have similar physical characteristics, mental exhaustion, and co-worker issues; they differ in onset and recovery.

    NURSING PROCESS STEP: Planning

    CATEGORY OF CLIENT NEED: Psychosocial Integrity

    KNOWLEDGE LEVEL: Knowledge

5. **ANSWER:** 2

    RATIONALE: Restful sleep is essential to cope with compassion fatigue. Medications, taking a leave of absence, and changing jobs are not essential.

    NURSING PROCESS STEP: Planning

    CATEGORY OF CLIENT NEED: Psychosocial Integrity

    KNOWLEDGE LEVEL: Knowledge

Index

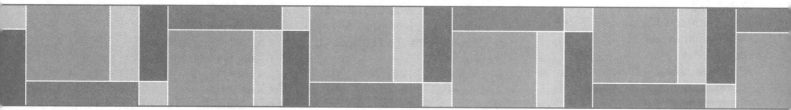